T0325743

ELECTRO-MAGNETIC
TISSUE PROPERTIES MRI

Modelling and Simulation in Medical Imaging

ISSN: 2045-0362

Series Editor: Habib Ammari *(Ecole Polytechnique, France)*

Vol. 1:   Electro-Magnetic Tissue Properties MRI
         by Jin Keun Seo, Eung Je Woo, Ulrich Katscher and Yi Wang

ELECTRO-MAGNETIC TISSUE PROPERTIES MRI

Jin Keun Seo
Yonsei University, Korea

Eung Je Woo
Kyung Hee University, Korea

Ulrich Katscher
Philips Technologie GmbH, Germany

Yi Wang
Cornell University, USA

Imperial College Press

ICP

Published by

Imperial College Press
57 Shelton Street
Covent Garden
London WC2H 9HE

Distributed by

World Scientific Publishing Co. Pte. Ltd.
5 Toh Tuck Link, Singapore 596224
USA office: 27 Warren Street, Suite 401-402, Hackensack, NJ 07601
UK office: 57 Shelton Street, Covent Garden, London WC2H 9HE

British Library Cataloguing-in-Publication Data
A catalogue record for this book is available from the British Library.

Modelling and Simulation in Medical Imaging — Vol. 1
ELECTRO-MAGNETIC TISSUE PROPERTIES MRI

ISBN 978-1-78326-339-4

Typeset by Stallion Press
Email: enquiries@stallionpress.com

Printed in Singapore

Preface

Recently, imaging techniques in science, engineering, and medicine have evolved to expand our ability to visualize internal information of an object such as the human body. In particular, there has been marked progress in magnetic resonance (MR)-based electromagnetic property imaging techniques which use magnetic resonance imaging (MRI) to provide cross-sectional images of conductivity, permittivity, and susceptibility distributions inside the human body. These electromagnetic material properties of biological tissues are important biomarkers since they reveal physiological and pathological conditions of body tissues and organs.

Magnetic resonance electrical impedance tomography (MREIT) is an MR-based conductivity imaging technique at low frequencies. In MREIT, we inject currents into an imaging object and measure induced magnetic flux density data from MR phase images. Quasistatic Maxwell equations provide a relation between the measured magnetic flux density and the conductivity from which we can reconstruct cross-sectional conductivity images. Magnetic resonance electrical properties tomography (MREPT) aims to reconstruct images of both conductivity and permittivity distributions inside the human body at MR frequency. In contrast to MREIT, MREPT does not require current injection since it is based on standard radio frequency (RF) field mapping techniques to measure the active magnetic RF field component. While MREIT and MREPT deal with electrical properties of conductivity and permittivity, quantitative susceptibility mapping (QSM) provides images of the magnetic susceptibility distribution inside the human body. Unlike susceptibility weighted imaging (SWI) methods, QSM utilizes MR phase images to produce absolute tissue susceptibility images by solving an inversion problem of magnetic sources.

In recent literature, theories, image reconstruction algorithms and experimental techniques of these MR-based electro-magnetic property imaging modalities have been developed to advance them to the stage of *in vivo* animal or human experiments. These modalities belong to interdisciplinary research areas incorporating mathematical theories and analyses of bioelectromagnetism, MR physics and imaging methods, inverse problems and image reconstruction algorithms, numerical analyses and experimental techniques. In order to facilitate clinical application studies as well as further technical refinements, we realized that an unmet need exists for a technical book dealing with MREIT, MREPT, and QSM.

In this book, we present their mathematical formulations to describe fundamental concepts and image reconstruction algorithms. We first introduce basics of bioelectromagnetism and MRI in the context of MREIT, MREPT, and QSM. We deal with each modality in a separate chapter where we explain associated measurement methods, interrelations between obtained MR data and image contrasts, image reconstruction algorithms, experimental techniques and potential biomedical applications. For researchers in applied mathematics, we also discuss mathematical theories including error estimates, uniqueness, and challenging open problems.

To facilitate technical progress, we will follow a kind of unified approach, as summarized below:

- Understanding underlying physical phenomena.
- Mathematical formulation of forward problems in such a way that we can deal with them systematically and quantitatively.
- Data collection method: practical limitations associated with measurement sensitivity and specificity, noise, artifacts, interface between target object and instrument, data acquisition time.
- Mathematical analysis explaining relations between those qualities and measurable data.
- Image reconstruction formulas and sensitivity analysis.
- Numerical implementation and *in vivo* experiments.
- Challenging problems and future research directions.

Expected readers of this book are graduate students and researchers in MR-based imaging science. Most of them will study or work in the areas of applied mathematics, biomedical engineering, and electrical engineering. The secondary audience will include scientist and engineers in universities and industry, who are interested in inverse problems in general.

Foreword

This is the first volume in the Imperial College Press series entitled Modelling and Simulation in Medical Imaging.

The purpose of the series is to publish high-level works describing advanced technologies in biomedical imaging and related mathematical problems and techniques. Its ultimate goal is to make mathematical modelling a more effective tool for biomedical imaging, leading to an enhancement of technological innovations.

This first volume is co-authored by a prominent mathematician and leading scientists from biomedical imaging. It covers recent advances on magnetic resonance electrical impedance tomography (MREIT). The mathematical problems that appear in this area are important and pose significant challenges to pure and applied mathematicians. They have also recently attracted a lot of attention from researchers.

The volume illustrates the interplay among many branches of mathematics and their applications in biomedical imaging. It highlights the benefits of sharing ideas among the fields of mathematics and medical imaging, and leads to very original mathematically based solutions to the most challenging problems in MREIT.

This impressive and timely volume is of interest not only to mathematicians working in the field of imaging, but also to physicists and engineers. We envision that it will stimulate much-needed progress in mathematical modelling for biomedical imaging.

Habib Ammari
Series Editor, Paris

Contents

Chapter 1

Introduction

Electro-magnetic tissue properties include electrical conductivity, permittivity and magnetic susceptibility. When properly probed by electric and/or magnetic means, their three-dimensional distributions in a subject become sources of magnetic field perturbations, which can be measured using a magnetic resonance imaging (MRI) scanner. Magnetic resonance (MR)-based electro-magnetic tissue property imaging is used to provide tomographic images of the tissue properties by investigating the sources of the magnetic field perturbations.

As the probing methods, we use externally applied electric and/or magnetic fields at direct current (dc) or radio frequency (RF). The applied fields induce distributions of internal current density and magnetization, which are determined by the tissue properties. Since the induced current density and magnetization perturb the main dc field and/or RF field of the MRI scanner, we can measure their effects from MR signals.

It is, therefore, important to understand the interactions among the external excitations, the tissue properties and the dc and RF fields of the MRI scanner. Based on this understanding, we can formulate forward problems to mathematically express the interactions. The external excitations will be considered as inputs and the MR signals as outputs of a system, of which characteristics are parameterized by the tissue properties. Since we control the external excitations and measure their responses from MR signals, the imaging problem turns out to be an inverse problem where the tissue properties are unknowns to be recovered.

1.1 Electro-magnetic Tissue Properties of Biological Tissues

The human body consists of electrolytes of various ions, molecules, cells, proteins and so on. The complicated structures and compositions of different biological tissues reveal their electro-magnetic properties through the conductivity, permittivity and susceptibility. We use the following notations to denote the intrinsic material properties and electro-magnetic vector quantities:

Symbol	Name	Unit	Relation
ϵ	permittivity	F/m	
σ	conductivity	S/m	
κ	admittivity	S/m	$\kappa = \sigma + i\omega\epsilon$
μ	permeability	H/m	
χ	(magnetic) susceptibility		$\mu = \mu_0(1 + \chi)$
ρ	charge density	C/m^3	

Symbol	Name	Unit	Relation
E	(time-harmonic) electric field intensity	V/m	
H	(time-harmonic) magnetic field intensity	A/m	
D	(time-harmonic) electric flux density	C/m^2	$\mathbf{D} = \epsilon\mathbf{E}$
B	(time-harmonic) magnetic flux density	T	$\mathbf{B} = \mu\mathbf{H}$
J	current density	A/m^2	$\mathbf{J} = \sigma\mathbf{E}$
M	magnetization of tissue in magnetic field		$\mathbf{M} = \chi\mathbf{H}$

The effective admittivity $\kappa = \sigma + i\omega\epsilon$ of a biological tissue under the influence of a time-harmonic electric field at an angular frequency ω, is determined by its ion concentrations in extra- and intracellular fluids, cellular structure and density, molecular compositions, membrane characteristics and other factors. While concentrations and mobilities of mobile ions and molecules affect an effective conductivity value, cell membranes contribute mostly to an effective permittivity value. Measured admittivity spectra of various biological tissues show frequency-dependent changes of conductivity and permittivity values.

For most biological tissues, $\kappa \approx \sigma$ at low frequencies below 10 kHz, whereas the $\omega\epsilon$ term is not negligible above 10 kHz due to the abundant membraneous structures in organisms. Since the admittivity values of tissues and organs change with their physiological and pathological conditions, they provide useful diagnostic information. For example, most cancerous tissues exhibit increased conductivity values. Cell swelling decreases conductivity values at low frequencies since low-frequency currents flow mostly through the extracellular space. Numerous diseases such as stroke, hemorrhage, edema, inflammation and others are known to alter tissue admittivity values. There are also trials to directly detect neural activities using a conductivity imaging method since they are accompanied by local changes of conductivity values. Many clinical applications such as electroencephalography (EEG) and magnetoencephalography (MEG) source imaging and therapeutic techniques using electric and magnetic stimulations require admittivity values of numerous biological tissues at different frequency ranges.

A biological tissue acquires a magnetic moment when it is put in a magnetic field $\mathbf{H}$. Magnetic susceptibility χ is defined through the relationship $\mathbf{M} = \chi\mathbf{H}$ where $\mathbf{M}$ is the magnetic moment per unit volume (magnetization) also referred to as the bulk magnetic moment. Magnetic susceptibility is an intrinsic property of the material, reflecting its electronic perturbation by the applied magnetic field. The strong intrinsic magnetic moment of unpaired electrons makes most material paramagnetic ($\chi > 0$), while the magnetic moment associated with electron orbits makes some materials diamagnetic. Physiology and disease processes involve changes in tissue magnetic susceptibilities. For example, the widely known functional MRI (fMRI) for studying brain function is based on the magnetic properties of oxyhemoglobin being paramagnetic and deoxyhemoglobin diamagnetic. Hemorrhage, neurodegenerative diseases and various other diseases affecting iron transport cause deposits of irons known to have large susceptibility. Depositions of calcium of negative susceptibility are associated with bone composition and breast cancer.

1.2   Three Electro-magnetic Tissue Property Imaging Modalities

This book focuses on three imaging techniques: magnetic resonance electrical impedance tomography (MREIT), electrical properties tomography (MREPT) and quantitative susceptibility mapping (QSM). All of these imaging methods are based on Maxwell's equations and MRI data acquisition techniques. The contrast information from these novel imaging modalities is unique since there is currently no other method to reconstruct high-resolution images of the electro-magnetic tissue properties of a biological tissue including the conductivity σ, permittivity ϵ and susceptibility χ.

Magnetic resonance electrical impedance tomography aims to provide conductivity images at dc or frequencies below a few kHz, whereas MREPT produces both conductivity and permittivity images at the Larmor frequency of 128 MHz at 3 T, for example. In MREIT, one injects currents into an imaging object after RF pulses and measures induced magnetic flux density data from MR phase images. MREIT relies on measured magnetic field data at low frequencies which are influenced by the low-frequency conductivity distribution. In contrast to MREIT, MREPT is based on standard RF field mapping techniques to measure the active magnetic RF field component, which is influenced by the admittivity distribution $\kappa = \sigma + i\omega\epsilon$ including both conductivity and permittivity distributions at the Larmor frequency. Due to the frequency-dependent behavior of the conductivity and permittivity values of biological tissues, MREIT and MREPT are supplementing each other providing different images of the same object in terms of its low- and high-frequency views, respectively. Implementation of MREPT on a clinical MRI scanner is easier since it does not require any additional instrumentation while MREIT requires attachment of surface electrodes and an interface to a constant current source.

Quantitative susceptibility mapping aims to provide susceptibility images from measured local field perturbations associated with the magnetization induced in the object. The component of the local field along the main magnetic field of the MR scanner can be expressed by a convolution of the susceptibility distribution with the magnetic field generated by a unit dipole. The inverse problem of QSM is ill-posed due to the presence of zeros at the magic cone in the Fourier representation of the unit dipole kernel.

1.3 Mathematical Frameworks

Mathematical techniques in science and engineering have evolved to expand our ability to visualize various physical phenomena of interest and their characteristics in detail. Carefully designed experimental studies are crucial to understand and solve these realistic model problems. Developing mathematical models with practical significance and value requires deep understanding of underlying physics and hands-on expertise of real imaging systems. This requires integrated knowledge and experience in biomedical science and engineering together with mathematics.

Mathematical models for MR-based electro-magnetic tissue property imaging can be described by suitable arrangements using Maxwell's equations, Bloch equations, and other constitutive laws of physical parameters:

- Maxwell's equations for time-harmonic fields:
  - Gauss's law: $\nabla \cdot \mathbf{E} = \rho/\epsilon$.
  - Gauss's law for magnetism: $\nabla \cdot \mathbf{B} = 0$.
  - Faraday's law of induction: $\nabla \times \mathbf{E} = -i\omega\mathbf{B}$.
  - Ampère's circuital law: $\nabla \times \mathbf{H} = \mathbf{J} + i\omega\mathbf{D}$.
- Bloch equation: $\frac{\partial}{\partial t}\underline{\mathbf{M}} = -\gamma\mathbf{B}_0 \times \underline{\mathbf{M}} - \frac{1}{T_2}\underline{\mathbf{M}}_{xy} - \frac{1}{T_1}(\underline{M}_z - M_0)\hat{\mathbf{z}}$.

In MREIT, we inject electrical current through a pair of electrodes $\mathcal{E}^+$ and $\mathcal{E}^-$ and measure the induced $B_z(\mathbf{r})$ by an MRI scanner with its main field in the z direction. The relation between B_z and σ is determined by the z-component of the Biot−Savart law:

$$B_z(\mathbf{r}) = \frac{\mu}{4\pi} \int \frac{\langle \mathbf{r} - \mathbf{r}', -\sigma(\mathbf{r}')\mathbf{E}(\mathbf{r}') \times \hat{\mathbf{z}} \rangle}{|\mathbf{r} - \mathbf{r}'|^3} \, d\mathbf{r}' + \text{harmonic term}$$

where $\mathbf{r} = (x, y, z)$, $\hat{\mathbf{z}} = (0, 0, 1)$, and the harmonic term is determined by the external lead wire currents outside the subject. The inverse problem is to reconstruct σ from the data B_z. This inverse problem is non-linear since the relationship between the conductivity and the measured data via the Biot–Savart law is non-linear. It is critical to properly analyze how σ influences B_z.

In MREPT, the input is an RF excitation by an external coil and the measurable data is the positive rotating magnetic field H^+ that is measured by a B1-mapping technique. The relation between κ and H^+ is determined by

$$-\nabla^2 \mathbf{H} = \frac{\nabla \kappa}{\kappa} \times [\nabla \times \mathbf{H}] - i\omega\kappa\mathbf{H}.$$

Analyzing the data of H^+ in terms of the admittivity κ is complicated due to the term $\frac{\nabla \kappa}{\kappa} \times [\nabla \times \mathbf{H}]$ in the governing equation.

In QSM, susceptibility imaging of an arbitrary distribution χ is performed by putting an imaging object in a known magnetic field $\mathbf{B}_0$ and measuring the field associated with the magnetization $\mathbf{M}$ induced in the object. The corresponding inverse problem is based on the fact that the measured data ψ is approximately the convolution of the tissue magnetic source χ with the dipole kernel d: $\psi = d * \chi$ where the dipole kernel is $d(\mathbf{r}) = \frac{1}{4\pi}\frac{2z^2-x^2-y^2}{|\mathbf{r}|^5}$. Unfortunately, the deconvolution to solve the inverse problem is ill-posed since the dipole kernel is zero on the magic cone $\{\mathbf{r} : 2z^2 = x^2 + y^2\}$ so that small errors in data near the cone produce large errors in the solution. Additional information is required to deal with the inherently ill-posed characteristic.

MREIT	MREPT	QSM
$\mathcal{E}_+$ $\sigma \rightsquigarrow \mathbf{B}$ $\sigma + \delta\sigma$ $\rightsquigarrow \mathbf{B} + \delta\mathbf{B}$ $\mathcal{E}_-$	$\kappa \rightsquigarrow \mathbf{B}$ $\kappa + \delta\kappa$ $\rightsquigarrow \mathbf{B} + \delta\mathbf{B}$ $I \sin \omega t$ RF coil	$\mathbf{N}$ $\chi \rightsquigarrow \delta\mathbf{B}$ $\mathbf{S}$ $\mathbf{B}_0$
$-\sigma\mathbf{E} = \nabla \times \mathbf{H}$ $\nabla \times \mathbf{E} = 0$	$-\kappa\mathbf{E} = \nabla \times \mathbf{H}$ $\nabla \times \mathbf{E} = -i\omega\mathbf{B}$	$\mathbf{M} = \chi\mathbf{H}_0$ $\mathbf{M} \rightsquigarrow \delta\mathbf{B}$

✶ $\mathbf{M}$ represents magnetization distribution of tissue in an MR scanner.

These studies are interdisciplinary in nature, involving mathematics, physics, engineering and biomedical science. We need to understand underlying physical laws, interrelations among the variables and measured data, constraints imposed on the problem, and uncertainties in models.

1.4 General Notations

For ease of explanation, we will use the following notations throughout this book:

Symbol	Explanation
Ω	three-dimensional domain to be imaged
$\partial\Omega$	boundary of Ω
$\mathbf{n}$	unit outward normal vector to the boundary
$\mathbf{r}$, i	position $\mathbf{r} = (x, y, z)$, $\mathrm{i} = \sqrt{-1}$
$\hat{\mathbf{x}}$, $\hat{\mathbf{y}}$, $\hat{\mathbf{z}}$	$\hat{\mathbf{x}} = (1, 0, 0)$, $\hat{\mathbf{y}} = (0, 1, 0)$, $\hat{\mathbf{z}} = (0, 0, 1)$
$d\mathbf{l}$, dS, dV	line, surface and volume elements, respectively
$\mathbb{R}$, $\mathbb{C}$	set of real numbers and complex numbers, respectively
$\mathbb{R}^n$	n-dimensional Euclidian space
$\propto$	By $f \propto g$, we mean $f = cg$ for a constant c.

Chapter 2

Electro-magnetism and MRI

Electro-magnetic tissue property imaging modalities combine advanced knowledge and techniques from a wide range of fields including partial differential equations, bioelectro-magnetism, magnetic resonance (MR) physics, scientific computing, and so on. For these studies, we need to understand underlying physical laws, interrelations among variables and measured data, constraints imposed on the problem, and uncertainties in modelings.

The human body can be regarded as a complex electro-magnetic conductor comprising many tissues that have distinct electromagnetic properties. The electrical properties of biological tissues can be described by the effective conductivity σ and the effective permittivity ϵ which depend on scale and applied frequency. The σ and ϵ of a biological tissue under the influence of a time-harmonic electric field at an angular frequency ω, is determined by its ion concentrations in extra- and intracellular fluids, cellular structure and density, molecular compositions, membrane characteristics and other factors. Cell membranes contribute to capacitance; the intracellular fluid gives rise to an intracellular resistance; the extracellular fluid contributes to effective resistance. As a result, biological tissues show a variable response over the frequency range from a few Hz to MHz. Hence, the effective conductivity and permttivity spectra of biological tissue can be used as a means of characterizing tissue structural information relating to the biological cell suspensions. The magnetic tissue property can be described as magnetic susceptibility that is an intrinsic property, reflecting the degree of magnetization of a material in response to an applied magnetic field. Physiology and disease processes involve changes in tissue magnetic susceptibilities.

In this chapter, we discuss the basic materials that will be used in those studies.

2.1 Basics of Electro-magnetism

2.1.1 *Maxwell's equations*

Maxwell's equations together with the Lorentz force describe the fundamentals of electro-magnetism in a concise manner. The Maxwell equations for time-varying and time-harmonic fields are the set of four fundamental equations using the electric field $\underline{\mathbf{E}}$, current density $\underline{\mathbf{J}}$, magnetic field $\underline{\mathbf{H}}$, and magnetic flux density $\underline{\mathbf{B}}$:

Name	Time-varying Field	Time-harmonic Field
Gauss's law	$\nabla \cdot \underline{\mathbf{E}} = \rho/\epsilon$	$\nabla \cdot \mathbf{E} = \rho/\epsilon$
Gauss's law for magnetism	$\nabla \cdot \underline{\mathbf{B}} = 0$	$\nabla \cdot \mathbf{B} = 0$
Faraday's law of induction	$\nabla \times \underline{\mathbf{E}} = -\frac{\partial}{\partial t}\underline{\mathbf{B}}$	$\nabla \times \mathbf{E} = -i\omega\mathbf{B}$
Ampère's circuital law	$\nabla \times \underline{\mathbf{H}} = \underline{\mathbf{J}} + \frac{\partial}{\partial t}\underline{\mathbf{D}}$	$\nabla \times \mathbf{H} = \mathbf{J} + i\omega\mathbf{D}$

✳ In the free space, $\epsilon = \epsilon_0 = 8.85 \times 10^{-12}$ and $\mu = \mu_0 = 4\pi \times 10^{-7}$.

If the time-varying fields $\underline{\mathbf{E}}$, $\underline{\mathbf{J}}$, $\underline{\mathbf{H}}$, and $\underline{\mathbf{B}}$ vary periodically and sinusoidally with time, phaser notations ($\mathbf{E}$, $\mathbf{J}$, $\mathbf{H}$, and $\mathbf{B}$) are convenient to work:

$$\underline{\mathbf{E}}(\mathbf{r}, t) = \mathrm{Re}\{\mathbf{E}(\mathbf{r})\, e^{i\omega t}\} \quad \underline{\mathbf{J}}(\mathbf{r}, t) = \mathrm{Re}\{\mathbf{J}(\mathbf{r})\, e^{i\omega t}\}$$

$$\underline{\mathbf{H}}(\mathbf{r}, t) = \mathrm{Re}\{\mathbf{H}(\mathbf{r})\, e^{i\omega t}\} \quad \underline{\mathbf{B}}(\mathbf{r}, t) = \mathrm{Re}\{\mathbf{B}(\mathbf{r})\, e^{i\omega t}\}$$

The Lorentz force describes the force acting on a charged particle q with its instantaneous velocity in the presence of the external fields $\underline{\mathbf{E}}$ and $\underline{\mathbf{B}}$. The force is described by

$$\underline{\mathbf{F}} = q(\underline{\mathbf{E}} + \mathbf{v} \times \underline{\mathbf{B}}). \tag{2.1}$$

We begin with studying electricity that can be divided into electrostatics (charges at rest) and current electricity (charges in motion).

2.1.2 *Electric field due to point charges in free space*

Electric charges are the source of electric fields, exerting electric force and responding to electric force. Coulomb's law states a force between two charged particles which is proportional to the product of the charges and inversely proportional to the square of the distance between them. Considering a space with charged particles, there exists an electric field with its intensity denoted by $\mathbf{E}$. To be precise, let q_1 and q_2 be stationary point charges located at $\mathbf{r}_1$ and $\mathbf{r}_2$, respectively. According to Coulomb's law, the force exerted on q_1 by q_2 is given by

$$\mathbf{F}_{q_2 \to q_1} = \frac{q_1 q_2}{\epsilon_0} \frac{\mathbf{r}_1 - \mathbf{r}_2}{4\pi |\mathbf{r}_1 - \mathbf{r}_2|^3}$$

where $\epsilon_0 = 8.85 \times 10^{-12}$ is the permittivity of the free space (see Figure 2.1). The force between q_1 and q_2 is repulsive if they have the same sign, and attractive if they have different signs.

The electric field $\mathbf{E}(\mathbf{r})$ is defined as the force that a stationary unit test charge at $\mathbf{r}$ will experience, where $\mathbf{E}(\mathbf{r})$ in an unbounded free space can be expressed as

$$\mathbf{E}(\mathbf{r}) = \sum_{j=1}^{2} \frac{q_j}{\epsilon_0} \frac{\mathbf{r} - \mathbf{r}_j}{4\pi |\mathbf{r} - \mathbf{r}_j|^3}. \tag{2.2}$$

This $\mathbf{E}$ in (2.2) can be expressed as:

$$\mathbf{E}(\mathbf{r}) = -\nabla u(\mathbf{r}) \tag{2.3}$$

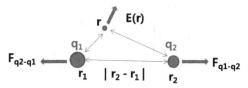

Fig. 2.1.   Forces between two point charges when q_1, $q_2 > 0$. Reciprocity requires $\mathbf{F}_{q_1 \to q_2} = -\mathbf{F}_{q_2 \to q_1}$.

where

$$u(\mathbf{r}) = \sum_{j=1}^{2} \frac{q_j}{\epsilon_0} \frac{1}{4\pi|\mathbf{r} - \mathbf{r}_j|}. \tag{2.4}$$

This scalar function u is said to be the electric potential, and it can be viewed as a solution of the Poisson equation:

$$-\nabla^2 u(\mathbf{r}) = \sum_{j=1}^{2} \frac{q_j}{\epsilon_0} \delta(\mathbf{r} - \mathbf{r}_j) \tag{2.5}$$

where $\delta(\mathbf{r})$ is the Dirac delta function.[1]

In general, $\mathbf{E}$ due to a certain charge distribution $\rho(\mathbf{r})$ in the subject Ω can be expressed as

$$\mathbf{E}(\mathbf{r}) = \frac{1}{\epsilon_0} \int_\Omega \frac{\mathbf{r} - \mathbf{r}'}{4\pi|\mathbf{r} - \mathbf{r}'|^3} \rho(\mathbf{r}') d\mathbf{r}'. \tag{2.6}$$

Here, $\rho(\mathbf{r})$ can be viewed as the signed net charge per unit volume at the point $\mathbf{r}$. Theorem 2.1 explains that the corresponding electric potential u is governed by Poisson's equation.

Theorem 2.1 (Poisson's equation). *Let Ω be a bounded domain in $\mathbb{R}^3$ with its smooth boundary $\partial\Omega$. For $\rho \in C(\mathbb{R}^3)$ (the set of continuous functions on the closure of the domain Ω), define*

$$u(\mathbf{r}) := \frac{1}{\epsilon_0} \int_\Omega \frac{1}{4\pi|\mathbf{r} - \mathbf{r}'|} \rho(\mathbf{r}') d\mathbf{r}'.$$

Then, the potential u satisfies $-\nabla u = \mathbf{E}$ where $\mathbf{E}$ is the electric field in 2.6. Moreover, $u(\mathbf{r}) = \epsilon_0 u(\mathbf{r})$ satisfies the Poisson equation:

$$-\nabla^2 u(\mathbf{r}) = \begin{cases} \dfrac{1}{\epsilon_0} \rho(\mathbf{r}) & \text{for } \mathbf{r} \in \Omega \\ 0 & \text{for } \mathbf{r} \notin \overline{\Omega} \end{cases}. \tag{2.7}$$

---

[1]The Dirac delta function $\delta(\mathbf{r})$ can be loosely thought of as the unit impulse function such that $\delta(\mathbf{r}) = 0$ for all $\mathbf{r} \neq 0$ and $\int_{\mathbb{R}^3} \delta(\mathbf{r}) d\mathbf{r} = 1$.

Proof. Set $v(\mathbf{r}) = \epsilon_0 u(\mathbf{r})$. Straightforward computation gives

$$\nabla^2 \left(\frac{1}{4\pi|\mathbf{r} - \mathbf{r}'|} \right) = 0 \quad \text{if } \mathbf{r} \neq \mathbf{r}'. \tag{2.8}$$

This proves that $-\nabla^2 v(\mathbf{r}) = 0$ for $\mathbf{r} \notin \overline{\Omega}$. From now on, let $\mathbf{r} \in \Omega$, and let D be a small sphere such that $D \subset \Omega$ and $\mathbf{r} \in D$. From (2.8),

$$\nabla^2 v(\mathbf{r}) = \nabla^2 \int_{\Omega} \frac{1}{4\pi|\mathbf{r} - \mathbf{r}'|} \rho(\mathbf{r}') d\mathbf{r}'$$

$$= \nabla^2 \int_{D} \frac{1}{4\pi|\mathbf{r} - \mathbf{r}'|} \rho(\mathbf{r}') d\mathbf{r}'. \tag{2.9}$$

Since the above identity holds true for an arbitrary small sphere D,

$$\nabla^2 \int_{D} \frac{1}{4\pi|\mathbf{r} - \mathbf{r}'|} (\rho(\mathbf{r}') - \rho(\mathbf{r})) d\mathbf{r}' = 0. \tag{2.10}$$

Therefore, it follows from (2.9) and (2.10) that

$$\nabla^2 v(\mathbf{r}) = \rho(\mathbf{r}) \nabla^2 \int_{D} \frac{1}{4\pi|\mathbf{r} - \mathbf{r}'|} d\mathbf{r}'. \tag{2.11}$$

Using the standard limiting process to handle singularity, (2.11) becomes

$$\nabla^2 v(\mathbf{r}) = \rho(\mathbf{r}) \lim_{s \downarrow 0} \int_{D} \nabla^2 \frac{1}{4\pi(|\mathbf{r} - \mathbf{r}'| + s)} d\mathbf{r}'$$

$$= \rho(\mathbf{r}) \lim_{s \downarrow 0} \int_{\partial D} \mathbf{n}(\mathbf{r}') \cdot \nabla \left(\frac{-1}{4\pi(|\mathbf{r} - \mathbf{r}'| + s)} \right) dS$$

$$= \rho(\mathbf{r}) \underbrace{\int_{\partial D} \mathbf{n}(\mathbf{r}') \cdot \nabla \left(\frac{-1}{4\pi|\mathbf{r} - \mathbf{r}'|} \right) dS}_{-1}$$

$$= -\rho(\mathbf{r}) \tag{2.12}$$

where $\mathbf{n}$ is the unit outward normal vector to the boundary. We refer to [Seo and Woo (2012)] for a detailed proof. □

Electric dipole, a pair of equal and opposite charges separated by a small distance, is more common than isolated charge. As shown

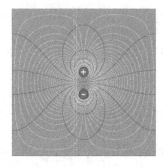

Fig. 2.2. The potential u due to a positive charge q at $\mathbf{r}_\oplus$ and negative charge at $\mathbf{r}_\ominus$.

in Figure 2.2, assume that a positive and a negative point charge, respectively, is placed at $\mathbf{r}_\oplus$ and $\mathbf{r}_\ominus$ in the free space. The charges create the electric field. The potential u due to a positive charge q at $\mathbf{r}_\oplus$ and negative charge at $\mathbf{r}_\ominus$ is

$$u(\mathbf{r}) = \frac{q}{\epsilon_0 4\pi} \left(\frac{1}{|\mathbf{r} - \mathbf{r}_\oplus|} - \frac{1}{|\mathbf{r} - \mathbf{r}_\ominus|} \right).$$

According to (2.7), the potential u satisfies

$$-\nabla^2 u(\mathbf{r}) = q(\delta(\mathbf{r} - \mathbf{r}_\oplus) - \delta(\mathbf{r} - \mathbf{r}_\ominus)). \tag{2.13}$$

If the distance $|\mathbf{r}_\oplus - \mathbf{r}_\ominus|$ is very small, then $\mathbf{p} := q(\mathbf{r}_\oplus - \mathbf{r}_\ominus)$ can be viewed as the electric dipole moment at the center position $\mathbf{r}_0 := (\mathbf{r}_\ominus + \mathbf{r}_\oplus)/2$, and it follows from the mean value theorem that the potential u can be expressed as

$$u(\mathbf{r}) = \frac{q}{\epsilon_0 4\pi} \left(\frac{1}{|\mathbf{r} - \mathbf{r}_\oplus|} - \frac{1}{|\mathbf{r} - \mathbf{r}_\ominus|} \right)$$

$$\approx \frac{1}{\epsilon_0 4\pi} \frac{\mathbf{r} - \mathbf{r}_0}{|\mathbf{r} - \mathbf{r}_0|^3} \cdot \underbrace{[q(\mathbf{r}_\oplus - \mathbf{r}_\ominus)]}_{\mathbf{p}}. \tag{2.14}$$

Hence, the electric potential u induced by the electric dipole moment $\mathbf{p} := q(\mathbf{r}_\ominus - \mathbf{r}_\oplus)$ can be expressed as

$$u(\mathbf{r}) = \frac{1}{\epsilon_0 4\pi} \frac{\mathbf{p} \cdot (\mathbf{r} - \mathbf{r}_0)}{|\mathbf{r} - \mathbf{r}_0|^3}, \tag{2.15}$$

and the corresponding electric field is

$$\mathbf{E}^{\mathbf{P}}(\mathbf{r}) = -\nabla u(\mathbf{r}) = \frac{1}{\epsilon_0 4\pi |\mathbf{r} - \mathbf{r}_0|^3} \left(3 \cos \theta^{\mathbf{p}}_{\mathbf{r}-\mathbf{r}_0} \frac{\mathbf{r} - \mathbf{r}_0}{|\mathbf{r} - \mathbf{r}_0|} - \mathbf{p} \right) \qquad (2.16)$$

where $\theta^{\mathbf{p}}_{\mathbf{r}-\mathbf{r}_0}$ is the angle between $\mathbf{p}$ and $\mathbf{r} - \mathbf{r}_0$.

Next, we consider the force on the dipole $\mathbf{p}$ when it is placed in an external electric field $\mathbf{E}$. Since opposite forces $q\mathbf{E}$ and $-q\mathbf{E}$ act at different points $\mathbf{r}_\oplus$ and $\mathbf{r}_\ominus$ (with the net force being approximately zero[2]), the dipole moment $\mathbf{p}$ in the field $\mathbf{E}$ experiences torque:

$$\boldsymbol{\tau} = \mathbf{r}_\oplus \times (q\mathbf{E}) + \mathbf{r}_\ominus \times (-q\mathbf{E}) = \mathbf{p} \times \mathbf{E}. \qquad (2.17)$$

The torque tends to rotate the dipole $\mathbf{p}$ to line up with $\mathbf{E}$ (see Figure 2.3). If $\mathbf{p}$ is aligned with $\mathbf{E}$, then $\mathbf{p} \times \mathbf{E} = 0$ and the torque is zero.

In material, there are many electric dipoles at each small volume element. There are three types of dipoles; induced dipole, instantaneous dipole, and permanent dipole. A molecule that has electric dipole in the absence of an external electric field is known as a polar molecule. Water, chloroform, and ammonia molecules are examples of polar molecules which possess permanent dipole moments. On the other hand, a molecule with equal distribution of electrons among its atoms is called a non-polar molecule, which does not have dipole in the absence of an external field. Oxygen, nitrogen, and carbon dioxide are examples of non-polar molecules that have no permanent dipole moments. In the presence of an external electric field $\mathbf{E}$, polar molecules generally polarize more strongly than non-polar molecules. For non-polar molecules, $\mathbf{E}$ produces induced dipole moments by distorting the charge distributions. For polar molecules,

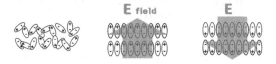

Fig. 2.3. Induced dipoles due to an external field.

---

[2]Under the influence of a uniform field $\mathbf{E}$, the net force $\mathbf{F} = q\mathbf{E} - q\mathbf{E}$ is zero. If $\mathbf{E}$ is non-uniform, the net force is $\mathbf{F} = q\mathbf{E}(\mathbf{r}_\oplus) - q\mathbf{E}(\mathbf{r}_\ominus) = \mathbf{p} \cdot \mathbf{E}(\mathbf{r}_0) \neq 0$. Hence, if $\mathbf{p}$ is parallel to $\mathbf{E}$, the net force is in the direction of increasing field. On the other hand, if $\mathbf{p}$ is antiparallel to $\mathbf{E}$, the net force is in the direction of decreasing field.

E tends to rotate the dipole **p** to line up the initially randomly oriented permanent dipole moments.

2.1.3 *Molecular polarization*

Consider a dielectric[3] material that is placed in the influence of an external electric field **E**. The external field **E** makes the dielectric polarized by producing induced dipole moments. The average dipole moment induced per unit volume is called polarization density, denoted by **P**. To be precise, if a small volume Δv centered at position $\mathbf{r}_0$ has electric dipoles $\{\mathbf{p}_j\}_{j=1}^{N}$, then the density of polarization **P** at $\mathbf{r}_0$ is defined by

$$\mathbf{P}(\mathbf{r}_0) = \frac{\sum_{j=1}^{N} \mathbf{P}_j}{\Delta v} \qquad \left[\frac{\text{Coulomb}}{m^3} \right]. \tag{2.18}$$

More generally, the electric potential due to the distribution of polarization density **P** over a domain Ω is

$$u(\mathbf{r}) = \frac{1}{4\pi\epsilon_0} \int_{\Omega} \frac{(\mathbf{r} - \mathbf{r}') \cdot \mathbf{P}(\mathbf{r}')}{|\mathbf{r} - \mathbf{r}'|^3} d\mathbf{r}'$$

$$= \frac{1}{4\pi\epsilon_0} \int_{\Omega} \frac{1}{|\mathbf{r} - \mathbf{r}'|} \underbrace{\nabla \cdot \mathbf{P}(\mathbf{r}')}_{-\rho_p} d\mathbf{r}'. \tag{2.19}$$

Here, the volume element $\mathbf{P}(\mathbf{r})d\mathbf{r}$ can be regarded as an electric dipole. According to the formula (2.7), $\rho_p = -\nabla \cdot \mathbf{P}$ behaves like the net charge unit volume, and hence $-\nabla \cdot \mathbf{P}$ is referred to as the polarization charge density.

From (2.19) and (2.7), the electric field $\mathbf{E}^{\mathbf{P}}$ induced by **P** is govern by

$$\mathbf{E}^{\mathbf{P}}(\mathbf{r}) = -\nabla u(\mathbf{r}) = \frac{1}{4\pi\epsilon_0} \int_{\Omega} \frac{\mathbf{r} - \mathbf{r}'}{|\mathbf{r} - \mathbf{r}'|^3} \nabla \cdot \mathbf{P}(\mathbf{r}') d\mathbf{r}'. \tag{2.20}$$

Hence, Gauss's law reads

$$\nabla \cdot \mathbf{E}(\mathbf{r}) = \frac{1}{\epsilon_0} \left(\rho(\mathbf{r}) - \underbrace{\nabla \cdot \mathbf{P}(\mathbf{r})}_{-\rho_p} \right). \tag{2.21}$$

---

[3]In dielectrics (or insulators), charges are bound and they do not have free charges.

The polarization **P** is known to be related to the external field **E** and the material property; the degree of **P** is somewhat proportional to the applied field **E**; different materials polarize to different degrees and in different ways. Electrical susceptibility, denoted by χ_e, is used to express the degree of polarization of the dielectric material due to the applied field **E**. For dielectrics having instantaneous response to change in **E**, **P** is related with **E** linearly:

$$\mathbf{P} = \epsilon_0 \chi_e \mathbf{E}. \tag{2.22}$$

The susceptibility is a macroscopic quantity, whereas polarizability (ability for a molecule to be polarized) expresses a microscopic quantity to measure the magnitude of the induced dipole moment. The electric displacement **D** in dielectric in the presence of $\mathbf{E}^{ext}$ is

$$\mathbf{D} = \epsilon_0 \mathbf{E} + \mathbf{P} = \underbrace{\epsilon_0 (1 + \chi_e)}_{\epsilon} \mathbf{E} \tag{2.23}$$

where $\epsilon = \epsilon_0 \epsilon_r$ and $\epsilon_r = 1 + \chi_e$ is called the relative permittivity of the material. We should note that this is a macroscopic expression connecting polarization.

2.1.4 *Electrical bioimpedance for cylindrical subjects*

This section considers an electrically conducting cylindrical object where metal electrodes are attached on its top and bottom surfaces. Assume that L and S are its length in meters (m) and cross-sectional area in m^2, respectively. We apply either current $I \cos \omega t$ or voltage $V \cos \omega t$ with an angular frequency ω through the electrodes. We confine the frequency $\frac{\omega}{2\pi}$ within the range of tens of Hz to several MHz.

2.1.4.1 *Conductivity and resistance at direct current*

If the cylinder is filled with a homogeneous saline solution including mobile ions, their migration under an external electric field characterizes its conductivity σ in Siemens per meter (S/m). As shown in Figure 2.4, the cylinder has the length of L and cross-sectional area of S. To measure the conductivity σ, we inject direct

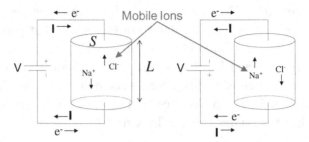

Fig. 2.4. Conductivity and resistance: Injecting a known current I and measuring the induced voltage V, we can find the conductivity σ of the cylindrical subject filled with homogeneous saline solution.

current(dc) I (Ampere, A) and measure the induced voltage V (Volt, V). The resistance R (Ohm, Ω) of the cylinder can be determined by Ohm's law $V = IR$.

Assuming that the cylinder has its axis along the z-axis (see Figure 2.4), the induced electric field $\mathbf{E}$ satisfies

$$\mathbf{E} = (0, 0, E_z), \quad |E_z| = \frac{V}{L} \tag{2.24}$$

where interfacial phenomena (contact impedance) between each electrode and the saline was neglected.

Next, we will define the current density $\mathbf{J}$ by considering the movements of each charged particle (such as ions) inside the cylinder due to the electric field $\mathbf{E}$. According to Newton's law, if the movement of a charged particle is not impeded by the molecular environment of the saline, its velocity $\mathbf{v}$ is expressed as

$$q\mathbf{E} = \underbrace{m}_{\text{mass}} \frac{d}{dt}\mathbf{v} \tag{2.25}$$

and therefore, in free space, the velocity increases linearly

$$\mathbf{v}(t) = \frac{q}{m} t\mathbf{E}. \tag{2.26}$$

However, in the saline as in the case of Figure 2.4, its movement is impeded by its molecular environment so that the particle's average drift velocity, denoted by $\langle \mathbf{v} \rangle_{ave}$, can be determined by the molecular structure of the saline:

$$\langle \mathbf{v} \rangle_{ave} = \underbrace{\frac{q}{m} t_{\mathrm{CA}}}_{\text{material property}} \mathbf{E} \qquad (2.27)$$

where t_{CA} is the characteristic time average of the charge particle traveling by the Coulomb force. With the use of the characteristic time t_{CA}, the current density $\mathbf{J}$ can be described by

$$\mathbf{J} = \rho \langle \mathbf{v} \rangle_{ave} = \rho \underbrace{\frac{q}{m} t_{\mathrm{CA}}}_{\sigma} \mathbf{E}$$

where ρ is the charge density.

Since the total injection current through the top surface is I, we have

$$I = \int_{\text{top}} |J_z| dA = |J_z| S = \sigma |E_z| S = \sigma \frac{V}{L} S.$$

Hence, the conductivity σ is

$$\sigma = \frac{L}{S} \frac{V}{I}. \qquad (2.28)$$

2.1.4.2 *Permittivity and capacitance*

Assume that the cylinder is a homogeneous perfect dielectric so that there is no mobile charge and its conductivity σ is zero. If we inject dc current I through the dielectric, we get zero dc voltage across it. Applying a dc voltage of V between top and bottom electrodes induces an electric field $\mathbf{E}$ inside the cylinder, but no dc current inside the perfect dielectric. The material contains immobile charges and their rotations or polarizations in the electric field produce surface charges Q and $-Q$ in Coulomb (C) (see Figure 2.5 which shows the section of the cylinder). The induced charge is proportional to the applied voltage; $Q \propto V$. The capacitance C (Coulomb per volt) is given by

$$C = \epsilon \frac{S}{L} = \frac{Q}{L} \qquad (2.29)$$

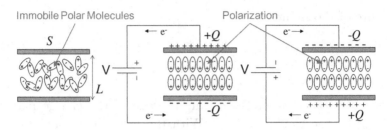

Fig. 2.5.   Polarization.

where ϵ is the permittivity in F/m. The permittivity is a material property determined by the polarization of the dielectric under an external electric field.

If we apply a sinusoidal voltage $\underline{V}(t) = V\cos\omega t$ with an angular frequency ω, there occurs an alternating current (ac) displacement current through the dielectric due to time-varying polarizations with the angular frequency ω:

$$\underline{I}(t) = C\frac{d}{dt}(V\cos\omega t) = -\omega CV\sin\omega t = \mathrm{Re}\{CVe^{\mathrm{i}(\omega t + \pi/2)}\}. \quad (2.30)$$

Note that the current and voltage are out of phase by 90° or the voltage is in the quadrature of the current.

2.1.4.3 *Admittivity of a material including both mobile and immobile charges*

We begin by considering the series resistor-capacitor (RC) circuit in Figure 2.6 (left). Applying a sinusoidal current $\underline{I}(t) = I\cos\omega t$, we can express the induced voltage $\underline{V}(t)$ as

$$\underline{V}(t) = IZ\cos(\omega t + \theta), \quad \tan\theta = \frac{\mathrm{Re}\{\mathbf{Z}\}}{\mathrm{Im}\{\mathbf{Z}\}} \quad (2.31)$$

where $Z = |\mathbf{Z}|$ and

$$\mathbf{Z} = Ze^{\mathrm{i}\theta} = R_1 + R_2 + \frac{1}{\mathrm{i}C_1} + \frac{1}{\mathrm{i}C_2}.$$

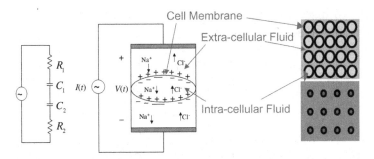

Fig. 2.6. Admittivity of a biological subject.

Next, we consider a cylinder filled with a material including both mobile and immobile charges such as a biological tissue. Assume that its electrical property is expressed as the admittivity $\kappa(\omega) = \sigma(\omega) + i\omega\epsilon(\omega)$ and is isotropic (see Figure 2.6). Note that $\sigma(\omega)$ and $\omega\epsilon(\omega)$ have the same unit of S/m. The impedance $\mathbf{Z}$ between the top and bottom surfaces is

$$\mathbf{Z} = \frac{1}{\sigma(\omega) + i\omega\epsilon(\omega)} \frac{L}{S} = \frac{L}{\sigma(\omega)S} \frac{1 - i\frac{\omega\epsilon(\omega)}{\sigma(\omega)}}{1 + \left(\frac{\omega\epsilon(\omega)}{\sigma(\omega)}\right)^2}. \quad (2.32)$$

If $\omega\epsilon(\omega) \ll \sigma(\omega)$, then $\mathbf{Z} \approx \frac{L}{\sigma(\omega)S} = R$ and the material is resistive.[4]

If $\sigma(\omega) \ll \omega\epsilon(\omega)$, then $\mathbf{Z} \approx -i\frac{L}{\omega\epsilon(\omega)S} = \frac{1}{i\omega C}$ and the material is reactive or capacitive. Most biological tissues are resistive at low frequencies of less than 10 kHz, and the capacitive term is not negligible beyond 10 kHz.

2.1.5 *Boundary value problems in electrostatics*

Assume that a biological subject occupies a domain Ω with its conductivity distribution σ. Assume that the diameter of Ω is less than 1 m. A pair of surface electrodes $\mathcal{E}^+$ and $\mathcal{E}^-$ are attached on the boundary $\partial\Omega$ to inject current of I at a fixed low angular frequency ω with $0 \leq \frac{\omega}{2\pi} \leq 500$ Hz (almost dc current). The injection

---

[4]The expression $0 < a \ll b$ means that $\frac{a}{b}$ is very close to zero.

current produces the time-independent fields **J**, **E**, **H** that satisfy the following boundary value problem:

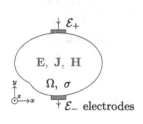

$$\nabla \times \mathbf{E} = 0 \quad \text{in } \Omega, \tag{2.33}$$

$$\nabla \times \mathbf{H} = \mathbf{J} = \sigma \mathbf{E} \quad \text{in } \Omega \tag{2.34}$$

with the boundary conditions of

$$\mathbf{J} \cdot \mathbf{n} = 0 \quad \text{on } \partial\Omega \setminus \overline{\mathcal{E}^+ \cup \mathcal{E}^-} \tag{2.35}$$

$$\mathbf{J} \times \mathbf{n} = 0 \quad \text{on } \mathcal{E}^+ \cup \mathcal{E}^- \tag{2.36}$$

$$I = -\int_{\mathcal{E}^+} \mathbf{J} \cdot \mathbf{n} \, dS = \int_{\mathcal{E}^+} \mathbf{J} \cdot \mathbf{n} \, dS. \tag{2.37}$$

The first boundary condition (2.35) comes from $\mathbf{J} = \sigma\mathbf{E} = 0$ in the air where $\sigma = 0$. The boundary condition (2.36) means that the vector **J** on each electrode is parallel or antiparallel to **n** since the electrodes are highly conductive. One may adopt the Robin boundary condition to include effects of the electrode-skin contact impedance.[5] The last boundary condition expresses that the total injection current spreads over each injection electrode.

The magnetic permeability μ of a biological tissue approximately equals to $\mu = \mu_0$. From the constitutive law $\mathbf{B} = \mu\mathbf{H}$, we may write (2.34) as

$$\frac{1}{\mu}\nabla \times \mathbf{B} = \mathbf{J} \quad \text{in } \Omega. \tag{2.38}$$

Since an isolated magnetic flux cannot exist, **B** always satisfies Gauss's law $\nabla \cdot \mathbf{B} = 0$.

Since $\nabla \times \mathbf{E} = 0$ (irrotational) by (2.33), it follows from Stokes's theorem that there exists a scalar potential u such that for any two points $\mathbf{r}_1$ and $\mathbf{r}_2$

$$u(\mathbf{r}_2) - u(\mathbf{r}_1) = -\int_{C_{\mathbf{r}_1 \to \mathbf{r}_2}} \mathbf{E} \cdot d\mathbf{l}$$

---

[5]When the electrode makes contact with the skin of a biological object, the interface can be modeled as a contact impedance and a contact potential in series. For details, we refer to [Seo and Woo (2012)].

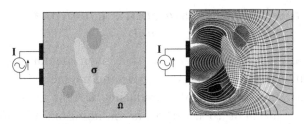

Fig. 2.7.   Voltage and current distribution due to injection current through the pair of electrodes.

where $C_{\mathbf{r}_1 \to \mathbf{r}_2}$ is a curve in Ω joining the starting point $\mathbf{r}_1$ to the ending point $\mathbf{r}_2$. The potential u can be expressed in terms of $\mathbf{E}$:

$$u(\mathbf{r}) = \int_\Omega \frac{1}{4\pi|\mathbf{r} - \mathbf{r}'|} \nabla \cdot \mathbf{E}(\mathbf{r}')d\mathbf{r}' + \text{harmonic term} \quad \text{for } \mathbf{r} \in \Omega.$$

Since $\nabla \times \mathbf{H} = \mathbf{J} = -\sigma \nabla u$ and $\nabla \cdot \nabla \times \mathbf{H} = 0$, u satisfies the following elliptic PDE:

$$-\nabla \cdot (\sigma(\mathbf{r})\nabla u(\mathbf{r})) = 0 \quad \text{for } \mathbf{r} \in \Omega. \tag{2.39}$$

Taking account of the boundary conditions (2.35)–(2.1.5), u is a solution of the following boundary value problem (see Figure 2.7):

$$
\begin{aligned}
\nabla \cdot (\sigma \nabla u) &= 0 & &\text{in } \Omega \\
\sigma \frac{\partial u}{\partial \mathbf{n}} &= 0 & &\text{on } \partial\Omega \backslash (\mathcal{E}^+ \cup \mathcal{E}^-) \\
\nabla u \times \mathbf{n} &= 0 & &\text{on } \mathcal{E}^+ \cup \mathcal{E}^- \\
I = \int_{\mathcal{E}^+} \sigma \frac{\partial u}{\partial \mathbf{n}}\, ds &= -\int_{\mathcal{E}^-} \sigma \frac{\partial u}{\partial \mathbf{n}} ds & &\text{on } \mathcal{E}^+ \cup \mathcal{E}^-.
\end{aligned}
\tag{2.40}
$$

The above non-standard boundary value problem is well posed and has a unique solution in the Sobolev space $H^1(\Omega)$ up to a constant. Here, $H^1(\Omega) = \{u : \|u\|_{H^1(\Omega)} < \infty\}$ where $\|u\|_{H^1(\Omega)} = \sqrt{\int_\Omega |u|^2 + |\nabla u|^2 d\mathbf{r}}$. We refer to [Seo and Woo (2012)] for details on the Sobolev space.

2.1.6 *Time-harmonic Maxwell's equations and eddy current model*

A sinusoidally time-varying source at a given angular frequency ω produces sinusoidal variations of electric and magnetic fields at every point $\mathbf{r}$ with the same angular frequency ω. For these sinusoidal fields, it is convenient to use the phasor notation. We denote the sinusoidally time-varying electric and magnetic fields by $\underline{\mathbf{E}}(\mathbf{r}, t)$ and $\underline{\mathbf{H}}(\mathbf{r}, t)$, respectively. As mentioned above, we express them using vector field phasors of $\mathbf{E}(\mathbf{r})$ and $\mathbf{H}(\mathbf{r})$ as

$$\underline{\mathbf{E}}(\mathbf{r}, t) = \mathrm{Re}\{\mathbf{E}(\mathbf{r})e^{i\omega t}\} \quad \text{and} \quad \underline{\mathbf{H}}(\mathbf{r}, t) = \mathrm{Re}\{\mathbf{H}(\mathbf{r})e^{i\omega t}\}.$$

Each component of $\mathbf{E}(\mathbf{r})$ (or $\mathbf{H}(\mathbf{r})$) is a complex-valued function (independent of time) that contains amplitude and phase information.

Assume that a coil C is placed outside a conducting domain Ω and $\sigma + i\omega\epsilon \approx 0$ outside Ω. If a sinusoidal current of I at an angular frequency ω, $0 \le \frac{\omega}{2\pi} \le 300\,\text{MHz}$, is applied to the coil C, the resulting time-harmonic fields satisfy time-harmonic Maxwell's equations:

$$\nabla \times \mathbf{E} = -i\omega\mathbf{B} \qquad (2.41)$$

$$\nabla \times \mathbf{H} = \underbrace{(\sigma + i\omega\epsilon)}_{\kappa}\mathbf{E} + \mathbf{J}_s \quad (2.42)$$

where $\mathbf{J}_s$ is the source current density at the coil C. Since $\mathbf{B}$ is divergence free, a vector magnetic potential $\mathbf{A}$ exists such that

$$\mathbf{B}(\mathbf{r}) = \nabla \times \mathbf{A}(\mathbf{r}), \quad \nabla \cdot \mathbf{A} = 0 \quad \text{(Coulomb gauge)}.$$

From (2.41) and the above identity, we have

$$\nabla \times (\mathbf{E} + i\omega\mathbf{A}) = 0.$$

Hence, it follows from Stoke's theorem that there exists a scalar potential u such that

$$-\nabla u(\mathbf{r}) = \mathbf{E}(\mathbf{r}) + i\omega\mathbf{A}(\mathbf{r}). \qquad (2.43)$$

This can be viewed as a Helmholtz decomposition of $\mathbf{E}$; according to the Helmholtz decomposition, $\mathbf{E}$ can be resolved into the sum of a curl-free vector field and a divergence-free vector field:

$$\mathbf{E}(\mathbf{r}) = \underbrace{-\nabla \int \frac{\nabla \cdot \mathbf{E}(\mathbf{r}')}{4\pi|\mathbf{r} - \mathbf{r}'|} d\mathbf{r}'}_{\text{curl-free} \Leftrightarrow -\nabla u} + \underbrace{\nabla \times \int \frac{\nabla \times \mathbf{E}(\mathbf{r}')}{4\pi|\mathbf{r} - \mathbf{r}'|} d\mathbf{r}'}_{\text{divergence-free} \Leftrightarrow -i\omega \mathbf{A}} + \text{Harmonic.}$$

$$(2.44)$$

See Remark 2.1 for detailed discussion on the identity (2.44).

Multiplying κ to both sides of the identity (2.43), we get

$$\underbrace{-\kappa(\mathbf{r})\nabla u(\mathbf{r})}_{\mathbf{J}_{\text{total}}} = \underbrace{\kappa(\mathbf{r})\mathbf{E}(\mathbf{r})}_{\mathbf{J}} + \underbrace{i\omega\kappa(\mathbf{r})\mathbf{A}(\mathbf{r})}_{\mathbf{J}_{\text{eddy}}}.$$

Hence, the total current density $\mathbf{J}_{\text{total}} = -\kappa\nabla u$ is decomposed into $\mathbf{J}$ and the eddy current $\mathbf{J}_{\text{eddy}} = i\omega\kappa\mathbf{A}$. Noting that $\nabla \cdot \mathbf{J} = 0$, we have

$$-\nabla \cdot [\kappa(\mathbf{r})\nabla u(\mathbf{r})] = i\omega\nabla \cdot [\kappa(\mathbf{r})\mathbf{A}(\mathbf{r})] = i\omega\nabla\kappa(\mathbf{r}) \cdot \mathbf{A}(\mathbf{r}). \quad (2.45)$$

This means that the eddy current $\mathbf{J}_{\text{eddy}}$ generates a source of charge where the admittivity κ changes.

Denoting $u_{\text{r}} = \text{Re}\{u\}$ and $u_{\text{i}} = \text{Im}\{u\}$, we have

$$\mathbf{J}_{\text{total}}(\mathbf{r}) = -[\sigma(\mathbf{r})\nabla u_{\text{r}}(\mathbf{r}) - \omega\epsilon(\mathbf{r})\nabla u_{\text{i}}(\mathbf{r})]$$
$$- i[\omega\epsilon(\mathbf{r})\nabla u_{\text{r}}(\mathbf{r}) + \sigma(\mathbf{r})\nabla u_{\text{i}}(\mathbf{r})]. \quad (2.46)$$

Noting that $-\nabla u_{\text{r}} = \text{Re}\{\mathbf{E}\} - \text{Im}\{\omega\mathbf{A}\}$ and $-\nabla u_{\text{i}} = \text{Im}\{\mathbf{E}\} + \text{Re}\{\omega\mathbf{A}\}$, we can interpret each term in (2.46) in the following ways:

- $-\sigma\nabla u_{\text{r}}$ is the sum of the conduction current by dc or ac electric field and the conduction eddy current by ac magnetic field induced by ac displacement current.
- $\omega\epsilon\nabla u_{\text{i}}$ is the sum of the displacement current by ac electric field induced by ac magnetic field and the displacement eddy current by ac magnetic field induced by ac conduction current.
- $-\omega\epsilon\nabla u_{\text{r}}$ is the sum of the displacement current by ac electric field and the displacement eddy current by ac magnetic field induced by ac displacement current.

- $-\sigma \nabla u_{\mathrm{i}}$ is the sum of the conduction current by ac electric field induced by ac magnetic field and the conduction eddy current by ac magnetic field induced by ac conduction current.

The primary field $\mathbf{E}_p = -\mathrm{i}\omega \mathbf{A}_{\mathrm{p}}$ generated by coil C is given by

$$\mathbf{E}_p(\mathbf{r}) = -\mathrm{i}\omega \mathbf{A}_{\mathrm{p}}(\mathbf{r}) = -\mathrm{i}\omega \frac{\mu_0 I}{4\pi} \int_C \frac{1}{|\mathbf{r} - \mathbf{r}'|} \mathrm{d}\mathbf{l}_{\mathbf{r}'}. \tag{2.47}$$

From (2.43), the secondary field $\mathbf{E}_s$ is

$$\mathbf{E}_s(\mathbf{r}) = \mathbf{E}(\mathbf{r}) - \mathbf{E}_p(\mathbf{r}) = -\mathrm{i}\omega \mathbf{A}_{\mathrm{s}}(\mathbf{r}) - \nabla u(\mathbf{r}) \tag{2.48}$$

where $\mathbf{A}_s = \mathbf{A} - \mathbf{A}_p$.

Substituting $\mathbf{H} = \frac{1}{\mu}\nabla \times \mathbf{A}$ and (2.43) into (2.42) yields

$$\nabla \times \left(\frac{1}{\mu}\nabla \times \mathbf{A}\right) + \kappa\left(i\omega\mathbf{A} + \nabla u\right) = \mathbf{J}_s. \tag{2.49}$$

Taking divergence to the above identity leads to

$$\nabla \cdot (\kappa \nabla u) = \nabla \cdot \mathbf{J}_s - i\omega \nabla \cdot (\kappa \mathbf{A}). \tag{2.50}$$

Inside the conducting medium Ω, the potential u satisfies

$$\nabla \cdot (\kappa(\nabla u + i\omega \mathbf{A}_{\mathrm{s}})) = -i\omega \nabla \kappa \cdot \mathbf{A}_{\mathrm{p}} \quad \text{in} \quad \Omega \tag{2.51}$$

with the boundary condition

$$\mathbf{n} \cdot (\kappa(\nabla u + i\omega \mathbf{A}_{\mathrm{s}}))|_{\partial\Omega} = -\mathbf{n} \cdot (i\omega\kappa \mathbf{A}_{\mathrm{p}})|_{\partial\Omega}. \tag{2.52}$$

Table 2.1 summarizes the induced current model.

Table 2.1.   Induced current model.

Governing Equation	
$\nabla \times (\mu^{-1}\nabla \times \mathbf{A}) + (\sigma + i\omega\epsilon)(i\omega\mathbf{A} + \nabla u) = \mathbf{J}_s$	in the entire region
$\nabla \times (\mu^{-1}\nabla \times \mathbf{A}) + (\sigma + i\omega\epsilon)(i\omega\mathbf{A} + \nabla u) = 0$	in conducting region
$\nabla \cdot ((\sigma + i\omega\epsilon)\nabla u) = 0$	in conducting region
$\left[\mathbf{n} \times \left(\frac{1}{\mu}\nabla \times \mathbf{A}\right)\right] = 0$	transmission boundary condition
$[\mathbf{n} \cdot ((\sigma + i\omega\epsilon)(i\omega\mathbf{A} + \nabla u))] = 0$	transmission boundary condition

Assuming that $i\omega\mathbf{A}_s$ is negligibly small compared to ∇u, (2.51) and (2.52) can be simplified into

$$\nabla \cdot (\kappa\nabla u) = -i\omega\nabla\kappa \cdot \mathbf{A}_p \quad \text{in } \Omega$$
$$\mathbf{n} \cdot (\kappa\nabla u)|_{\partial\Omega} = -i\omega\mathbf{n} \cdot (\kappa\mathbf{A}_p)|_{\partial\Omega}. \tag{2.53}$$

We can compute the boundary value problem (2.53), and its solution is a good approximation of the true potential u up to a constant.

Lemma 2.1 (Helmholtz decomposition). *Helmholtz's theorem is known as the fundamental theorem of vector calculus. It states that any smooth vector field $\mathbf{F}$ in a smooth bounded domain Ω can be rewritten as the sum of a divergence-free (solenoidal) vector field and a curl-free (irrotational) vector field. Every vector field $\mathbf{F}(\mathbf{r}) = (F_1(\mathbf{r}), F_2(\mathbf{r}), F_3(\mathbf{r})) \in [L^2(\Omega)]^3$ can be decomposed into*

$$\mathbf{F}(\mathbf{r}) = -\nabla u(\mathbf{r}) + \nabla \times \mathbf{A}(\mathbf{r}) + Harmonic \quad in \ \Omega \tag{2.54}$$

where Harmonic is a vector field whose Laplacian is zero in Ω. Moreover, u and $\mathbf{A}$ can be uniquely determined up to harmonic functions:

$$u(\mathbf{r}) = -\int_\Omega \frac{\nabla \cdot \mathbf{F}(r')}{4\pi|\mathbf{r} - \mathbf{r}'|}d\mathbf{r}' + Harmonic \tag{2.55}$$

and

$$\mathbf{A}(\mathbf{r}) = \int_\Omega \frac{\nabla \times \mathbf{F}(\mathbf{r}')}{4\pi|\mathbf{r} - \mathbf{r}'|}d\mathbf{r}' + Harmonic. \tag{2.56}$$

Proof. We write the vector field $\mathbf{F}$ as

$$\mathbf{F}(\mathbf{r}) = \int_\Omega \delta(\mathbf{r} - \mathbf{r}')\mathbf{F}(\mathbf{r}')d\mathbf{r}' = -\int_\Omega \nabla^2\left(\frac{1}{4\pi|\mathbf{r} - \mathbf{r}'|}\right)\mathbf{F}(\mathbf{r}')d\mathbf{r}'.$$

Integration by parts yields

$$\mathbf{F}(\mathbf{r}) = -\int_\Omega \frac{1}{4\pi|\mathbf{r} - \mathbf{r}'|}\nabla^2\mathbf{F}(\mathbf{r}')d\mathbf{r}' + \int_{\partial\Omega} \Psi_1(\mathbf{r}, \mathbf{r}')dS_{\mathbf{r}'}, \quad \mathbf{r} \in \Omega \tag{2.57}$$

where

$$\Psi_1(\mathbf{r}, \mathbf{r}') = -\frac{\partial}{\partial\mathbf{n}}\left(\frac{1}{4\pi|\mathbf{r} - \mathbf{r}'|}\right)\mathbf{F}(\mathbf{r}') + \frac{1}{4\pi|\mathbf{r} - \mathbf{r}'|}\frac{\partial}{\partial\mathbf{n}}\mathbf{F}(\mathbf{r}').$$

Due to the property $\nabla_{\mathbf{r}}^2 \left(\frac{-1}{4\pi|\mathbf{r}-\mathbf{r}'|} \right) = \delta(\mathbf{r} - \mathbf{r}')$, we have

$$\nabla_{\mathbf{r}}^2 \Psi_1(\mathbf{r}, \mathbf{r}') = 0 \quad \text{for } \mathbf{r} \in \Omega, \quad \mathbf{r}' \in \partial\Omega.$$

Using the vector identity $-\nabla^2 \mathbf{F} = \nabla \times (\nabla \times \mathbf{F}) - \nabla(\nabla \cdot \mathbf{F})$, we can express (2.57) as

$$\mathbf{F}(\mathbf{r}) = \int_\Omega \frac{1}{4\pi|\mathbf{r} - \mathbf{r}'|} \left[\nabla \times (\nabla \times \mathbf{F}) - \nabla(\nabla \cdot \mathbf{F}) \right] dV$$

$$+ \int_{\partial\Omega} \Psi_1(\mathbf{r}, \mathbf{r}') dS, \quad \mathbf{r} \in \Omega. \tag{2.58}$$

Integrating by parts again yields

$$\mathbf{F}(\mathbf{r}) = \nabla \times \int \frac{\nabla \times \mathbf{F}(\mathbf{r}')}{4\pi|\mathbf{r} - \mathbf{r}'|} dV - \nabla \int \frac{\nabla \cdot \mathbf{F}(\mathbf{r}')}{4\pi|\mathbf{r} - \mathbf{r}'|} d\mathbf{r}'$$

$$+ \int_{\partial\Omega} \Psi_1(\mathbf{r}, \mathbf{r}') + \Psi_2(\mathbf{r}, \mathbf{r}') dS$$

where Ψ_2 is a function satisfying $\nabla_{\mathbf{r}}^2 \Psi_2(\mathbf{r}, \mathbf{r}') = 0$ for $\mathbf{r} \in \Omega$ and $\mathbf{r}' \in \partial\Omega$. This completes the proof of Helmholtz's decomposition. $\square$

2.1.7 *Magnetic field created by magnetic moment*

In this subsection, we evaluate the magnetic field due to magnetization represented by a current carrying circular loops. Here, we take account of the magnetic moment of an equivalent current due to a circulation of charges along a small circle.

We begin with reviewing the relation among $\mathbf{B}$ and $\mathbf{J}$. According to Helmholtz's decomposition in (2.44) with $\mathbf{E}$ replaced by $\mathbf{B}$, a vector magnetic potential $\mathbf{A}$ exists such that

$$\mathbf{B} = \nabla \times \mathbf{A} \quad \text{and} \quad \nabla \cdot \mathbf{A} = 0. \tag{2.59}$$

Here, we use the fact that $\nabla \cdot \mathbf{B} = 0$. We should note that $\mathbf{A}$ in (2.59) is different from that in (2.43). Since $\nabla \times \mathbf{B} = \nabla \times \nabla \times \mathbf{A} = \nabla\nabla \cdot \mathbf{A} - \nabla^2 \mathbf{A} = -\nabla^2 \mathbf{A}$, the vector magnetic potential $\mathbf{A}$ can be viewed as the solution of the Poisson equation

$$-\nabla^2 \mathbf{A} = \mu \mathbf{J}.$$

Since $\frac{1}{4\pi|\mathbf{r}-\mathbf{r}'|}$ is the fundamental solution of the Laplacian, we have

$$-\nabla^2 \left(\frac{1}{4\pi|\mathbf{r}-\mathbf{r}'|} \right) = \delta(\mathbf{r}-\mathbf{r}'),$$

where δ is the Dirac delta function. We can express $\mathbf{A}$ as

$$\mathbf{A}(\mathbf{r}) = \frac{\mu}{4\pi} \int \frac{1}{|\mathbf{r}-\mathbf{r}'|} \mathbf{J}(\mathbf{r}') \, d\mathbf{r}' + \text{Harmonic} \quad \text{in } \Omega \qquad (2.60)$$

where *Harmonic* is a vector field whose Laplacian is zero. From the relation $\mathbf{B} = \nabla \times \mathbf{A}$, we have

$$\mathbf{B}(\mathbf{r}) = -\frac{\mu}{4\pi} \int \frac{\mathbf{r}-\mathbf{r}'}{|\mathbf{r}-\mathbf{r}'|^3} \times \mathbf{J}(\mathbf{r}') \, d\mathbf{r}' + \text{Harmonic.} \qquad (2.61)$$

The following proposition explains the magnetic field produced by a current in a small circular loop such as $\mathcal{C} = \{\mathbf{r} : |\mathbf{r}-\mathbf{r}_0| = r, \ z = z_0\}$.

Proposition 2.1. *Let $\mathcal{C}$ be a circular coil $\mathcal{C} = \{\mathbf{r} : |\mathbf{r}-\mathbf{r}_0| = r, \ z = z_0\}$ with its radius $r \approx 0$. In the presence of a current of I mA along the coil $\mathcal{C}$, the induced magnetic potential $\mathbf{A}$ in free space can be approximated as*

$$\mathbf{A}(\mathbf{r}) \approx \frac{\mu_0 I}{4\pi} \int_{\mathcal{C}} \frac{1}{|\mathbf{r}-\mathbf{r}'|} d\mathbf{l}_{\mathbf{r}'} \qquad (2.62)$$

where $d\mathbf{l}$ is the line element. Writing $\mathbf{M} = I\pi r^2 \hat{\mathbf{z}}$, called the magnetic moment, we have

$$\mathbf{A}(\mathbf{r}) \approx \frac{\mu_0}{4\pi} \frac{\mathbf{M} \times (\mathbf{r}-\mathbf{r}_0)}{|\mathbf{r}-\mathbf{r}_0|^3}. \qquad (2.63)$$

In general, the magnetic potential due to a distribution of magnetization can be expressed as

$$\mathbf{A}^{\mathrm{M}}(\mathbf{r}) \approx \frac{\mu_0}{4\pi} \int \mathbf{M}(\mathbf{r}') \times \frac{\mathbf{r}-\mathbf{r}'}{|\mathbf{r}-\mathbf{r}'|^3} d\mathbf{r}'. \qquad (2.64)$$

Proof. Assume that $r \approx 0$, it follows from Stoke's theorem that

$$
\hat{\mathbf{z}} \times \mathbf{A}(\mathbf{r}) = \frac{\mu_0 I}{4\pi} \hat{\mathbf{z}} \times \oint_C \frac{1}{|\mathbf{r} - \mathbf{r}'|} d\mathbf{l}_{\mathbf{r}'}
$$

$$
= \frac{\mu_0 I}{4\pi} \hat{\mathbf{z}} \times \oint_C \frac{1}{|\mathbf{r} - \mathbf{r}'|} (\hat{\mathbf{x}}(\hat{\mathbf{x}} \cdot d\mathbf{l}_{\mathbf{r}'}) + \hat{\mathbf{y}}(\hat{\mathbf{y}} \cdot d\mathbf{l}_{\mathbf{r}'}))
$$

$$
= \frac{\mu_0 I}{4\pi} \sum_{j=1}^{2} \hat{\mathbf{z}} \times \hat{\mathbf{r}}_j \int_{C_{area}} \nabla \times \frac{\hat{\mathbf{r}}_j}{|\mathbf{r} - \mathbf{r}'|} \cdot \hat{\mathbf{z}} \, dS_{\mathbf{r}'}
$$

$$
(\hat{\mathbf{r}}_1 = \hat{\mathbf{x}}, \ \hat{\mathbf{r}}_2 = \hat{\mathbf{y}})
$$

$$
\approx -\frac{\mu_0}{4\pi} (I\pi r^2) \sum_{j=1}^{2} \left[\hat{\mathbf{r}}_j \cdot \nabla \frac{1}{|\mathbf{r} - \mathbf{r}_0|} \right] \hat{\mathbf{r}}_j.
$$

Since $\mathbf{A}$ is orthogonal to $\mathbf{n} = \hat{\mathbf{z}}$, we have $\hat{\mathbf{z}} \times (\hat{\mathbf{z}} \times \mathbf{A}) = \hat{\mathbf{z}}(\hat{\mathbf{z}} \cdot \mathbf{A}) - (\hat{\mathbf{z}} \cdot \hat{\mathbf{z}})\mathbf{A} = -\mathbf{A}$ and

$$
\mathbf{A}(\mathbf{r}) \approx \frac{-\mu_0}{4\pi} (I\pi r^2) \sum_{j=1}^{2} \left[\hat{\mathbf{r}}_j \cdot \nabla \frac{1}{|\mathbf{r} - \mathbf{r}_0|} \right] \hat{\mathbf{z}} \times \mathbf{e}_j
$$

$$
= \frac{\mu_0}{4\pi} (I\pi r^2 \hat{\mathbf{z}}) \times \left[\frac{\mathbf{r} - \mathbf{r}_0}{|\mathbf{r} - \mathbf{r}_0|^3} \right].
$$

This leads to (2.63). □

From the approximation (2.64), the magnetic field induced by the distribution of the magnetic dipoles can be expressed as

$$
\mathbf{B}^{\mathrm{M}}(\mathbf{r}) = \nabla \times \mathbf{A}^{\mathrm{M}}(\mathbf{r}) \approx \frac{\mu_0}{4\pi} \nabla \times \int \mathbf{M}(\mathbf{r}') \times \frac{\mathbf{r} - \mathbf{r}'}{|\mathbf{r} - \mathbf{r}'|^3} d\mathbf{r}'.
$$

$$
\approx \frac{\mu_0}{4\pi} \int \frac{1}{|\mathbf{r} - \mathbf{r}'|^3} \left[\frac{3[\mathbf{M}(\mathbf{r}') \cdot (\mathbf{r} - \mathbf{r}')](\mathbf{r} - \mathbf{r}')}{|\mathbf{r} - \mathbf{r}'|^2} - \mathbf{M}(\mathbf{r}') \right] d\mathbf{r}'.
$$

$$(2.65)$$

Under the assumption that $\mathbf{M} = M_z \hat{\mathbf{z}}$ has only z-component, (2.65) can be simplified into

$$
B_z^{\mathrm{M}}(\mathbf{r}) \approx \frac{\mu_0}{4\pi} \int \frac{2(z - z')^2 - (x - x')^2 - (y - y')^2}{|\mathbf{r} - \mathbf{r}'|^5} M_z(\mathbf{r}') d\mathbf{r}'.
$$

$$(2.66)$$

Tissue magnetic susceptibility reflects the degree of biomaterials being magnetized by the applied magnetic field $\mathbf{B}_0$. In a conducting medium, steady-state Maxwell's equations for $\mathbf{B}$ due to magnetic polarization $\mathbf{M}$ can be expressed as

$$\frac{1}{\mu_0}\nabla \times \mathbf{B} = \mathbf{J} + \nabla \times \mathbf{M}. \tag{2.67}$$

Hence, we can write

$$\mathbf{H} = \frac{1}{\mu_0}\mathbf{B} - \mathbf{M}. \tag{2.68}$$

2.2 Magnetic Resonance Imaging

An MR scanner can non-invasively measure magnetic moments inside the human body in a form of cross-sectional image. MRI makes use of the hydrogen atoms inside the biological tissue to create magnetization; hydrogen nuclei become polarized by the external magnetic field, and then produce magnetic fields in the detecting coil of the MR scanner. In the human body, the amount of hydrogen would be the major factor for the net magnetization vector $\underline{\mathbf{M}}$. MRI uses nuclear magnetic resonance (NMR) phenomenon and linear gradient field to localize $\underline{\mathbf{M}}$ to provide a cross-sectional image of the density of $\underline{\mathbf{M}}$ inside the human body. This section focuses on electro-magnetic fields interacting with biological tissue in an MRI system.

MRI uses several sources of magnetic fields which can be classified into two groups; (1) external fields generated by the MRI scanner and (2) internal field emitted via the nuclear resonance of the subject Ω. The external fields include the main field $\mathbf{B}_0$, RF field, and gradient field $G = (G_x, G_y, G_z)$. To obtain the desired image, the internal field (i.e., the "MR signal") is measured after turning off the RF field and proper application of the gradient field (which will be described later). Appropriate and efficient use of notations is very important for the quick understanding of the fundamental concepts of MRI. The following provides a rough outline of this section:

- The human body when being imaged occupies the three-dimensional domain Ω. The subject Ω is placed inside the MR scanner which generates the main magnetic field $\mathbf{B}_0$. Magnetic moments in $\mathbf{B}_0$ will tend to align with the direction of $\mathbf{B}_0$.

- We choose the direction of the main magnetic field of the MRI scanner as $\hat{\mathbf{z}}$ direction. We assume that its main magnetic field is

$$\mathbf{B}_0 = (0, 0, B_0) = B_0\hat{\mathbf{z}}$$

where $B_0 > 0$ is a constant and field inhomogeneities (e.g., from system imperfections) are neglected.

- In the presence of the external magnetic field $\mathbf{B}(\mathbf{r}, t) = \mathbf{B}_0 + [G \cdot \mathbf{r}]\hat{\mathbf{z}}$, it causes $\underline{\mathbf{M}}$ to precess around $\hat{\mathbf{z}}$-axis with the angular velocity

$$\boldsymbol{\omega} = -\gamma\mathbf{B} = \underbrace{-\gamma(B_0 + G \cdot \mathbf{r})\hat{\mathbf{z}}}_{:=\omega(\mathbf{r})}$$

where γ is the gyromagnetic ratio depending on the regarded type of nucleus.[6] In this section, we assume $\gamma > 0$ and $\mu = \mu_0$ in Ω.

- The RF field is applied to excite the nuclear spins in the body in order to tilt $\underline{\mathbf{M}}$ from its equilibrium position $\underline{\mathbf{M}}^{\text{equm}}$.

- After turning off the RF field, we receive RF signals from the spins. The magnetization $\underline{\mathbf{M}}(\mathbf{r}, t)$ as a source of the signal is governed by the Bloch equation (after turning off the RF field):

$$\frac{\partial}{\partial t}\underline{\mathbf{M}}(\mathbf{r}, t) = \underbrace{-\gamma(\mathbf{B}_0 + G(t) \cdot \mathbf{r})}_{:=\omega(\mathbf{r},t)} \times \underline{\mathbf{M}}(r, t) + \text{relaxation effects}$$

$$(2.69)$$

where the gradient field G depends on time t. The time-varying magnetic moments $\underline{\mathbf{M}}(\mathbf{r}, t)$ produce a time-varying magnetic field. By placing a coil near the body, we can receive the signal produced by the distribution of $\underline{\mathbf{M}}(\mathbf{r}, t)$. The voltage signal in the coil (electromotive force) is governed by Faraday's law.

- These received signals are converted into voltages that are often measured by the same coil used to create the excitation of the RF field. These voltage signals provide so-called k-space data, whose

---

[6]For instance, $\gamma = 2\pi \times 42.576 \times 10^6$ rad/s/T is positive for ^1H, while $\gamma < 0$ for ^{17}O. For a 1.5 T MRI system, the frequency of $\frac{\omega_0}{2\pi} := \frac{\gamma B_0}{2\pi}$ is approximately 63 MHz for ^1H.

inverse Fourier transform results in a tomographic image of the patient or the imaged object.

There are many well-organized books about the basics of MRI. For a fundamental understanding of MRI, we recommend reading [Haacke *et al.* (1999); Wang (2012)].

2.2.1 *MR signal and Larmor precession of spins ignoring relaxation effects*

2.2.1.1 *Larmor precession of* $\underline{\mathbf{M}}$ *in an external field* $\mathbf{B}$

The strong field $\mathbf{B}(\mathbf{r}) = (0, 0, B(\mathbf{r}))$ produces a distribution of net magnetization $\underline{\mathbf{M}}(\mathbf{r}, t)$ in Ω by aligning protons inside the human body where $\underline{\mathbf{M}}(\mathbf{r}, t) = (\underline{M}_x(\mathbf{r}, t), \underline{M}_y(\mathbf{r}, t), \underline{M}_z(\mathbf{r}, t))$ depends on time t, position $\mathbf{r}$, and the initial magnetization $\underline{\mathbf{M}}(\mathbf{r}, 0)$. The interaction of $\mathbf{M}$ with the external magnetic field $\mathbf{B}$ is dictated by the Bloch equation (ignoring relaxation effects):

$$\frac{\partial}{\partial t}\underline{\mathbf{M}} = -\gamma \mathbf{B} \times \underline{\mathbf{M}} = \begin{vmatrix} \hat{\mathbf{x}} & \hat{\mathbf{y}} & \hat{\mathbf{z}} \\ M_x & M_y & M_z \\ 0 & 0 & \omega \end{vmatrix} \tag{2.70}$$

where

$$\omega(\mathbf{r}) = \gamma B(\mathbf{r}). \tag{2.71}$$

The equation (2.70) tells

$$\underline{\mathbf{M}} \cdot \frac{\partial}{\partial t}\underline{\mathbf{M}} = 0 \quad \& \quad \mathbf{B} \cdot \frac{\partial}{\partial t}\underline{\mathbf{M}} = 0 \tag{2.72}$$

which mean that the vector $\frac{\partial}{\partial t}\underline{\mathbf{M}}$ is perpendicular to both $\underline{\mathbf{M}}$ and $\mathbf{B}$.

Proposition 2.2. *Denoting* $\underline{M}_\perp(\mathbf{r}, t) := \underline{M}_x(\mathbf{r}, t) + \mathrm{i}\underline{M}_y(\mathbf{r}, t)$, *the equation* (2.70) *is equivalent to the simple ODE:*

$$\frac{\partial}{\partial t}\underline{M}_\perp(\mathbf{r}, t) = -\mathrm{i}\omega_0 \underline{M}_\perp(\mathbf{r}, t). \tag{2.73}$$

The solution of ODE (2.73) *is*

$$\underline{M}_\perp(\mathbf{r}, t) = M_\perp^0(\mathbf{r})\, e^{-\mathrm{i}\omega t} \tag{2.74}$$

where $M_\perp^0(\mathbf{r}) := \underline{M}_\perp(\mathbf{r}, 0)$ is the initial magnetization (see Figure 2.8). The transversal component $\mathbf{M}_{xy} = \underline{M}_x\hat{\mathbf{x}} + \underline{M}_y\hat{\mathbf{y}}$ can be expressed as

$$\mathbf{M}_{xy} = Re\{M_\perp^0 e^{-i\omega t}\, \mathbf{a}^+\} = Re\{(M_\perp^0)^* e^{i\omega t}\, \mathbf{a}^-\} \tag{2.75}$$

where $(M_\perp^0)^*(\mathbf{r}) = M_x(\mathbf{r}, 0) - iM_y(\mathbf{r}, 0)$ (the harmonic conjugate), $\mathbf{a}^+$ and $\mathbf{a}^-$, respectively, are the positive and negative rotating phaser given by vectors

$$\mathbf{a}^+ = \hat{\mathbf{x}} - i\hat{\mathbf{y}} \quad \& \quad \mathbf{a}^- = \hat{\mathbf{x}} + i\hat{\mathbf{y}}. \tag{2.76}$$

Proof. The Bloch equation (2.72) can be written as

$$\frac{\partial}{\partial t}\begin{pmatrix} M_x \\ M_y \\ M_z \end{pmatrix} = \begin{vmatrix} \hat{\mathbf{x}} & \hat{\mathbf{y}} & \hat{\mathbf{z}} \\ \underline{M}_x & \underline{M}_y & \underline{M}_z \\ 0 & 0 & \omega \end{vmatrix} = \begin{pmatrix} \omega\underline{M}_y \\ -\omega\underline{M}_x \\ 0 \end{pmatrix} \tag{2.77}$$

which leads to (2.74).

The expression (2.75) comes from (2.74) and the simple identities

$$\alpha\hat{\mathbf{x}} + \beta\hat{\mathbf{y}} = \Re\left\{(\alpha + i\beta)\mathbf{a}^+\right\} = \Re\left\{(\alpha + i\beta)^*\mathbf{a}^-\right\} \quad (\forall \alpha, \beta \in \mathbb{R}) \qquad \square$$

The expression (2.75) explains the behavior of $\underline{\mathbf{M}}$ intuitively. Noting that

$$Re\{\mathbf{a}^\pm e^{-i\omega t}\} = \begin{pmatrix} \cos\omega t \\ \mp\sin\omega t \\ 0 \end{pmatrix}, \quad \mathbf{a}^\pm \cdot \mathbf{a}^\pm = 0, \quad \mathbf{a}^+ \cdot \mathbf{a}^- = 2, \tag{2.78}$$

we have

$$Re\{(\alpha + i\beta)e^{-i\omega t}\mathbf{a}^\pm\} = \Theta_{\mp\omega t}\begin{pmatrix} \alpha \\ \beta \\ 0 \end{pmatrix} \quad (\forall \alpha, \beta \in \mathbb{R})$$

where $\Theta_{\pm\omega t}$ is the rotation matrix given by

$$\Theta_{\pm\omega t} = \begin{pmatrix} \cos\omega t & \mp\sin\omega t & 0 \\ \pm\sin\omega t & \cos\omega t & 0 \\ 0 & 0 & 1 \end{pmatrix}.$$

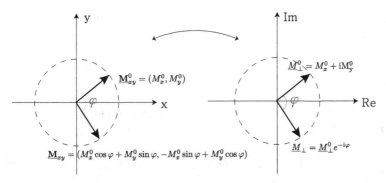

Fig. 2.8. The complex plane and Euler's formula $e^{i\varphi} = \cos\varphi + i\sin\varphi$. The complex plane allows a convenient geometric description of the motion of $\underline{\mathbf{M}}_{xy}$. In Cartesian coordinate, $\underline{\mathbf{M}}_{xy} = (M_x^0\cos\varphi - M_y^0\sin\varphi, M_x^0\sin\varphi + M_y^0\cos\varphi)$ where $\varphi = \omega t$. With the complex plain, $\underline{M}_\perp = M_\perp^0 e^{i\varphi}$.

Hence, (2.75) explains that the transversal component $\underline{\mathbf{M}}_{xy} = M_x\hat{\mathbf{x}} + M_y\hat{\mathbf{y}}$ rotates clockwise at the angular frequency $\omega = \gamma B$ for $\gamma > 0$. That is, (2.74) explains how $\mathbf{B}$ causes $\underline{M}$ to precess about z-axis with the angular velocity $-\omega\hat{\mathbf{z}} = -\gamma B\hat{\mathbf{z}}$. For a 1.5 T MRI system, the frequency of $\frac{\omega}{2\pi}$ is approximately 63 MHz for ^1H.

We will use the facts of Proposition 2.2 many times. For the reader's convenience, we will rewrite it in the following general form:

Proposition 2.3. *Let* $\underline{\mathbf{V}}(t) = (V_x(t), V_y(t), V_z(t))$ *be a vector depending on time t and denote its transversal component* $(V_x(t), V_y(t))$ *as the complex form* $V_\perp(t) = V_x(t) + iV_y(t)$. *Then, the following are equivalent:*

(i) $\dfrac{d}{dt}\underline{\mathbf{V}}(t) = \pm(\omega\hat{\mathbf{z}}) \times \underline{\mathbf{V}}(t)$ \hfill (2.79)

(ii) $V_\perp(t) = V_\perp(0)e^{\pm i\omega t}$ & $V_z(t) = V_z(0)$ \hfill (2.80)

(iii) $\underline{\mathbf{V}}(t) = \Theta_{\pm\omega t}\underline{\mathbf{V}}(0)$. \hfill (2.81)

It is convenient to introduce a rotating frame (the viewpoint of an observer riding along on a rotating axis) in which the xy-plane is rotating at the angular frequency $\omega_0 = \gamma B_0$:

$$\underline{\mathbf{x}}^\pm := \Theta_{\pm\omega_0 t}\hat{\mathbf{x}} \quad \text{and} \quad \underline{\mathbf{y}}^\pm := \Theta_{\pm\omega_0 t}\hat{\mathbf{y}}, \tag{2.82}$$

assuming $\omega_0 > 0$, $\underline{\mathbf{x}}^+$ and $\underline{\mathbf{y}}^+$ are rotating counterclockwise. The rotating axes $\underline{\mathbf{x}}^\pm$ and $\underline{\mathbf{y}}^\pm$ satisfy

$$\frac{d\underline{\mathbf{x}}^\pm}{dt} = \pm(\omega_0\hat{\mathbf{z}}) \times \underline{\mathbf{x}}^\pm \quad \& \quad \frac{d\underline{\mathbf{y}}^\pm}{dt} = \pm(\omega_0\hat{\mathbf{z}}) \times \underline{\mathbf{y}}^\pm. \tag{2.83}$$

With the use of the rotating axes, the $\underline{\mathbf{M}}_{xy}(\mathbf{r}, t) = \underline{M}_x(\mathbf{r}, t)\hat{\mathbf{x}} + \underline{M}_y(\mathbf{r}, t)\hat{\mathbf{y}}$ satisfying (2.70) with $\mathbf{B} = \mathbf{B}_0$ can be expressed as

$$\underline{\mathbf{M}}_{xy}(\mathbf{r}, t) = M_x^-(\mathbf{r})\, \underline{\mathbf{x}}^- + M_y^-(\mathbf{r})\, \underline{\mathbf{y}}^- \tag{2.84}$$

for some time-independent functions $M_x^-(\mathbf{r})$ and $M_y^-(\mathbf{r})$.

Remark 2.1. Let us briefly discuss equilibrium magnetization $M_0(\mathbf{r})$. Assume that the patient's body is exposed only to the main field $\mathbf{B}_0 = B_0\hat{\mathbf{z}}$. Considering the protons in the body as tiny magnets, they align either along or against the main field $\mathbf{B}_0$. The average magnetic moment at equilibrium precesses around the $\hat{\mathbf{z}}$-axis with the Larmor frequency $\omega_L \approx \gamma B_0$. In the human body, the local magnetic field acting on $\mathbf{M}$ will be slightly different from $\mathbf{B}_0$ since electrons in atoms tend to oppose $\mathbf{B}_0$. The local field can be expressed as

$$\mathbf{B}_0 - \Delta\mathbf{B} = (1 - \chi)\mathbf{B}_0$$

and different molecules having different χ. For example, water and fat have different χ. Indeed, $0 < \chi_{[\text{water}]} < \chi_{[\text{fat}]}$, and therefore the corresponding Larmor frequencies ω_L satisfy

$$\gamma B_0 > \underbrace{\gamma(1 - \chi_{[\text{water}]})B_0}_{\omega_L[\text{water}]} > \underbrace{\gamma(1 - \chi_{[\text{fat}]})B_0}_{\omega_L[\text{fat}]}.$$

The effect of χ, the chemical shift, is very small compared to $\mathbf{B}_0$. For example,

$$\frac{\omega_{L[\text{fat}]} - \omega_{L[\text{water}]}}{\gamma B_0} \approx 10^{-6} \quad \text{at 3T MRI.}$$

2.2.1.2 *MR signal ignoring relaxation effects*

Noting that the magnitude of the net magnetization $|M_\perp^0(\mathbf{r})| = |\underline{M}_\perp(\mathbf{r}, t)|$ is independent of time t and depends on the amount of hydrogen, the natural question is how we visualize $|M_\perp^0(\mathbf{r})| = |\underline{M}_\perp(\mathbf{r},t)|$. According to (2.65), the magnetic field induced by the distribution of $\mathbf{M}$ is expressed as

$$\underline{\mathbf{B}}^{\mathbf{M}}(\mathbf{r},t) \approx \frac{\mu_0}{4\pi} \nabla \times \int_\Omega \underline{\mathbf{M}}(\mathbf{r}',t) \times \frac{\mathbf{r} - \mathbf{r}'}{|\mathbf{r} - \mathbf{r}'|^3} \, d\mathbf{r}'. \qquad (2.85)$$

By placing a sensing coil near the precessing spins (with its surface normal vector being $\hat{z}$), we can measure the induced electromotive force due to $\frac{\partial}{\partial t}\mathbf{B}^{\mathbf{M}}$ along the coil; according to Faraday's law, we can measure

$$\text{Signal}\,(t) = \int_{\text{coil surface}} \frac{\partial}{\partial t}\underline{\mathbf{B}}^{\mathbf{M}}(\mathbf{r},t) \cdot dS$$

and therefore it follows from Stoke's theorem that

$$\text{Signal}\,(t) = \int_{\text{coil}} \left[\frac{\mu_0}{4\pi} \int_\Omega \frac{\partial}{\partial t}\underline{\mathbf{M}}(\mathbf{r}',t) \times \frac{\mathbf{r} - \mathbf{r}'}{|\mathbf{r} - \mathbf{r}'|^3} \, d\mathbf{r}' \right] \cdot d\mathbf{l_r}. \qquad (2.86)$$

By changing the order of integration, (2.86) can be simplified into

$$\text{Signal}\,(t) \approx \int_\Omega \frac{\partial}{\partial t}\underline{\mathbf{M}}(\mathbf{r},t) \cdot \mathbf{B}^{coil}(\mathbf{r}) \, d\mathbf{r} \qquad (2.87)$$

where $\mathbf{B}^{coil}(\mathbf{r})$ is the magnetic field induced by the unit current coil

$$\mathbf{B}^{coil}(\mathbf{r}) = \frac{-\mu_0}{4\pi} \int_{\text{coil}} \frac{\mathbf{r} - \mathbf{r}'}{|\mathbf{r} - \mathbf{r}'|^3} \times dl_{|r'}.$$

Using the notation $\underline{M}_\perp$, (2.87) leads to (see Figure 2.9)

$$\text{Signal}\,(t) \approx \int_\Omega \frac{\partial}{\partial t}\underline{M}_\perp(\mathbf{r},t) \, \mathfrak{S}(\mathbf{r}) \, d\mathbf{r} \qquad (2.88)$$

where $\mathfrak{S}(\mathbf{r})$ is the coil sensitivity determined by $\mathbf{B}^{coil}(\mathbf{r})$, which will be explained later.

2.2.1.3 *MR signal with gradient field*

Assume that $M_\perp^0(\mathbf{r})$ is the magnetization vector at the time right after terminating the RF pulse (this will be explained later). Assume

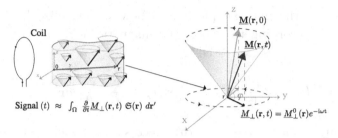

Fig. 2.9.   MR signal detection. According to Faraday's law, rotating magnetiza-tion $\underline{\mathbf{M}}_{xy}$ induces a signal.

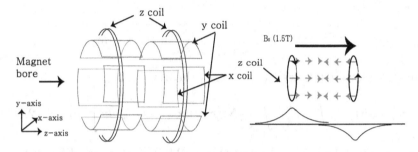

Fig. 2.10.   Gradient coils. The main magnetic field is aligned in z-direction.

that the gradient field $G = (G_x, G_y, G_z) \in \mathbb{R}^3$ is a constant vector and $\mathbf{B}$ is given by

$$\mathbf{B}(\mathbf{r}) = (B_0 + G \cdot \mathbf{r})\hat{\mathbf{z}} = (B_0 + G_x x + G_y y + G_z z)\hat{\mathbf{z}}.$$

This gradient field is generated by $x, y, z-$gradient coils as shown in Figure 2.10.

Then, the signal (2.88) is

$$\text{Signal}(t) \approx \int_\Omega \underbrace{-\mathrm{i}(B_0 + G \cdot \mathbf{r})M_\perp^0(\mathbf{r})\, e^{-\mathrm{i}\gamma(B_0 + G \cdot \mathbf{r})t}}_{\frac{\partial}{\partial t}\underline{M}_\perp(\mathbf{r},t)}\, \mathfrak{S}(\mathbf{r})\, d\mathbf{r}.$$

$$(2.89)$$

Note that $G \cdot \mathbf{r}$ is much smaller than B_0. Assuming that $\frac{|G \cdot \mathbf{r}|}{B_0} \approx 0$, Signal($t$) in (2.89) can be approximated into

$$\text{Signal}(t) \approx -iB_0 e^{-\mathrm{i}\gamma B_0 t} \int_\Omega \underbrace{\left[\mathfrak{S}(\mathbf{r})M_\perp^0(\mathbf{r})\right]}_{:= \mathfrak{m}_\perp(\mathbf{r})}\, e^{-\mathrm{i}\gamma G \cdot \mathbf{r}t}\, d\mathbf{r}. \qquad (2.90)$$

Denoting

$$\mathfrak{m}(\mathbf{r}) := \mathfrak{S}(\mathbf{r})M_\perp^0(\mathbf{r}) \quad \text{and} \quad \mathfrak{s}(\mathbf{k}(t)) := \frac{1}{-iB_0}e^{i\gamma B_0 t}\,\text{Signal}(t),$$

the measurable signal as a function of time t and G is

$$\mathfrak{s}(\mathbf{k}(t)) \approx \int_\Omega \mathfrak{m}(\mathbf{r})\, e^{-2\pi i \mathbf{k}(t)\cdot\mathbf{r}}\, d\mathbf{r} \quad \text{where} \quad \mathbf{k}(t) := \frac{\gamma G t}{2\pi}. \qquad (2.91)$$

In general, we can design the gradient G as a function of time t, and the measurable signal with the time-dependent gradient field $G(t)$ is given by

$$\mathfrak{s}\bigg(\underbrace{\frac{\gamma}{2\pi}\int_0^t G(t')dt'}_{:=\mathbf{k}(t)}\bigg) \approx \int_\Omega \mathfrak{m}(\mathbf{r})\, e^{-2\pi i \mathbf{k}(t)\cdot\mathbf{r}}\, d\mathbf{r}. \qquad (2.92)$$

Figure 2.11 is an example of gradient field $G(t)$ and the corresponding $\mathbf{k}(t)$.

In order to reconstruct the image of $\mathfrak{m}(\mathbf{r})$ using (discrete) inverse Fourier transform, we need a suitable design of $\mathbf{k}(t)$ (via frequency encoding and phase encoding) and accurate sampling (taking account of the Nyquist criterion or Whittaker−Shannon sampling theorem). These will be discussed later. For the basics of Fourier transform and sampling theorem, we refer to [Seo and Woo (2012)].

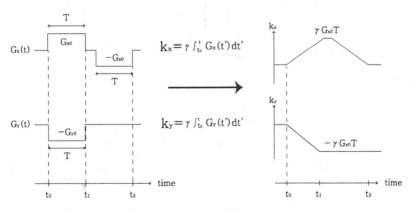

Fig. 2.11. Gradient pulse and $\mathbf{k}(t)$ as a function of time t.

2.2.1.4 *One-dimensional imaging with frequency encoding*

In this subsection, we consider the one-dimensional case where

$$\Omega = \{\mathbf{r} : |x| < N, |y| < 1, |z| < 1\} \quad \& \quad \mathfrak{m}(\mathbf{r}) = \mathfrak{m}(x).$$

Here, the voxel size is $1 \times 1 \times 1$ and $\mathfrak{m}(\mathbf{r}) = \mathfrak{m}(x)$ means that $\mathfrak{m}(\mathbf{r})$ in (2.92) depends only on x-variable. Assuming $G = (G_x, 0, 0)$ (the frequency encoding gradient), the signal in (2.92) leads to (see Figure 2.12)

$$\mathfrak{s}(k_x(t)) = \int_{-N}^{N} \mathfrak{m}(x) \, e^{-2\pi i k_x(t) x} \, dx \quad \& \quad k_x(t) := \frac{\gamma}{2\pi} G_x t. \quad (2.93)$$

Writing $\mathfrak{m}_n = \mathfrak{s}(n)$, the x-variable function $\mathfrak{m}(x)$ can be expressed as the following vector form:

$$\vec{\mathfrak{m}} := \begin{pmatrix} \mathfrak{m}_{-N} \\ \vdots \\ \mathfrak{m}_0 \\ \vdots \\ \mathfrak{m}_N \end{pmatrix} = \begin{pmatrix} \mathfrak{m}(-N) \\ \vdots \\ \mathfrak{m}(0)) \\ \vdots \\ \mathfrak{m}(N) \end{pmatrix}. \quad (2.94)$$

Similarly, writing $\mathfrak{s}_{n-N} = \mathfrak{s}(k_x(n\Delta t))$ (where Δt is time interval), the digital signal $\mathfrak{s}(k_x(t))$ can be expressed as the following vector form:

$$\vec{\mathfrak{s}} := \begin{pmatrix} \mathfrak{s}_{-N} \\ \vdots \\ \mathfrak{s}_0 \\ \vdots \\ \mathfrak{s}_N \end{pmatrix} = \begin{pmatrix} \mathfrak{s}(0) \\ \vdots \\ \mathfrak{s}(N\Delta k_x) \\ \vdots \\ \mathfrak{s}(2N\Delta k_x) \end{pmatrix} \quad \& \quad \Delta k_x = k_x(\Delta t)). \quad (2.95)$$

Then, the equation (2.101) can be written as the following linear system:

$$\vec{\mathfrak{s}} = \underbrace{\begin{pmatrix} 1 & 1 & 1 & \cdots & 1 \\ 1 & e & e^2 & \cdots & e^{2N} \\ 1 & e^2 & e^4 & \cdots & e^{4N} \\ \vdots & \vdots & \vdots & \ddots & \vdots \\ 1 & e^{2N} & e^{4N} & \cdots & e^{(2N)^2} \end{pmatrix}}_{:= \mathfrak{F}} \vec{\mathfrak{m}} \quad (2.96)$$

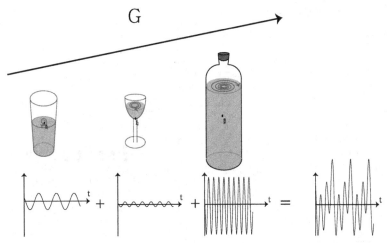

Fig. 2.12.   Frequency encoding by applying gradient field during reading of the signal. From the signal, we can recover the amount of water at three different positions.

where $\mathfrak{e} := e^{-2\pi i \Delta k_x}$.

It is important to observe that $\vec{\mathfrak{s}}$ can be viewed as the DFT (discrete Fourier transform) of $\vec{\mathfrak{m}}$ if the time interval Δt is chosen such that $\mathfrak{e}$ is the $2N + 1$ th principle root of 1, that is,

$$\mathfrak{e} = e^{-2\pi i/(2N+1)} \quad \text{or equivalently} \quad \frac{1}{2N+1} = \frac{\gamma}{2\pi}\, G_x \Delta t. \qquad (2.97)$$

With this special choice of Δt, the inverse of the matrix $\mathfrak{F}$ is a multiple of its transpose, and $\vec{\mathfrak{m}}$ is reconstructed via the inverse DFT:

$$\vec{\mathfrak{m}} = \underbrace{\frac{1}{2N+1}\, \mathfrak{F}^*\mathfrak{F}}_{\text{Identity matrix}}\, \vec{\mathfrak{m}} = \frac{1}{2N+1}\mathfrak{F}^*\vec{\mathfrak{s}} \qquad (2.98)$$

where $\mathfrak{F}^*$ is the transpose of $\mathfrak{F}$.

2.2.1.5   *Two-dimensional imaging with phase and frequency encoding*

In this subsection, we consider the two-dimensional case where

$$\Omega = \{\mathbf{r} : |x| < N, |y| < N, |z| < 1\} \quad \& \quad \mathfrak{m}(\mathbf{r}) = \mathfrak{m}(x, y).$$

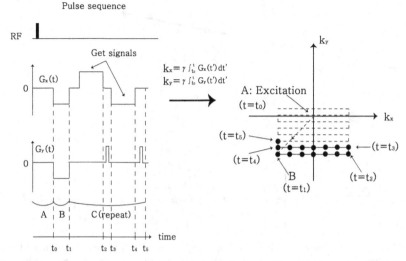

Fig. 2.13. Gradient pulse and **k**-space trajectory. Fourier transform of time domain signal (**k**-space data) → frequency (image) domain signal.

Then, the signal in (2.92) can be expressed as

$$\mathfrak{s}(k_x(t), k_y(t)) = \int_{-N}^{N} \int_{-N}^{N} \mathfrak{m}(x, y) \ e^{-2\pi i [k_x(t)x + k_y(t)y]} \ dxdy. \quad (2.99)$$

In Figure 2.13, we apply a phase encoding gradient in y-direction before frequency encoding in x-direction. We should note that the signal is collected during the frequency encoding gradient (readout gradient). In Figure 2.13, $G_y(t)$ is chosen in the following way

$$\underbrace{\Delta k_y}_{constant} = \frac{\gamma}{2\pi} \int_{t_3}^{t_4} G_y(t')dt'$$

$$= \frac{\gamma}{2\pi} \int_{t_5}^{t_6} G_y(t')dt' = -\frac{1}{N}\frac{\gamma}{2\pi} \int_{t_0}^{t_1} G_y(t')dt'.$$

Hence, in Figure 2.13, $k_y(t)$ during the frequency encoding period is given by

$$k_y(t) = \begin{cases} -N\Delta k_y & \text{if } t_1 < t < t_2 \\ 1 - N\Delta k_y & \text{if } t_3 < t < t_4 \\ 2 - N\Delta k_y & \text{if } t_5 < t < t_6 \end{cases} \quad (2.100)$$

With this $k_y(t)$, the signal $\mathfrak{s}(k_x(t), k_y(t))$ in (2.99) is

$$
\mathfrak{s}(k_x(t), k_y(t)) = \begin{cases} \mathfrak{s}(k_x(t), -N\Delta k_y) & \text{if } t_1 < t < t_2 \\ \mathfrak{s}(k_x(t), 1 - N\Delta k_y) & \text{if } t_3 < t < t_4 \ . \\ \mathfrak{s}(k_x(t), 2 - N\Delta k_y) & \text{if } t_5 < t < t_6 \end{cases} \quad (2.101)
$$

We perform frequency encoding as in (2.96) with multiple phase encodings to collect a set of k-space data of

$$
\mathfrak{s}(n\Delta k_x, m\Delta k_y) \quad \text{for } n, m = -N, 1 - N, \ldots, N. \quad (2.102)
$$

As in section 2.2.1.5, the inverse DFT provides the image of $\mathfrak{m}(x, y)$.

Remark 2.2. In MRI, the data acquisition time is roughly proportional to the number of phase-encoding lines due to the time-consuming phase encoding which separates signals from different y-positions within the image $m(x, y)$. Hence, to accelerate the acquisition process, we can skip phase-encoding lines in the k-space. Reduction in k-space data violating the Nyquist criterion is associated with an aliasing in the image space. If we use sub-sampled k-space data by a factor of R in phase-encoding direction (y-direction), according to Poisson summation formula, the corresponding inverse Fourier transform produces a fold-over artifact. Parallel imaging (PI) deals with this fold-over artifact by using multiple receiver coils and its supplementary spatial information in the image space. Great attention has been received for PI since the works by [Sodickson and Manning (1997); Sodickson *et al.* (1999); Pruessmann *et al.* (1999)] were published. In PI, we skip phase-encoding lines in the k-space during MRI acquisition in order to reduce the number of time-consuming phase-encoding steps. In the image reconstruction step, we compensate the skipped k-space data by the use of space-dependent properties of multiple receiver coils. Numerous parallel reconstruction algorithms such as SENSE, SMASH, and GRAPPA have been suggested, aiming for the smallest possible amount of phase-encoding lines, while eliminating aliasing which is a consequence of violating Nyquist criteria due to skipping the data. We refer to [Jakob *et al.* (1998); Kyriakos *et al.* (2000); Heidemann *et al.* (2001); Pruessmann *et al.* (2001); Bydder *et al.* (2002); Griswold *et al.*

(2002)] for pMRI algorithms and to [Larkman and Nunes (2001)] for the review.

2.2.2   On-resonance RF excitation to flip $\underline{\mathbf{M}}$ toward the xy-plane

According to (2.74), the strong magnetic field $\mathbf{B} = \omega\hat{\mathbf{z}}$ causes $\underline{\mathbf{M}}$ to precess clockwise around the $\hat{\mathbf{z}}$-direction at the angular frequency $\omega = \gamma|\mathbf{B}|$. To extract a signal of $\underline{\mathbf{M}}$ in the region $\Omega_0 := \{\mathbf{r} \in \Omega :$ $\omega(\mathbf{r}) = \omega_0 = \gamma B_0\}$, we flip $\underline{\mathbf{M}}$ toward the transversal direction to produce its xy-component. Flipping $\underline{\mathbf{M}}$ toward the xy-plane requires a second magnetic field $\underline{\mathbf{B}}_1$ perpendicular to $\mathbf{B}_0$. We can flip $\underline{\mathbf{M}}$ toward the xy-plane by using an RF magnetic field $\underline{\mathbf{B}}_1$ that is generated by an RF coil where we inject a sinusoidal current of I mA at the Larmor frequency $\omega_0 = \gamma B_0$.

Then, $\underline{\mathbf{M}}(\mathbf{r}, t)$ satisfies the generalized Bloch equation

$$\frac{\partial}{\partial t}\underline{\mathbf{M}} = -\gamma\underline{\mathbf{B}} \times \underline{\mathbf{M}} - \frac{1}{T_2}\underline{\mathbf{M}}_{xy} + \text{relaxation effects}. \qquad (2.103)$$

where $\underline{\mathbf{M}}_{xy} = \underline{M}_x\hat{\mathbf{x}} + \underline{M}_y\hat{\mathbf{y}}$ and

$$\underline{\mathbf{B}}(\mathbf{r}, t) = (B_0 + G \cdot \mathbf{r})\hat{\mathbf{z}} + \underline{\mathbf{B}}_1(\mathbf{r}, t).$$

Throughout this subsection, we will neglect relaxation effects in (2.103) so that $\underline{\mathbf{M}}$ satisfies

$$\frac{\partial}{\partial t}\underline{\mathbf{M}}(\mathbf{r}, t) = -\gamma((B_0 + G \cdot \mathbf{r})\hat{\mathbf{z}} + \underline{\mathbf{B}}_1(\mathbf{r}, t)) \times \underline{\mathbf{M}}(\mathbf{r}, t). \qquad (2.104)$$

2.2.2.1   *Time-harmonic RF field* $\mathbf{B}_1$

For ease of understanding, we treat the RF field excited by an RF coil as a time-harmonic electro-magnetic field. The following are about $\underline{\mathbf{B}}_1(\mathbf{r}, t)$:

- Using an RF coil, we inject a sinusoidal current of I with the RF frequency $\omega_{RF} \approx \omega_0 = \gamma B_0$ to generate a sinusoidally time-varying field $\underline{\mathbf{B}}_1(\mathbf{r}, t)$ inside the sample occupying the three-dimensional domain Ω.
- For simplicity, we assume $\omega_{RF} = \omega_0$.

- The RF field $\underline{\mathbf{B}}_1(\mathbf{r}, t)$ is perpendicular to $\mathbf{B}_0 = \omega_0 \hat{\mathbf{z}}$ direction.
- Let $\mathbf{B}_1(\mathbf{r})$ be the corresponding time-harmonic field:

$$\underline{\mathbf{B}}_1(\mathbf{r}, t) = \text{the real part of } \mathbf{B}_1(\mathbf{r})e^{i\omega_0 t}. \qquad (2.105)$$

Denote by $\phi_x(\mathbf{r})$ and $\phi_y(\mathbf{r})$, respectively, the phase angles of B_{1x} and B_{1y}:

$$B_{1x}(\mathbf{r}) = |\underline{B}_{1x}(\mathbf{r})| \, e^{i\phi_x(\mathbf{r})} \quad \& \quad B_{1y}(\mathbf{r}) = |\underline{B}_{1y}(\mathbf{r})| \, e^{i\phi_y(\mathbf{r})}. \qquad (2.106)$$

- The magnitude of $\underline{\mathbf{B}}_1$ is much smaller than B_0. Assume $|\mathbf{B}_1| \leq 10^{-5}|\mathbf{B}_0|$.

The time-harmonic $\mathbf{B}_1$ field depends on the admittivity distribution $\sigma(\mathbf{r}) + i\omega_0\epsilon(\mathbf{r})$ at angular frequency $\omega_0 = \gamma B_0$ and at the position $\mathbf{r} \in \Omega$. The governing equation of $\mathbf{B}_1$ is described in Theorem 2.2.

Theorem 2.2. *The time-harmonic field $\mathbf{B}_1$ is dictated by*

$$-\nabla^2 \mathbf{B}_1 = \frac{\nabla(\sigma + i\omega_0\epsilon)}{\sigma + i\omega_0\epsilon} \times (\nabla \times \mathbf{B}_1) - i\omega_0(\sigma + i\omega_0\epsilon)\mathbf{B}_1 \qquad (2.107)$$

within the subject Ω.

Proof. Denote $\mathbf{H} = \frac{1}{\mu_0}\mathbf{B}_1$. According to Maxwell's equations,

$$\nabla \times \mathbf{E} = -i\omega_0\mu_0\mathbf{H} \quad \& \quad \nabla \times \mathbf{H} = (\sigma + i\omega_0\epsilon)\mathbf{E}. \qquad (2.108)$$

Applying the curl operation to $\nabla \times \mathbf{H} = (\sigma + i\omega_0\epsilon)\mathbf{E}$, we get

$$
\begin{aligned}
\nabla \times \nabla \times \mathbf{H} &= \nabla \times ((\sigma + i\omega_0\epsilon)\mathbf{E}) \\
&= \nabla(\sigma + i\omega_0\epsilon) \times \mathbf{E} + (\sigma + i\omega_0\epsilon)\nabla \times \mathbf{E} \\
&= \frac{\nabla(\sigma + i\omega_0\epsilon)}{\sigma + i\omega_0\epsilon} \times (\nabla \times \mathbf{H}) - i\omega_0\mu_0(\sigma + i\omega_0\epsilon)\mathbf{H}.
\end{aligned}
$$

$$(2.109)$$

Then, the identity (2.107) follows from

$$\nabla \times \nabla \times \mathbf{H} = -\nabla^2\mathbf{H} - \nabla\nabla \cdot \mathbf{H} = -\nabla^2\mathbf{H}. \qquad \square$$

The RF field can be regarded as a stationary field with respect to the rotating frame that is rotating at the angular frequency ω_0. We assume that z-component of $\mathbf{B}_1$ is zero. Indeed, the time-varying field $\mathbf{B}_1$ can be expressed by a combination of stationary functions and the rotating axes $\mathbf{x}^\pm$, $\mathbf{y}^\pm$.

Proposition 2.4 ($\mathbf{B}_1^\pm$ field in the rotating frame). $\mathbf{B}_1$ *can be decomposed into*

$$\underline{B}_{1x}\hat{\mathbf{x}} + \underline{B}_{1y}\hat{\mathbf{y}} = B_{1x}^+\mathbf{x}^+ + B_{1x}^-\underline{\mathbf{x}}^- + B_{1y}^+\underline{\mathbf{y}}^+ + B_{1y}^-\underline{\mathbf{y}}^- \qquad (2.110)$$

where $B_{1x}^\pm$ and $B_{1y}^\pm$ are time-independent functions given by

$$\begin{pmatrix} B_{1x}^\pm \\ B_{1y}^\pm \end{pmatrix} = \frac{|B_{1x}|}{2}\begin{pmatrix} \cos\phi_x \\ \pm\sin\phi_x \end{pmatrix} + \frac{|B_{1y}|}{2}\begin{pmatrix} \mp\sin\phi_y \\ \cos\phi_y \end{pmatrix}. \qquad (2.111)$$

Moreover, we have the following identities:

$$B_{1x} + iB_{1y} = B_{1x}^+ + iB_{1y}^+ \quad \& \quad B_{1x} - iB_{1y} = B_{1x}^- + iB_{1y}^-. \qquad (2.112)$$

Proof. Note that

$$e^{i\omega t}\hat{\mathbf{x}} = \underbrace{\frac{\mathbf{x}^+ + \mathbf{x}^-}{2}}_{\cos\omega t\hat{\mathbf{x}}} - i\underbrace{\frac{\mathbf{y}^+ - \mathbf{y}^-}{2}}_{-\sin\omega t\hat{\mathbf{x}}} \quad \text{and}$$

$$e^{i\omega t}\hat{\mathbf{y}} = i\underbrace{\frac{\mathbf{x}^+ - \mathbf{x}^-}{2}}_{\sin\omega t\hat{\mathbf{y}}} + \underbrace{\frac{\mathbf{y}^- + \mathbf{y}^+}{2}}_{\cos\omega t\hat{\mathbf{y}}},$$

the transversal components of $\mathbf{B}_1(\mathbf{r}, t) = \text{Re}\{\mathbf{B}_1(\mathbf{r})e^{i\omega t}\}$ can be expressed as

$$\underline{B}_{1x}\hat{\mathbf{x}} = |B_{1x}|\left(\cos\phi_x\frac{\mathbf{x}^+ + \mathbf{x}^-}{2} + \sin\phi_x\frac{\mathbf{y}^+ - \mathbf{y}^-}{2}\right)$$

$$\underline{B}_{1y}\hat{\mathbf{y}} = |B_{1y}|\left(-\sin\phi_y\frac{\mathbf{x}^+ - \mathbf{x}^-}{2} + \cos\phi_y\frac{\mathbf{y}^+ + \mathbf{y}^-}{2}\right).$$

Then the proof follows from the definition (2.105). $\qquad\qquad\square$

2.2.2.2 *Time-harmonic RF excitation and flip angle*

To compute the flip angle as a function of the strength of $\underline{\mathbf{B}}_1(\mathbf{r}, t)$ and duration of the RF pulse, we need to solve the equation (2.104). With the above conditions on $\underline{\mathbf{B}}_1(\mathbf{r}, t)$ during RF excitation, the equation (2.104) can be expressed as

$$\frac{\partial}{\partial t} \begin{pmatrix} \underline{M}_x \\ \underline{M}_y \\ \underline{M}_z \end{pmatrix} = -\gamma \begin{vmatrix} \hat{\mathbf{x}} & \hat{\mathbf{y}} & \hat{\mathbf{z}} \\ \underline{B}_{1x} & \underline{B}_{1y} & B_0 + G \cdot \mathbf{r} \\ \underline{M}_x & \underline{M}_y & \underline{M}_z \end{vmatrix}. \tag{2.113}$$

Direct computation of (2.113) leads to the following expression of the transverse component $\underline{M}_\perp = \underline{M}_x + i\underline{M}_y$:

$$\frac{\partial}{\partial t}\underline{M}_\perp(\mathbf{r}, t) = -i\omega(\mathbf{r})\,\underline{M}_\perp(\mathbf{r}, t) + i\gamma\underline{B}_{1\perp}(\mathbf{r}, t)\,\underline{M}_z(\mathbf{r}, t) \tag{2.114}$$

where $\omega(\mathbf{r}) := \omega_0 + \gamma G \cdot \mathbf{r}$ and

$$\underline{B}_{1\perp} := \underline{B}_{1x} + i\underline{B}_{1y}.$$

Proposition 2.5. *If the initial magnetic moment is* $\mathbf{M}(\mathbf{r}, 0) = (0, 0, M_0(\mathbf{r}))$ *the solution of ODE* (2.114) *is*

$$\underline{M}_\perp(\mathbf{r}, t) = i\gamma e^{-i\omega(\mathbf{r})t} \int_0^t (e^{i\omega(\mathbf{r})t'} \underline{B}_{1\perp}(\mathbf{r}, t')\,\underline{M}_z(\mathbf{r}, t'))dt'. \tag{2.115}$$

The flip angle $\alpha(t)$ *as a function of position* $\mathbf{r}$ *and time* t *is given by*

$$\sin\alpha(\mathbf{r}, t) = \gamma \left| \int_0^t e^{i\omega(\mathbf{r})t'} \underline{B}_{1\perp}(\mathbf{r}, t')\frac{M_z(\mathbf{r}, t')}{M_0(\mathbf{r})}dt' \right| \tag{2.116}$$

provided $\alpha \leq \frac{\pi}{2}$.

The proof of the above proposition is straightforward, so we omit the proof. Let us briefly discuss the flip angle α in (2.115). If $\alpha(\mathbf{r}, t)$ is suffuciently small, then

$$\sin\alpha(\mathbf{r}, t) \approx \alpha(\mathbf{r}, t) \quad \& \quad \frac{M_z(\mathbf{r}, t')}{M_0(\mathbf{r})} \approx 1,$$

and therefore (2.116) can be simplified into

$$\alpha(\mathbf{r}, t) \approx \gamma \left| \int_0^t e^{i\gamma G \cdot \mathbf{r} t'} \underbrace{e^{i\omega_0 t'} \underline{B}_{1\perp}(\mathbf{r}, t')}_{:=\mathfrak{B}(\mathbf{r}, t)} dt' \right|. \tag{2.117}$$

In particular, (2.117) becomes

$$\alpha(\mathbf{r}, t) \approx \gamma \left| \int_0^t \mathfrak{B}(\mathbf{r}, t') \, dt' \right| \quad \text{for } \mathbf{r} \in \Omega_0 := \{\mathbf{r} \in \Omega : \gamma G \cdot \mathbf{r} = 0\} \tag{2.118}$$

where $\mathfrak{B}(\mathbf{r}, t) = e^{i\omega_0 t} \underline{B}_{1\perp}(\mathbf{r}, t)$ that can be decomposed into a stationary term and a high-frequency term with the angular frequency $2\omega_0$. With (2.117), slice selective excitation (selecting Ω_0) can be understood.

To understand the flip angle in detail, let us study the behavior of $\underline{\mathbf{M}}$ in the selected slice $\Omega_0 := \{\mathbf{r} \in \Omega : \gamma G \cdot \mathbf{r} = 0\}$.

Proposition 2.6. *Let $M_x^-(\mathbf{r}, t)$ and $M_y^-(\mathbf{r}, t)$ be functions such that*

$$\underline{\mathbf{M}}(\mathbf{r}, t) = M_x^-(\mathbf{r}, t)\underline{\mathbf{x}}^- + M_y^-(\mathbf{r}, t)\underline{\mathbf{y}}^- + M_z(\mathbf{r}, t)\hat{\mathbf{z}}. \tag{2.119}$$

Then $\mathbf{M}^- := (M_x^-, M_y^-, M_z)$ in Ω_0 satisfies

$$\gamma \underline{\mathbf{B}}_1 \times \underline{\mathbf{M}} = \frac{\partial M_x^-}{\partial t} \underline{\mathbf{x}}^- + \frac{\partial M_y^-}{\partial t} \underline{\mathbf{y}}^- + \frac{\partial M_z}{\partial t} \hat{\mathbf{z}}. \tag{2.120}$$

Moreover,

$$\underbrace{\begin{pmatrix} \dfrac{\partial M_x^-}{\partial t} \\[2mm] \dfrac{\partial M_y^-}{\partial t} \\[2mm] \dfrac{\partial M_z}{\partial t} \end{pmatrix}}_{\partial_t \mathbf{M}^-} = \underbrace{-\gamma \begin{pmatrix} 0 & 0 & B_{1y}^- \\ 0 & 0 & -B_{1x}^- \\ -B_{1y}^- & B_{1x}^- & 0 \end{pmatrix} \begin{pmatrix} M_x^- \\ M_y^- \\ M_z \end{pmatrix}}_{-\gamma \mathbf{B}_1^- \times \mathbf{M}^-} + \mathcal{R}(\cos 2\omega_0 t, \sin 2\omega_0 t) \tag{2.121}$$

where $\mathbf{B}_1^- = (B_{1x}^-, B_{1y}^-, 0)$ and $\mathcal{R}(\cos 2\omega_0 t, \sin 2\omega_0 t)$ is the term involving $\cos(2\omega_0 t)$ or $\sin(2\omega_0 t)$.

Proof. From (2.83),

$$\frac{\partial}{\partial t}\mathbf{M} = \frac{\partial M_x^-}{\partial t}\mathbf{x}^- + \frac{\partial M_y^-}{\partial t}\mathbf{y}^- + \frac{\partial M_z}{\partial t}\hat{\mathbf{z}} - \underbrace{\gamma\mathbf{B}_0 \times \left(M_x^-\mathbf{x}^- + M_y^-\mathbf{y}^-\right)}_{\gamma\mathbf{B}_0\times\underline{\mathbf{M}}}.$$

$$(2.122)$$

Since $\partial_t\underline{\mathbf{M}} = -\gamma(\mathbf{B}_0 + \underline{\mathbf{B}}_1) \times \underline{\mathbf{M}}$ in the slice Ω_0, the above identity (2.122) leads to

$$\underbrace{\partial_t\underline{\mathbf{M}} + \gamma\mathbf{B}_0 \times \underline{\mathbf{M}}}_{\gamma\underline{\mathbf{B}}_1\times\underline{\mathbf{M}}} = \frac{\partial M_x^-}{\partial t}\mathbf{x}^+ + \frac{\partial M_y^-}{\partial t}\underline{\mathbf{y}}^+ + \frac{\partial M_z}{\partial t}\hat{\mathbf{z}} \qquad (2.123)$$

which proves (2.120).

Next, (2.121) follows from a direct computation of

$$\begin{aligned}\underline{\mathbf{B}}_1 \times \underline{\mathbf{M}} &= \left(B_{1x}^+\mathbf{x}^+ + B_{1x}^-\underline{\mathbf{x}}^- + B_{1y}^+\underline{\mathbf{y}}^+ + B_{1y}^-\underline{\mathbf{y}}^-\right) \\ &\quad \times \left(M_x^-\underline{\mathbf{x}}^- + M_y^-\underline{\mathbf{y}}^- + M_z\hat{\mathbf{z}}\right)\end{aligned}$$

with the following identities:

$$\begin{aligned}\underline{\mathbf{x}}^- \times \underline{\mathbf{y}}^- &= \hat{\mathbf{z}}, \quad \underline{\mathbf{x}}^\pm \times \hat{\mathbf{z}} = -\underline{\mathbf{y}}^\pm, \quad \underline{\mathbf{y}}^\pm \times \hat{\mathbf{z}} = \underline{\mathbf{x}}^\pm \\ \underline{\mathbf{x}}^- &\times \underline{\mathbf{x}}^- = 0, \quad \underline{\mathbf{y}}^- \times \underline{\mathbf{y}}^- = 0 \\ -\sin(2\omega_0 t)\hat{\mathbf{z}} &= \underline{\mathbf{x}}^+ \times \underline{\mathbf{x}}^- = \underline{\mathbf{y}}^+ \times \underline{\mathbf{y}}^- \\ \cos(2\omega_0 t)\hat{\mathbf{z}} &= \underline{\mathbf{x}}^+ \times \underline{\mathbf{y}}^- = -\underline{\mathbf{y}}^+ \times \underline{\mathbf{x}}^-.\end{aligned}$$

$\square$

The above proposition explains that only the negatively rotating field $\underline{\mathbf{B}}_1^- = B_{1x}^-\underline{\mathbf{x}}^- + B_{1y}^-\underline{\mathbf{y}}^-$ produces a time-averaged torque on the magnetization. In the rotating frame, the behavior of $\mathbf{M}^- = (M_x^-, M_y^-, M_z)$ can be described by

$$\frac{\partial}{\partial t}\mathbf{M}^- = -(\gamma\,\mathbf{B}_1^-) \times \mathbf{M}^-.$$

Since $|\mathbf{B}_1| \leq 10^{-5}|\mathbf{B}_0|$, the time change of $\mathbf{M}^-$ is negligibly low when compared with the rotating speed of $\underline{\mathbf{M}}$. This is the reason why we use the notation $\mathbf{M}^-$ (without underline) instead of $\underline{\mathbf{M}}^-$.

Theorem 2.3 (Interrelation between $\mathbf{B}_1$ and $\mathbf{M}$). *Assume that* $\mathbf{M}^- := (M_x^-, M_y^-, M_z)$ *satisfies*

$$\frac{\partial}{\partial t}\mathbf{M}^-(\mathbf{r}) = -\gamma\,\mathbf{B}_1^-(\mathbf{r}) \times \mathbf{M}^-(\mathbf{r}, t) \quad \& \quad \mathbf{M}^-(\mathbf{r}, 0) = M_0(\mathbf{r})\hat{\mathbf{z}},$$

$$(2.124)$$

then we have

$$M_x^-(\mathbf{r}, \tau) - iM_y^-(\mathbf{r}, \tau) = M_0(\mathbf{r})\,\sin\left(\gamma|B_{1,\perp}^-(\mathbf{r})|\,\tau\right)\frac{-iB_{1\perp}^-(\mathbf{r})}{|B_{1\perp}^-(\mathbf{r})|}$$

$$(2.125)$$

where $B_{1\perp}^- = \frac{1}{2}(B_{1x} - iB_{1y})$.

Proof. We begin by considering the case of $\mathbf{B}_1^-(\mathbf{r}) = (B_{1,x}^-(\mathbf{r}), 0, 0)$ that points to the direction of $\underline{\mathbf{x}}^-$-axis in the rotating frame. It is convenient to write (2.124) as the single equation of

$$\frac{\partial}{\partial t}(M_z^- + iM_y^-) = i\gamma B_{1,x}^-(M_z^- + iM_y^-).$$

$$(2.126)$$

The solution at time $t = \tau$ is

$$M_z^-(\mathbf{r}, \tau) + iM_y^-(\mathbf{r}, \tau) = \underbrace{\left(M_z^-(\mathbf{r}, 0) + iM_y^-(\mathbf{r}, 0)\right)}_{=M_0(\mathbf{r})} e^{i\gamma B_{1,x}^-(\mathbf{r})\,\tau}.$$

This leads to

$$M_y^-(\mathbf{r}, \tau) = M_0(\mathbf{r})\sin\left(\gamma|B_{1,x}^-(\mathbf{r})|\,\tau\right)\frac{B_{1,x}^-(\mathbf{r})}{|B_{1,x}^-(\mathbf{r})|}.$$

$$(2.127)$$

Similarly, if $\mathbf{B}_1^- = \left(0, B_{1,y}^-, 0\right)$, then (2.124) leads to

$$\frac{\partial}{\partial t}(M_z^- + iM_x^-) = -i\gamma B_{1,y}^-(M_z^- + iM_x^-)$$

$$(2.128)$$

and its solution at time $t = \tau$ is

$$M_x^-(\mathbf{r}, \tau) = M_0(\mathbf{r})\sin\left(\gamma|B_{1,y}^-(\mathbf{r})|\,\tau\right)\frac{-B_{1,y}^-(\mathbf{r})}{|B_{1,y}^-(\mathbf{r})|}.$$

$$(2.129)$$

Hence, for the general case of $\mathbf{B}_1^- = (B_{1,x}^-, B_{1,y}^-, 0)$, we obtain

$$M_x^-(\mathbf{r}, \tau) - iM_y^-(\mathbf{r}, \tau) = M_0(\mathbf{r}) \sin(\gamma |\mathbf{B}_1^-(\mathbf{r})| \, \tau) \frac{-B_{1,y}^-(\mathbf{r}) - iB_{1,x}^-(\mathbf{r})}{|\mathbf{B}_1^-(\mathbf{r})|}.$$

$$(2.130)$$

This gives (2.125).   □

2.2.3 *Signal detection and RF reciprocity principle*

Magnetic resonance signal detection is based on Faraday's law and the reciprocity principle. A receiver coil outside the body detects MR signals from the body. We may use the same or different RF coils for RF excitation and signal reception. In this section, we will describe the coil sensitivity $\mathfrak{S}$ in (2.88) and RF reciprocity principle. For detailed explanations of the RF reciprocity principle, please refer to [Landau and Lifshitz (1960); Hoult and Richards (1976); Haacke *et al.* (1999); Hoult (2000); Scott (1993); Wang (2012)].

According to Proposition 2.3, the B1 field ($\mathbf{B}_1$) at the Larmor frequency flips the spins in the slice Ω_0 toward the xy-plane, and the flip angle α of $\underline{\mathbf{M}}$ toward the xy-plane is determined by $\mathbf{B}_1$ and the duration of the RF pulse. Assume that the RF field duration is τ.

After turning off the RF field, $\underline{\mathbf{M}}$ starts going back to its equilibrium position along $\mathbf{B}_0$. Assume that the magnetization is exposed to a main field $\mathbf{B}(\mathbf{r}) = (B_0 + G \cdot \mathbf{r})\hat{\mathbf{z}}$ right after turning off the RF field. Note that the gradient G of each occurrence may be different. With the field $\mathbf{B}$, $\underline{\mathbf{M}}$ will rotate around the $\hat{\mathbf{z}}$-axis at the angular frequency $\omega = \gamma|\mathbf{B}|$. $\underline{\mathbf{M}}$ is governed by the Bloch equation

$$\frac{\partial}{\partial t}\underline{\mathbf{M}} = -\mathbf{B} \times \underline{\mathbf{M}} - \frac{1}{T_2}\underline{\mathbf{M}}_{xy} + \frac{1}{T_1}(\underline{M}_z - M_0)\hat{\mathbf{z}} \qquad (2.131)$$

where M_0 is the equilibrium magnetic moment distribution and $\underline{\mathbf{M}}_{xy} = \underline{M}_x\hat{\mathbf{x}} + \underline{M}_y\hat{\mathbf{y}}$. Here, T1 is the time constant involved in longitudinal (or spin−lattice) relaxation to reach the thermal equilibrium distribution following RF excitation, and T2 is the time constant involved in transversal (or spin–spin) relaxation that corresponds to a decoherence of nuclei in a local area. Since free precession speed with its angular frequency ω is at a much faster rate than the spin relaxation T1 and T2, we again ignore the last two terms of (2.131) involving T1 and T2.

From (2.92) and Proposition 2.6, the measurable signal due to $\mathbf{M}$ in (2.131) (ignoring relaxation effects) is

$$\underbrace{s(t)}_{s(\mathbf{k}(t))} \approx \int_\Omega \underbrace{\mathfrak{S}(\mathbf{r})M_\perp(\mathbf{r},0)}_{s(\mathbf{r})} \underbrace{e^{-i\gamma G \cdot \mathbf{r}t}}_{e^{-2\pi i\mathbf{k}(t)\cdot\mathbf{r}}} \, d\mathbf{r}' \qquad (2.132)$$

where $t = 0$ is the time right after turning off the RF pulse. In this section, we will evaluate the term $\mathfrak{S}(\mathbf{r})M_\perp(\mathbf{r},0)$ precisely using the reciprocity relation.

2.2.3.1 *RF reciprocity principle*

Now we are ready to explain the RF reciprocity principle. For ease of understanding, we assume that $\mathbf{B} = \mathbf{B}_0$ (or $G = 0$) in (2.131) and the relaxation effects are neglected. Then $\underline{\mathbf{M}}(\mathbf{r},t)$ in (2.131) (with $G = 0$ and neglecting relaxation effects) satisfies

$$\underline{\mathbf{M}}(\mathbf{r},t) = M_x^\diamond(\mathbf{r})\underline{\mathbf{x}}^- + M_y^\diamond(\mathbf{r})\underline{\mathbf{y}}^- + M_z^\diamond(\mathbf{r})\hat{\mathbf{z}} \qquad (2.133)$$

where $M_x^\diamond(\mathbf{r}) - iM_y^\diamond(\mathbf{r})$ is $M_x^-(\mathbf{r},\tau) - iM_y^-(\mathbf{r},\tau)$ in (2.125). That is:

$$M_x^\diamond(\mathbf{r}) - iM_y^\diamond(\mathbf{r}) = M_0(\mathbf{r}) \, \sin\left(\gamma|B_{1,\perp}^-(\mathbf{r})| \, \tau\right) \frac{-i(B_{1\perp}^-(\mathbf{r}))}{|B_{1\perp}^-(\mathbf{r})|}. \qquad (2.134)$$

Here, τ is the duration of the RF pulse, and (2.134) is given by (2.125).

Proposition 2.7. *Let* $\mathbf{M}_{xy}(\mathbf{r})$ *be the time-harmonic expression of the* $\underline{\mathbf{M}}_{xy}(\mathbf{r},t) = M_x^\diamond(\mathbf{r})\underline{\mathbf{x}}^- + M_y^\diamond(\mathbf{r})\underline{\mathbf{y}}^-$, *i.e.,* $\underline{\mathbf{M}}_{xy}(\mathbf{r},t) = \Re\{\mathbf{M}_{xy}(\mathbf{r})e^{i\omega_0 t}\}$. *Then,*

$$\mathbf{M}_{xy}(\mathbf{r}) = \left(M_x^\diamond(\mathbf{r}) - iM_y^\diamond(\mathbf{r})\right) \mathbf{a}^-. \qquad (2.135)$$

Proof. Since $e^{i\omega t}\hat{\mathbf{x}} = \frac{\mathbf{x}^+ + \mathbf{x}^-}{2} - i\frac{\mathbf{y}^+ - \mathbf{y}^-}{2}$ and $e^{i\omega t}\hat{\mathbf{y}} = i\frac{\mathbf{x}^+ - \mathbf{x}^-}{2} + \frac{\mathbf{y}^+ + \mathbf{y}^-}{2}$, we have $e^{i\omega t}(\hat{\mathbf{x}} + i\hat{\mathbf{y}}) = \underline{\mathbf{x}}^- + i\underline{\mathbf{y}}^-$. Hence,

$$\underline{\mathbf{M}}_{xy} = \mathrm{Re}\Big\{ \underbrace{(M_x^\diamond - iM_y^\diamond)(\hat{\mathbf{x}} + i\hat{\mathbf{y}})\, e^{i\omega t}}_{\mathbf{M}_{xy}} \Big\}. \qquad \square$$

From Faraday's law and (2.86), the induced RF signal at the coil $\mathcal{C}$ due to the magnetization $\underline{\mathbf{M}}$ is

$$\underbrace{\oint_{\mathcal{C}} \underline{\mathbf{E}}^{\mathrm{M}}(\mathbf{r}, t) \cdot dl}_{\text{emf signal}} = -\underbrace{\int_{\text{coil surface}} \frac{\partial}{\partial t}\underline{\mathbf{B}}^{\mathrm{M}}(\mathbf{r}, t) \cdot dS}_{\text{changing magentic flux over time}} \qquad (2.136)$$

where $\underline{\mathbf{B}}^{\mathrm{M}}$ and $\underline{\mathbf{E}}^{\mathrm{M}}$, respectively, are the induced magnetic field and electrical field due to $\underline{\mathbf{M}}$. The corresponding time-harmonic fields $\mathbf{B}^{\mathrm{M}}$ and $\mathbf{E}^{\mathrm{M}}$ are governed by

$$\nabla \times \mathbf{E}^{\mathrm{M}} = -\mathrm{i}\omega\mu_0(\mathbf{H}^{\mathrm{M}} + \mathbf{M}), \quad \nabla \times \mathbf{H}^{\mathrm{M}} = (\sigma + \mathrm{i}\omega\epsilon)\mathbf{E}^{\mathrm{M}}.$$

$$(2.137)$$

Theorem 2.4. *Assume* $\underline{\mathbf{M}}$ *is given by (2.133) in the region* Ω. *Let* $\mathbf{B}_1$ *be the time-harmonic magnetic flux density produced by the current* $Ie^{i\omega_0 t}$ *through the RF coil* $\mathcal{C}$. *The induced RF signal in (2.136) is expressed as*

$$\oint_{\mathcal{C}} \mathbf{E}^{\mathrm{M}}(\mathbf{r}) \cdot d\mathbf{l_r} = -\mathrm{i}\frac{\omega}{I} \int_{\Omega} \mathbf{B}_1(\mathbf{r}) \cdot \mathbf{M}(\mathbf{r}) d\mathbf{r} \qquad (2.138)$$

Proof. Let $\mathbf{H} = \frac{1}{\mu_0}\mathbf{B}_1$. Denote by $\mathbf{J}_c$ the filamentary current flow along the coil so that $\nabla \times \mathbf{H} - \kappa\mathbf{E} = \mathbf{J}_c$. Then, we have

$$I \oint_{\mathcal{C}} \mathbf{E}^{\mathrm{M}}(\mathbf{r}) \cdot d\mathbf{l_r} = \int_{\mathbb{R}^3} \mathbf{E}^{\mathrm{M}} \cdot \mathbf{J}_c d\mathbf{r} = \int_{\mathbb{R}^3} \mathbf{E}^{\mathrm{M}} \cdot (\nabla \times \mathbf{H} - \kappa\mathbf{E})d\mathbf{r}$$

$$= \int_{\mathbb{R}^3} \Big[\mathbf{E}^{\mathrm{M}} \cdot \nabla \times \mathbf{H} - \underbrace{\nabla \times \mathbf{H}^{\mathrm{M}}}_{\kappa\mathbf{E}^{\mathrm{M}}} \cdot \mathbf{E}\Big] d\mathbf{r}$$

$$= \underbrace{\int_{\mathbb{R}^3} \nabla \cdot (\mathbf{E}^{\mathrm{M}} \times \mathbf{H} - \mathbf{E} \times \mathbf{H}^{\mathrm{M}})d\mathbf{r}}_{=0}$$

$$- \int_{\mathbb{R}^3} [\nabla \times \mathbf{E}^M \cdot \mathbf{H} - \nabla \times \mathbf{E} \cdot \mathbf{H}^M] dr$$

$$= \int_{\mathbb{R}^3} \left[\underbrace{(i\omega\mu_0(\mathbf{H}^M + \mathbf{M})) \cdot \mathbf{H}}_{-\nabla \times \mathbf{E}^M} - \underbrace{i\omega_0\mu_0 \mathbf{H} \cdot \mathbf{H}^M}_{\nabla \times \mathbf{E}} \right] dr$$

$$= i\omega_0\mu_0 \int_{\mathbb{R}^3} \mathbf{M} \cdot \mathbf{H} dr.$$

This completes the proof of (2.138).   □

Theorem 2.5. *Under the assumptions of Theorem 2.4, we have*

$$\oint_C \mathbf{E}^M(\mathbf{r}) \cdot d\mathbf{l_r} = \frac{2\omega_0}{I} \int_\Omega M_0(\mathbf{r}) \ B_\perp^+(\mathbf{r}) \sin\left(\gamma |B_{1,\perp}^-(\mathbf{r})| \ \tau\right) \frac{B_{1\perp}^-(\mathbf{r})}{|B_{1\perp}^-(\mathbf{r})|} dr \tag{2.139}$$

where $B_{1\perp}^\pm = \frac{1}{2}(B_{1x} \pm iB_{1y})$.

Proof. From (2.135) and the identity $\mathbf{B}_1 = B_{1\perp}^+ \mathbf{a}^+ + B_{1\perp}^- \mathbf{a}^-$, we have

$$\int_\Omega \mathbf{B}_1 \cdot \mathbf{M} \ dr = \int_\Omega \left(B_{1\perp}^+ \mathbf{a}^+ + B_{1\perp}^- \mathbf{a}^-\right) \cdot \left[\left(M_x^\diamond - iM_y^\diamond\right) \mathbf{a}^-\right] dr. \tag{2.140}$$

The result follows from (2.134), $\mathbf{a}^+ \cdot \mathbf{a}^+ = 0$ and $\mathbf{a}^+ \cdot \mathbf{a}^- = 2$.   □

Note that

$$\underline{\mathbf{M}}_{xy}(\mathbf{r}, t) = \text{Re}\{(M_x^-(\mathbf{r}) - iM_y^-(\mathbf{r}))\mathbf{a}_- e^{i\omega t}. \tag{2.141}$$

Remark 2.3. In this remark, we briefly discuss the method of determining $B_{1\perp}^-$. From (2.139), we may assume that the following signal is a measurable quantity for each $\alpha > 0$:

$$\xi(\tau) := M_0 B_{1\perp}^+ \sin\left(\gamma\tau|B_{1\perp}^-|\right) \frac{B_{1\perp}^-}{|B_{1\perp}^-|}. \tag{2.142}$$

One simple method to extract $|B_{1\perp}^-|$ is the double-angle method [Stollberger and Wach (1996)], which uses

$$\frac{\xi(2\tau)}{\xi(\tau)} = \frac{\sin\left(\gamma\tau|B_{1\perp}^-|\right)}{\sin\left(\gamma\tau|B_{1\perp}^-|\right)} = 2\cos\left(\gamma\tau|B_{1\perp}^-|\right). \tag{2.143}$$

The phase of $B_{1\perp}^-$ can be measured by assuming $\frac{B_{1\perp}^-}{|B_{1\perp}^-|} \approx \frac{B_{1\perp}^-}{|B_{1\perp}^-|}$. This B_1 map is influenced by the admittivity at the Larmor frequency [Haacke *et al.* (1999)]. Since we can obtain the B_1 map without using surface electrodes, admittivity imaging at the Larmor frequency using the B_1 map can be implemented without adding any extra hardware to an existing MRI scanner. For details on the B_1 mapping techniques, we refer to numerous publications [Akoka *et al.* (1993); Stollberger and Wach (1996); Van de Moortele *et al.* (2005); Wang *et al.* (2005); Yarnykh *et al.* (2007); Sacolick *et al.* (2010); Nehrke and Börnert (2012)].

2.2.4 *Relaxation effects*

In this section, we briefly discuss relaxation effects that were ignored in the previous section. Radio frequency excitation into a transverse plane causes the spin system to deviate from its thermal equilibrium state, and after turning off the RF field, the magnetization **M** starts going back to its equilibrium distribution. The k-space signals are measured during the return of the magnetization back to the equilibrium distribution. For the proper signal detections, we need to understand the relaxation process. There are two major relaxation processes: spin−lattice relaxation (termed T_1 relaxation) and spin–spin relaxation (termed T_2 relaxation).

Roughly speaking, the following Bloch equation explains how the spins return to the equilibrium states (macroscopically and microscopically) under the influence of the external field **B** (right after turning off the RF field):

$$\frac{\partial}{\partial t} \underbrace{\begin{pmatrix} M_x \\ M_y \\ M_z \end{pmatrix}}_{\mathbf{M}} = \gamma \underbrace{\begin{vmatrix} \hat{\mathbf{x}} & \hat{\mathbf{y}} & \hat{\mathbf{z}} \\ M_x & M_y & M_z \\ B_x & B_y & B_z \end{vmatrix}}_{-\mathbf{B}\times\mathbf{M}} - \begin{pmatrix} \frac{1}{T_2} M_x \\ \frac{1}{T_2} M_y \\ \frac{1}{T_2}(M_z - M_0) \end{pmatrix}. \quad (2.144)$$

Here, T_1 and T_2 are the relaxation times that are different between tissues. Table 2.2 shows relaxation times (1.5 T) for tissues and tumors [Wang (2012)].

Table 2.2.   NMR relaxation times for tissues and tumors.

Tissue type	T1 (ms)	T2 (ms)
White matter (brain)	560–787	82–92
Gray matter (brain)	921–110	92–101
CSF (brain)	3000	1500–2000
Fat (muscle)	200–250	100
Blood (venous)	1300	240
Tumor (muscle)	1300	240
Tumor (brain)	1073	121, 170–200

Note that $T_1 > T_2$. To understand T_1 and T_2 relaxation effects quickly, we imagine for a moment that $\mathbf{B} = 0$ in (2.144). Under the assumption of $\mathbf{B} = 0$, the system (2.144) is decoupled, and we have

$$\frac{\partial}{\partial t}\underline{M}_\perp = \frac{-1}{T_2}\underline{M}_\perp \Leftrightarrow \underline{M}_\perp(\mathbf{r},t) = \underline{M}_\perp(\mathbf{r},0)\,e^{\frac{-t}{T_2}}$$

$$\frac{\partial}{\partial t}\underline{M}_z = \frac{M_0 - \underline{M}_z}{T_2} \Leftrightarrow \underline{M}_z(\mathbf{r},t) = \underline{M}_z(\mathbf{r},0)e^{\frac{-t}{T_1}} + M_0(\mathbf{r})\left(1 - e^{\frac{-t}{T_1}}\right).$$

Hence, the transverse component $\underline{M}_\perp$ has T_2 decay, and the longitudinal component $\underline{M}_z$ has T_1 growth to the equilibrium value M_0. These are the reasons why T_1 and T_2 are called the longitudinal relaxation time and transverse relaxation time, respectively. Note that $\underline{M}_z(\mathbf{r},T_2) \approx 0.37\,\underline{M}_\perp(\mathbf{r},0)$ and $\underline{M}_z(\mathbf{r},T_1) \approx 0.37\,\underline{M}_\perp(\mathbf{r},0) + 0.63M_0(\mathbf{r})$.

For a detailed explanation of relaxation effects including T_1, T_2, T_2*, we refer to [Wang (2012)].

2.3   Fourier Transform

Joseph Fourier (1768–1830) showed that a general signal can be decomposed into a linear combination of basic harmonics (pure tones), sines or cosines, that are easier to analyze. The Fourier transform can be viewed as a prism in the sense that a signal $f(x)$ can be split into $f(x) = \sum_n a_n e^{2\pi i n x}$. Moreover, the Fourier transform is a reversible operation due to the Fourier inversion formula in Theorem 2.145 that will be explained later in this section.

Let us provide a brief description of the Fourier transform. We use the following notations:

- If f is integrable over $\mathbb{R}$, its Fourier transform is defined by

$$\widehat{f}(k) := (\mathcal{F}f)(k) = \int_{-\infty}^{\infty} f(x)e^{-2\pi ikx} \, dx.$$

- The convolution of two functions f and g is given by

$$f * g(x) = \int_{-\infty}^{\infty} f(x - x')g(x') \, dx'.$$

The following Fourier inversion provides that f can be recovered from its Fourier transform $\widehat{f}$.

Theorem 2.6 (Fourier inversion formula). *Assume f and $\hat{f}$ are continuous and integrable. Then*

$$f(x) = \int_R \hat{f}(k)e^{2\pi ikx} \, dk. \tag{2.145}$$

Proof. The inverse Fourier transform of $\widehat{f}$ can be expressed as

$$\int_{\mathbb{R}} \hat{f}(k)e^{2\pi ikx}dk = \int_{\mathbb{R}} \hat{f}(k)e^{2\pi ikx} \underbrace{\lim_{\epsilon \to 0}[\exp(-\pi\epsilon^2 k^2)]}_{=1} \, dk$$

$$= \lim_{\epsilon \to 0} \int_{\mathbb{R}} \left[\int_{\mathbb{R}} e^{2\pi i(x-x')k}\exp(-\pi\epsilon^2 k^2)dk \right] f(x')dx'. \tag{2.146}$$

The last identity can be obtained by interchanging the order of the integration. From the identity $\widehat{e^{-\pi x^2}}(k) = e^{-\pi k^2}$ and the scaling property $\widehat{f(ax)}(k) = \frac{1}{a}\widehat{f}(\frac{k}{a})$, the last quantity in (2.146) can be expressed as

$$\left[\int_{\mathbb{R}} e^{2\pi i(x-x')k}\exp(-\pi\epsilon^2 k^2)dk \right] = \underbrace{\frac{1}{\epsilon}\exp\left(\frac{-\pi(x - x')^2}{\epsilon^2} \right)}_{\phi_\epsilon(x-x')}.$$

Then, the identity (2.146) can be simplified into

$$\int_{\mathbb{R}} \hat{f}(k)e^{2\pi ikx}dk = \lim_{\epsilon \to 0} \phi_\epsilon * f(x).$$

Since $\lim_{\epsilon \to 0} \phi_\epsilon(x) = 0$ for all $x \neq 0$ and $\int_\mathbb{R} \phi_\epsilon(x)dx = 1$, we have

$$\lim_{\epsilon \to 0} \phi_\epsilon * f(x) = \int_\mathbb{R} \delta(x - x')f(x')dy = f(x).$$

For the detailed proof, we refer to [Seo and Woo (2012)]. □

The following Poisson summation formula indicates that the T−periodic summation of f is expressed as the discrete samples of its Fourier transform $\widehat{f}$ with the sampling distance $\frac{1}{T}$.

Theorem 2.7 (Poisson summation formula). *For $f \in C(\mathbb{R}) \cap L^1(\mathbb{R})$, we have*

$$\sum_{n=-\infty}^{\infty} f(x - nT) = \frac{1}{T} \sum_{n=-\infty}^{\infty} \widehat{f}\left(\frac{n}{T}\right) e^{2\pi i \frac{n}{T} x}. \qquad (2.147)$$

In particular,

$$supp\,(f) \subset [0, T] \Rightarrow f(x) = \frac{1}{T} \sum_{n=-\infty}^{\infty} \widehat{f}\left(\frac{n}{T}\right) e^{2\pi i \frac{n}{T} x} \quad for\; x \in [0, T]$$

$$supp\,(f) \subset [0, 2T] \Rightarrow f(x) + f(x + T) = \frac{1}{T} \sum_{n=-\infty}^{\infty} \widehat{f}\left(\frac{n}{T}\right) e^{2\pi i \frac{n}{T} x}$$

$$for\; x \in [0, 2T].$$

For the proof of the Poisson summation formula (2.147), we refer to [Seo and Woo (2012)].

The bandlimited function f with bandwidth B, that is, $supp(\widehat{f}) \subset [-B, B]$, does not contain sinusoidal waves at frequencies higher than B. This means that f cannot oscillate rapidly within a distance less than $\frac{1}{2B}$. Hence, the bandlimited f can be represented by means of its uniformly spaced discrete sample $\{f(n\Delta x) : n = 0, \pm 1, \pm 2, \cdots\}$ provided that the sampling interval Δx is sufficiently small. Indeed, the following sampling theorem (2.8) says that if $\Delta x \leq \frac{1}{2B}$, then the discrete sample $\{f(n\Delta x) : n = 0, \pm 1, \pm 2, \cdots\}$ contains the complete information of f. This $2B$ is called the Nyquist rate.

Theorem 2.8 (Whittaker–Shannon sampling theorem). *Suppose $f \in C(\mathbb{R}) \cap L^1(\mathbb{R})$ and $supp(\widehat{f}) \subset [-B, B]$. The original data f*

can be reconstructed by the interpolation formula

$$f(x) = \sum_{n=-\infty}^{\infty} f\left(\frac{1}{2B}n\right) sinc\left(2B\left(x - \frac{1}{2B}n\right)\right)$$

where $sinc(x) = \frac{\sin(\pi x)}{\pi x}$.

The one-dimensional definition of the Fourier transform can be extended to multiple dimensions. The Fourier transform of a two-dimensional function $f(x, y)$, denoted by $F(k_x, k_y)$, is defined by

$$F(k_x, k_y) = \int_{-\infty}^{\infty} \int_{-\infty}^{\infty} f(x, y)e^{-2\pi i(k_x x + k_y y)} \, dx \, dy.$$

We can generalize all the results in the one-dimensional Fourier transform to the two-dimensional case because the two-dimensional Fourier transform can be expressed as two one-dimensional Fourier transforms along x and y variables:

$$F(k_x, k_y) = \int_{-\infty}^{\infty} \underbrace{\left(\int_{-\infty}^{\infty} f(x, y)e^{-2\pi i k_x x}dx\right)}_{=(\mathcal{F}f(\cdot, y))(k_x)} e^{-2\pi i k_y y} \, dy.$$

If $f(x, y)$ and $F(k_x, k_y)$ are a Fourier transform pair, we have the Fourier inversion formula:

$$f(x, y) \propto \int_{-\infty}^{\infty} \int_{-\infty}^{\infty} F(k_x, k_y)e^{2\pi i(k_x x + k_y y)} \, dk_x \, dk_y.$$

A two-dimensional sampling theorem can be stated as follows: If $supp(S) \subset [-B, B] \times [-B, B]$, then the original data $\rho(x, y)$ can be reconstructed by the interpolation formula

$$f(x, y) = \sum_{n=-\infty}^{\infty} \sum_{m=-\infty}^{\infty} f\left(\frac{n}{2B}, \frac{m}{2B}\right) sinc\left(2B\left(x - \frac{n}{2B}\right)\right)$$

$$\times sinc\left(2B\left(y - \frac{m}{2B}\right)\right).$$

2.4 Image Processing

In MR-based electro-magnetic property imaging, we need to deal with noisy MR data; the measured data tend to have lower SNR (signal-to-noise ratio) and usually get degraded in their accuracy due to the non-ideal data acquisition of an MR scanner. This demands innovative data processing methods as well as improved measurement techniques to maximize SNR for a given data collection time.

Data denoising for medical images aims to eliminate the random and systematic noise in the data while preserving important features. Image segmentation techniques are useful tools in improving the detectability of diagnostic features. Numerous algorithms for image denoising and segmentation are based on mathematical models with partial differential equations, level set methods, regularization, energy functionals, and others. Recently, geometric properties of images have been incorporated in noise-removal partial differential equations (PDEs) by regarding the intensity image as a two-dimensional surface in a three-dimensional space with the gray level assigned to the z-axis. Then, geometric properties of images can be interpreted using the distribution of its gradient, Laplacian, curvature, and so on. For example, noise is usually characterized as having a local high curvature, and edges are extracted by using gradient magnitude. We refer to [Aubert and Kornprobst (2002); Osher *et al.* (2002); Seo and Woo (2012)].

2.4.1   *Diffusion techniques for denoising: L^1 vs. L^2 minimization*

Let $u(x, y)$ be the intensity function of an image or signal. Assume that the measured image f and the true image u are related by

$$f = \mathcal{L}u + Noise \qquad (2.148)$$

where $\mathcal{L}$ is an operator including blurring, shifting, and others. Introducing a new coordinate z, and assigning the gray level of the image to this z-coordinate, the image $u(x, y)$ can be viewed as a surface $z = u(x, y)$. Then the noise is usually characterized as having a local high (mean) curvature.

Standard smoothing methods (such as low-pass filtering) eliminate highly oscillating noise, while edges having high frequencies are also smeared at the same time. A typical way of denoising (or image restoration) is to find the best function by minimizing the functional:

$$\Phi(u) = \frac{1}{2} \iint |\mathcal{L}u - f|^2 dxdy + \frac{\lambda}{p} \iint |\nabla u|^p \, dxdy, \qquad (2.149)$$

where $1 \leq p \leq \infty$. The first term in (2.149), called the fidelity term, forces the residual $\mathcal{L}u - f$ to be small; the second term, called the regularization term, enforces the regularity of u; and λ, called the regularization parameter, controls the trade-off between the residual norm and the regularity.

If u is a minimizer of the functional (2.149), then

$$\Phi(u) \leq \Phi(v) \quad \text{for all } v \in \mathcal{A}, \qquad (2.150)$$

where $\mathcal{A}$ is an admissible class. Assuming that $\mathcal{A}$ is a Banach space,[7] u satisfying (2.150) can be viewed as a critical point in the sense that

$$\frac{\partial}{\partial t} \Phi(u + t\phi)|_{t=0} = 0 \quad \text{for all } \phi \text{ satisfying } u + t\phi \in \mathcal{A}. \qquad (2.151)$$

If $\mathcal{L}$ is a linear operator, (2.150) leads to the corresponding Euler−Lagrange equation:

$$-\nabla \cdot (|\nabla u|^{p-2} \nabla u) + \frac{1}{\lambda} \mathcal{L}^*(\mathcal{L}u - f) = 0 \qquad (2.152)$$

where $\mathcal{L}^*$ is the dual of $\mathcal{L}$. The above PDE (2.152) is non-linear except $p = 2$. To solve the equation (2.152) with a suitable boundary condition, one may use the following gradient descent method by introducing the time variable t:

$$\frac{\partial}{\partial t} u(x, y, t) = -\left[-\nabla \cdot (|\nabla u|^{p-2} \nabla u) + \frac{1}{\lambda} \mathcal{L}^*(\mathcal{L}u - f) \right] \qquad (2.153)$$

with the initial data $u(x, y, 0) = f(x, y)$. Diffusion PDE in (2.153) can act as a smoothing tool for removing high-frequency noise in the surface $z = f(x, y)$. When $p = 2$ (L^2-minimization), the minimizer u of (2.149) is a solution of the linear PDE $-\nabla^2 u = \lambda^{-1} \mathcal{L}^*(\mathcal{L}u - f)$. The Laplace operator ∇^2 has isotropic smoothing properties

---

[7]A Banach space is a vector space that is equipped with a norm $\| \cdot \|$ and which is complete with respect to that norm. For example, $L^p(\Omega) = \{f : \|f\|_p < \infty\}$ ($1 < p < \infty$) is a Banach space equipped with the norm $\|f\|_p := \left(\int_\Omega |f|^p \right)^{1/p}$.

eliminating highly oscillatory noise, but it also smears edges having high frequencies at the same time. When $p = 1$ (L^1 minimization), the term $\nabla \cdot \left(\frac{1}{|\nabla u|} \nabla u \right)$ performs the diffusion process by smoothing the surface $z = f(x, y)$ except cliffs and preventing diffusion across cliffs. This is the reason why L^1-minimization has been widely used in the image-processing community.

To compare the performance of L^1 minimization with L^2 minimization, we begin with considering the following sequence f_n defined on the interval $[-1, 1]$:

$$f_n(x) := \begin{cases} n\,x & \text{if } -1 \leq x < 1/n \\ 1 & \text{if } 1/n \leq x \leq 1. \end{cases} \tag{2.154}$$

Then, the sequence f_n converges to the Heaviside step function[8] in a pointwise sense (except $x = 0$), but

$$\lim_{n \to \infty} \|f_n\|_1 = \lim_{n \to \infty} \underbrace{\int_{-1}^{1} \left| \frac{d}{dx} f_n(x) \right| dx}_{=1} = 1$$

$$\tag{2.155}$$

and $\quad \lim_{n \to \infty} \|f_n\|_2 = \lim_{n \to \infty} \underbrace{\sqrt{\int_{-1}^{1} \left| \frac{d}{dx} f_n(x) \right|^2 dx}}_{=\sqrt{n}} = \infty.$

This explains that the L^2-distance between $f_n(x)$ and the Heaviside step function $H(x)$ is infinite, whereas the corresponding L^1-distance is 1. This implies that edges (or jump discontinuities) cannot be preserved when using L^2 minimization, whereas L^1 minimization is able to preserve edges.

Now, we explain TV (total variation) regularization with its corresponding time-marching algorithm $p = 1$ in (2.153):

$$\begin{cases} \dfrac{\partial u}{\partial t} = \lambda \nabla \cdot \left(\dfrac{\nabla u}{|\nabla u|} \right) - \mathcal{L}^*(\mathcal{L}u - f) & \text{in } \Omega \times (0, T] \\ u(x, y, t) = f(\mathbf{r}), \quad \mathbf{r} \in \Omega \\ \dfrac{\partial u}{\partial \mathbf{n}} = 0 \quad \text{on } \partial\Omega \times (0, T]. \end{cases} \tag{2.156}$$

---

[8]The Heaviside step function is the unit step function $H(x)$ whose value is 0 if $x < 0$ and 1 if $x > 0$.

As above, f is a given noisy image defined in a two-dimensional domain Ω.

Since $\nabla \cdot \left(\frac{\nabla u}{|\nabla u|} \right)$ is the mean curvature of level curve $u = $ constant, the time-marching algorithm of (2.156) removes smaller-scaled noise quicker than noise with high curvature. Note that $\mathbf{n} := \frac{\nabla u}{|\nabla u|}$ is the normal vector to its level curve $u = $ constant, $T = \frac{(-u_y, u_x)}{|\nabla u|}$ is the tangent vector, and $|\nabla u| = \frac{\nabla u}{|\nabla u|} \cdot \nabla u = \mathbf{n} \cdot \nabla u$. Since $\nabla^2 u = (\mathbf{n} \cdot \nabla)^2 u + (T \cdot \nabla)^2 u$, the leading order term $\nabla \cdot \left(\frac{\nabla u}{|\nabla u|} \right)$ can be written as

$$\nabla \cdot [|\nabla u|^{-1} \nabla u] = |\nabla u|^{-1} \nabla^2 u - \underbrace{|\nabla u|^{-2} \nabla u}_{|\nabla u|^{-1} \mathbf{n}} \cdot \underbrace{\nabla(|\nabla u|)}_{=\mathbf{n} \cdot \nabla u}$$

$$= |\nabla u|^{-1} (T \cdot \nabla)^2 u. \tag{2.157}$$

This is the reason why the time-marching algorithm of (2.156) permits diffusion along the edges while also preserving them.

2.4.2 *Segmentation*

Let f be a given image defined in a two-dimensional domain. Segmentation of a target object (imaged by f) in the form of a closed curve has many potential applications in medical imaging because it provides quantitative information related to the target object's size and shape. The curve evolution method is one of the most widely used segmentation techniques. It is based on the minimization problem of an energy functional and is often implemented under the level set terminology for robust and fine segmentation. By representing a contour by level set $\mathcal{C}_\phi = \{(x, y) : \phi(x, y) = 0\}$, the segmentation problem may be converted to finding a closed curve $\mathcal{C}_\phi$ that minimizes the energy functional represented as

$$\Phi[\mathcal{C}_\phi] := \mathbf{Reg}[\mathcal{C}_\phi] + \lambda \, \mathbf{Fit}[\mathcal{C}_\phi, f] \tag{2.158}$$

where $\mathbf{Reg}[\mathcal{C}_\phi]$ is a regularization term for penalizing non-smoothness of the contour $\mathcal{C}_\phi$ and $\mathbf{Fit}[\mathcal{C}_\phi, f]$ is a fitting term for attracting the contour $\mathcal{C}_\phi$ toward the target object in the image f; λ is a tunable fitting parameter which controls the balance between those two terms. There exists a variety of fitting models such as edge-based methods [Caselles *et al.* (1993, 1997); Kichenassamy *et al.*

(1995); Malladi *et al.* (1995); Goldenberg *et al.* (2001)], region-based methods [Paragios *et al.* (1998); Yezzi *et al.* (1999); Chan and Vese (2001)], the methods by the prior information [Chen *et al.* (2002)] and so on. These fitting models are mostly combined with the standard regularization term penalizing the arc length of the contour $\mathcal{C}$.

Edge-based methods use the strength of the image gradient along the boundary between target object and the background in order to evolve an active contour toward the boundary of the target region; the direction of the velocity of the active contour is the negative direction of the gradient of the energy functional. To be precise, we begin with considering a minimization problem of finding a closed curve $\mathcal{C}$ that minimizes the fitting term

$$\mathbf{Fit}[\mathcal{C}] = \int_{\mathcal{C}} w(|\nabla f|) \, ds \qquad (2.159)$$

where $w : \mathbb{R} \to \mathbb{R}$ is a function such that

- w is a decreasing function with $w(0) = 1$
- $w(|\nabla f|) \approx 0$ for large $|\nabla f|$. (With this setting, $\mathcal{C}$ may settle on the boundary of the target since $|\nabla f| \approx \infty$ on edges.)

For example, one may choose $w(|\nabla f|) = \frac{1}{1+|\nabla f|}$. We hope that minimization of the fitting term in (2.159) results in the contour $\mathcal{C}$ that separates the target from the background in the image f.

For computation of a local minimum $\mathcal{C}$, we may start from an initial contour $\mathcal{C}^0$. We need to construct a minimizing sequence $\mathcal{C}^1, \mathcal{C}^2, \cdots$ such that

$$\mathbf{Fit}[\mathcal{C}^0] > \mathbf{Fit}[\mathcal{C}^1] > \cdots > \mathbf{Fit}[\mathcal{C}^n] \to \mathbf{Fit}[\mathcal{C}].$$

To calculate the next curve $\mathcal{C}^{n+1}$ from $\mathcal{C}^n$, we may use the gradient descent method based on the Fréchet gradient $-\nabla \mathbf{Fit}[\mathcal{C}^n]$.

The contour $\mathcal{C}^n$ can be parameterized by $\mathbf{r}(s, n) = x(s, n)\hat{\mathbf{x}} + y(s, n)\hat{\mathbf{y}}, 0 < s < 1$:

$$\mathcal{C}^n = \{\mathbf{r}(s, n) = x(s, n)\hat{\mathbf{x}} + y(s, n)\hat{\mathbf{y}} \mid 0 < s < 1\}.$$

For ease of explanation, it is convenient to use the time variable t with considering time-varying contour $\mathcal{C}^t$ instead of $\mathcal{C}^n$:

$$\mathcal{C}^t = \{\mathbf{r}(s, t) := x(s, t)\hat{\mathbf{x}} + y(s, t)\hat{\mathbf{y}} \mid 0 < s < 1\} \quad t > 0.$$

Writing

$$\mathbf{Fit}[\mathcal{C}^t] = \int_0^1 \underbrace{w(|\nabla f(\mathbf{r}(s,t))|)}_{:=g(\mathbf{r}(s,t))} \, |\mathbf{r}_s(s,t)| ds,$$

the time derivative of $\mathbf{Fit}[\mathcal{C}^t]$ is

$$\frac{d}{dt}\mathbf{Fit}[\mathcal{C}^t] = \int_0^1 |\mathbf{r}_s|[\nabla g \cdot \mathbf{r}_t]ds + \int_0^1 g\left[\frac{\mathbf{r}_s}{|\mathbf{r}_s|} \cdot \mathbf{r}_{ts}\right]ds$$

$$= \int_0^1 |\mathbf{r}_s|[\nabla g \cdot \mathbf{r}_t]ds - \int_0^1 \left\langle g\left[\frac{\mathbf{r}_s}{|\mathbf{r}_s|}\right]_s + [\nabla g \cdot \mathbf{r}_s]\frac{\mathbf{r}_s}{|\mathbf{r}_s|}, \mathbf{r}_t\right\rangle ds$$

$$= \int_0^1 |\mathbf{r}_s|\,\mathbf{r}_t \cdot [\nabla g - \kappa g\mathbf{n} - \langle T, \nabla g\rangle T]ds$$

where $\mathbf{r}_t = \frac{\partial \mathbf{r}}{\partial t}$, $\mathbf{r}_s = \frac{\partial \mathbf{r}}{\partial s}$, $\mathbf{n} = \mathbf{n}(s,t)$ the unit normal to the curve $\mathcal{C}^t$, and $T = T(s,t)$ the unit tangent vector. Hence, the direction for which $\mathbf{Fit}[\mathcal{C}^t]$ decreases most rapidly is given by the steepest descent direction

$$\mathbf{r}_t = -[\nabla g - \kappa g\mathbf{n} - \langle T, \nabla g\rangle T]. \tag{2.160}$$

Decomposing $\nabla g = \langle \nabla g, \mathbf{n}\rangle \mathbf{n} + \langle \nabla g, T\rangle T$, the equation (2.160) becomes $\mathbf{r}_t = (\kappa g - \langle \nabla g, \mathbf{n}\rangle)$ which is equivalent to

$$\frac{\partial}{\partial t}\mathcal{C}^t = \underbrace{(\kappa \, w(|\nabla f|) - \nabla w(|\nabla f|) \cdot \mathbf{n})}_{speed} \mathbf{n}. \tag{2.161}$$

This means that the curve $\mathcal{C}^t$ moves along its normal direction with the speed $\kappa \, w(|\nabla f|) - \nabla w(|\nabla f| \cdot \mathbf{n}$. Hence, we can update $\mathcal{C}^{n+1}$ by

$$\mathbf{r}(s, n+1) = \mathbf{r}(s,n) + \alpha \underbrace{(\kappa \, w(|\nabla f|) - \nabla w(|\nabla f|) \cdot \mathbf{n})}_{speed} \mathbf{n}(s,n)$$

$$\tag{2.162}$$

where $0 < \alpha < 1$ is a step size.

The active contour scheme using the explicit expression $\mathcal{C}^t = \{\mathbf{r}(s,t) : 0 \leq s \leq 1\}$ is not appropriate for segmenting multiple targets whose locations are unknown. Using an auxiliary function $\phi(\mathbf{r}, t)$, the propagating contour $\mathcal{C}^t$ changing its topology (splitting multiple closed curves) can be expressed effectively by the implicit expression of the zero level set

$$\mathcal{C}^t = \{\mathbf{r} : \phi(\mathbf{r}, t) = 0\}.$$

With the level set method [Osher *et al.* (2002)], the motion of the active contour with the explicit expression (2.161) is replaced by the motion of the level set. Using the property

$$\phi(\mathbf{r}(s, t), t) = 0,$$

we have the equation of ϕ containing the embedded motion of $\mathcal{C}^t$; for a fixed s,

$$0 = \frac{d}{dt}\phi(\mathbf{r}(s, t), t) = \frac{\partial}{\partial t}\phi(\mathbf{r}, t) + \frac{\partial}{\partial t}\mathbf{r}(s, t) \cdot \nabla\phi(\mathbf{r}(s, t), t).$$

Since $\frac{\partial}{\partial t}\mathbf{r}(s, t) = F(\mathbf{r}(s, t), t)\mathbf{n}(s, t)$ and $\mathbf{n}(s, t) = \frac{\nabla\phi(\mathbf{r}(s,t),t)}{|\nabla\phi(\mathbf{r}(s,t),t)|}$, the above identity leads to

$$\frac{\partial}{\partial t}\phi(\mathbf{r}, t) + F(\mathbf{r}, t)|\nabla\phi(\mathbf{r}, t)| = 0. \tag{2.163}$$

With the use of the level set expression, the geodesic active contour model (2.161) can be expressed as

$$\phi_t(\mathbf{r}, t) = \left(w(|\nabla f|)\left[\nabla \cdot \frac{\nabla\phi}{|\nabla\phi|}\right] + \frac{\nabla\phi}{|\nabla\phi|} \cdot \nabla w(|\nabla f|)\right)|\nabla\phi|. \tag{2.164}$$

The convection term $\langle \nabla g, \nabla\phi \rangle$ increases the attraction of the deforming contour toward the boundary of objects.

For example, [Chan and Vese (2001)] use the following energy functional (Chan–Vese model):

$$\Phi(\phi) = \int |\nabla H(\phi(\mathbf{r}))|d\mathbf{r} + \lambda_1 \int H(\phi(\mathbf{r}))|u(\mathbf{r}) - ave_{\{\phi \geq 0\}}|^2 d\mathbf{r}$$

$$+ \lambda_2 \int H(-\phi(\mathbf{r}))|u(\mathbf{r}) - ave_{\{\phi < 0\}}|^2 d\mathbf{r} \tag{2.165}$$

where λ_1, λ_2 are non-negative parameters, ϕ is the level set function, and $ave_{\{\phi \geq 0\}}, ave_{\{\phi < 0\}}$ are the average values of $f(s, y)$ in the two-dimensional regions $\{\phi < 0\}$ and $\{\phi > 0\}$, respectively. Here, $H(\phi)$ is the one-dimensional Heaviside function with $H(s) = 1$ if $s \geq 0$, and

$H(s) = 0$ if $s < 0$. To compute a minimizer ϕ for the minimization problem (2.165), the following parabolic equation is solved to the steady state:

$$\frac{\partial \phi}{\partial t} = |H'(\phi)| \left[\nabla \cdot \left(\frac{\nabla \phi}{|\nabla \phi|} \right) - \lambda_1 (f - ave_{\{\phi \geq 0\}})^2 + \lambda_2 (f - ave_{\{\phi < 0\}})^2 \right]$$

(2.166)

with an appropriate initial level set function. After the evolution has come to a converged state, the zero level set of ϕ becomes the contour that separates the object from the background.

We refer to [Seo and Woo (2012)] for a detailed explanation.

2.4.3 *Sparse sensing*

Let $\mathbf{A}$ be an $m \times N$ matrix. We consider a linear system of equations $\mathbf{Ax} = \mathbf{b}$. If it has more equations than unknowns (that is, $m > N$), it is overdetermined and may not have any solution. On the other hand, if it has fewer equations than unknowns (that is, $m < N$), it is underdetermined and has an infinite number of solutions. In these cases, we need to seek a best solution of $\mathbf{Ax} = \mathbf{b}$ in an appropriate sense.

In this section, we consider the underdetermined linear system $A\mathbf{x} = \mathbf{b}$:

$$\underbrace{\begin{pmatrix} a_{11} & a_{12} & \cdots & \cdots & a_{1,N} \\ \vdots & \vdots & & & \vdots \\ a_{m1} & a_{m2} & \cdots & \cdots & a_{m,N} \end{pmatrix}}_{\mathbf{A}} \underbrace{\begin{pmatrix} x_1 \\ x_2 \\ \vdots \\ \vdots \\ x_N \end{pmatrix}}_{\mathbf{x}}$$

$$= \underbrace{\begin{pmatrix} b_1 \\ \vdots \\ b_m \end{pmatrix}}_{\mathbf{b}} \quad \text{and} \quad m < N.$$

(2.167)

If $A\mathbf{x} = \mathbf{b}$ has a solution, then an infinite number of solutions $\mathbf{x} = (x_1, \ldots, x_N)$ exist such that

$$x_1 \mathbf{a}_1 + \cdots + x_N \mathbf{a}_N = \mathbf{b}$$

where $\mathbf{a}_j = (a_{1j}, \ldots, a_{mj})^T$ is the j-th column vector of $\mathbf{A}$. Applying an SVD (singular value decomposition), $\mathbf{A}$ can be expressed as

$$\mathbf{A} = \begin{pmatrix} \mathbf{u}_1 \cdots \mathbf{u}_r \end{pmatrix} \begin{pmatrix} \lambda_1 & & \\ & \ddots & \\ & & \lambda_r \end{pmatrix} \begin{pmatrix} \mathbf{v}_1^T \\ \vdots \\ \mathbf{v}_r^T \end{pmatrix}, \qquad (2.168)$$

where $\lambda_1 > \cdots > \lambda_r > 0 = \lambda_{r+1} = \cdots = \lambda_N$ are eigenvalues of $\mathbf{A}^T\mathbf{A}$, $\mathbf{v}_1, \ldots, \mathbf{v}_N$ are orthonormal eigenvectors of $\mathbf{A}^T\mathbf{A}$, and $\mathbf{u}_j = \frac{1}{\lambda_j}\mathbf{A}\mathbf{v}_j$. Hence, the null space of $\mathbf{A}$ is the vector space spanned by vectors $\mathbf{v}_{r+1}, \ldots, \mathbf{v}_N$, that will be denoted by $\mathrm{Span}\{\mathbf{v}_{r+1}, \ldots, \mathbf{v}_N\}$. Writing

$$\mathbf{x}^\dagger = \underbrace{\frac{1}{\lambda_1}\langle \mathbf{b}, \mathbf{u}_1 \rangle \mathbf{v}_1}_{x_1^\dagger} + \cdots + \underbrace{\frac{1}{\lambda_j}\langle \mathbf{b}, \mathbf{u}_r \rangle \mathbf{v}_r}_{x_r^\dagger} \qquad (2.169)$$

we have

$$\mathbf{b} = \mathbf{A}(\mathbf{x}^\dagger) = \mathbf{A}(\mathbf{x}^\dagger + \mathbf{y}) \quad \text{for all } \mathbf{y} \in \mathrm{Span}\{\mathbf{v}_{r+1}, \ldots, \mathbf{v}_N\}.$$

Hence, without having some knowledge of the true solution such as sparsity (having a few non-zero entries of the solution), there is no hope of solving the underdetermined linear system (2.167). However, if the true solution, denoted by $\mathbf{x}_{true}$, is sufficiently sparse, then we have a chance to extract the true solution $\mathbf{x}_{true} = \mathbf{x}^\dagger$.

[Donoho and Elad (2003)] studied the uniqueness problem of the underdetermined linear system by enforcing the sparsity constraint. Define

$$\|\mathbf{x}\|_0 = \sharp\{j : x_j \neq 0\} \quad \text{(the number of non-zero entries of } \mathbf{x})$$

and

$$\mathrm{spark}(A) = \underbrace{\min\{\|\mathbf{x}\|_0 : A\mathbf{x} = 0 \ \& \ \|\mathbf{x}\|_2 = 1\}}_{\text{the smallest number of linearly dependent columns of } A}.$$

[Donoho and Elad (2003)] found the following:

- Let $W_S := \{\mathbf{x} \in \mathbb{R}^N : \|\mathbf{x}\|_0 \leq S\}$. The underdetermined linear system (2.167) has at most one solution within the restricted set W_S for $S < \frac{\mathrm{spark}(A)}{2}$.

To see this, let $\mathbf{x}, \mathbf{x}' \in W_S$ with $S \leq \frac{\text{spark}(A)}{2}$ and let $A\mathbf{x} = A\mathbf{x}'$. Then, the uniqueness $(\mathbf{x} = \mathbf{x}')$ follows from the definition of spark that

$$\text{either} \quad \mathbf{x} = \mathbf{x}' \quad \text{or} \quad \|\mathbf{x} - \mathbf{x}'\|_0 \geq \text{spark}(A)$$

and noting that

$$\text{spark}(A) > \|\mathbf{x}\|_0 + \|\mathbf{x}'\|_0 \geq \|\mathbf{x} - \mathbf{x}'\|_0.$$

In order to solve the underdetermined linear system (2.167) subject to the sparsity constraint, one may consider the following sparse optimization problem:

$$(P_0): \quad \min \|\mathbf{x}\|_0 \quad \text{subject to } A\mathbf{x} = \mathbf{b}. \tag{2.170}$$

Let $\mathbf{x}_0$ be a solution of the ℓ_0-minimization problem (P_0). Unfortunately, finding $\mathbf{x}_0$ via ℓ_0-minimization is extremely difficult. It is non-deterministic Polynomial-time hard (NP-hard) due to lack of convexity; we cannot use Newton's iteration.

Instead of solving the NP-hard problem (P_0), one can consider the relaxed ℓ_1-minimization problem which is the closest convex minimization problem to (P_0):

$$P_1: \quad \min \|\mathbf{x}\|_1 \quad \text{subject to } A\mathbf{x} = \mathbf{b}. \tag{2.171}$$

Let $\mathbf{x}^1$ be a solution of the ℓ_1-minimization problem (P_1). Then, the major question is under what condition can the sparsest solution of (P_0) be the solution of (P_1). [Donoho and Elad (2003)] observe that it could be $\mathbf{x}^0 = \mathbf{x}^1$ when $\|\mathbf{x}^0\|_0$ is sufficiently small and A has incoherent columns. Here, the mutual coherence of A measures the largest correlation between different columns from A (see [Donoho and Huo (1999)]).

For robustness of compressed sensing, [Candès and Tao (2005)] used a notion of the restricted isometry property (RIP) condition: A is said to have RIP of order S if there exists an isometry constant $\delta_S \in (0, 1)$ such that

$$(1 - \delta_S)\|\mathbf{x}\|_2^2 \leq \|A\mathbf{x}\|_2^2 \leq (1 + \delta_S)\|\mathbf{x}\|_2^2, \quad \forall \mathbf{x} \in W_S. \tag{2.172}$$

If A has a RIP of order $2S$, then the underdetermined linear system (2.167) has "well-distinguishability" within the S-sparse set W_S:

$$(1 - \delta_{2S}) \leq \frac{\|A(\mathbf{x} - \mathbf{x}')\|_2^2}{\|\mathbf{x} - \mathbf{x}'\|_2^2} \leq (1 + \delta_{2S}), \quad \forall \mathbf{x}, \mathbf{x}' \in W_S.$$

If $\delta_{2S} < 1$, then the map A is injective within the set W_S. If δ_{2S} is close to 0, the transformation A roughly preserves the distance between any two different points.

[Candès *et al.* (2006b)] observe that the sparse solution of the problem (P_0) can be found by solving (P_1) under the assumption that A obeys $2S$-restricted isometry property (RIP) condition with δ_{2S} not being close to one [Candès and Tao (2005); Candès *et al.* (2006a)].

Theorem 2.9. [Candès *et al.* (2006b)] *Let* $\mathbf{x}^{exact}$ *be a solution of the underdetermined linear system* (2.167). *Assume that A has RIP of order* $2S$ *with the isometry constant* $\delta_{2S} < \sqrt{2} - 1$. *Then there exists a constant* C_0 *such that*

$$\|\mathbf{x}^{exact} - \mathbf{x}^1\|_1 + \sqrt{S}\, \|\mathbf{x}^{exact} - \mathbf{x}^1\|_2 \leq C_0 \min_{\mathbf{x} \in W_S} \|\mathbf{x}^{exact} - \mathbf{x}\|_1.$$

$$(2.173)$$

Most inverse problems in medical imaging are used to recover three-dimensional images of tissue properties from knowledge of the relationship between input data and output data. To solve inverse problems, we usually develop a linearized system $A\mathbf{x} = \mathbf{b}$ where $\mathbf{x}$ is the image to be recovered, $\mathbf{b}$ is measured data, and A is the sensitivity matrix made from a suitable arrangement of the governing equation. The j-th column of A represents the response change due to unit perturbation of the j-th element of $\mathbf{x}$. When measurable data are either insufficient for uniqueness or insensitive to local perturbation of the parameter to be imaged, we need to deal with an underdetermined linear system (or ill-posed problem) $A\mathbf{x} = \mathbf{b}$. In order to obtain stable reconstructions, one must incorporate *a priori* information on the solution $\mathbf{x}$. Regularization is an important tool to deal with an ill-posed problem by imposing *a priori* information on the solution. Sparsity regularization is one of the common uses of *a priori* information on sparse gradient images.

References

Akoka S, Franconi F, Seguin F and Le Pape A (1993). *Radiofrequency map of an NMR coil by imaging, Magn. Reson. Imag.*, Vol. 11, pp. 437–441.

Aubert G and Kornprobst P (2002). *Mathematical problems in image processing: partial differential equations and the calculus of variations,* Second edition, Applied Mathematical Sciences Series, Vol. 147, Springer Verlag, Berlin.

Aubert G and Vese L (1997). *A variational method in image recovery, SIAM J. Numer. Anal.*, Vol. 34, no. 5, pp. 1948–1979.

Bracewell RN (1956). *Strip integration in radioastronomy, J. Phys.*, Vol. 9, pp. 198–217.

Bracewell RN and Riddle AC (1967). *Inversion of fan-beam scans in radion astronomy, Astrophys J.*, Vol. 150, pp. 427–434.

Brooks RA and Chiro GD (1976). *Beam hardening in x-ray reconstructive tomography, Phys. Med. Biol.*, Vol. 21, pp. 390–398.

Bydder M, Larkman DJ and Hajnal JV (2002). *Generalized SMASH imaging, Magn. Reson. Med.*, Vol. 47, pp. 160–170.

Calder J and Mansouri A (2011). *Anisotropic image sharpening via well-posed Sobolev gradient flows, SIAM J. Math. Analysis,* Vol. 43, pp. 1536–1556.

Candès EJ and Tao T (2005). *Decoding by linear programming, IEEE Trans. Inform. Theory,* Vol. 51, no. 12, pp. 4203–4215.

Candès EJ, Romberg J and Tao T (2006a). *Robust uncertainty principles: exact signal reconstruction from highly incomplete frequency information, IEEE Trans. Inform. Theory,* Vol. 52, no. 2, pp. 489–509.

Candès EJ, Romberg JK and Tao T (2006b). *Stable signal recovery from incomplete and inaccurate measurements, Comm. Pure Appl. Math.*, Vol. 59, pp. 1207–1223.

Candès EJ and Tao T (2006c). *Near-optimal signal recovery from random projections: universal encoding strategies, IEEE Trans. Inform. Theory,* Vol. 52, pp. 5406–5425.

Candès EJ and Tao T (2008). *Reflections on compressed sensing, IEEE Trans. Inform. Theory,* Vol. 58, pp. 20–23.

Canny JA (1986). *Computational approach to edge detection, IEEE Trans. Pattern Anal.*, Vol. 8, no. 6, pp. 679–698.

Carr H and July YH (2004). *Field gradients in early MRI, Physics Today (American Institute of Physics),* Vol. 57, no. 7, p. 83.

Caselles V, Catte F, Coll T and Dibos F (1993). *A geometric model for active contours in image processing, Numerische Mathematik,* Vol. 66, no. 1, pp. 1–31.

Caselles V, Kimmel R and Sapiro G (1997). *Geodesic active contours, Int. J. Comp. Vis.*, Vol. 22, no. 1, pp. 61–79.

Chan TF and Vese LA (2001). *Active contours without edges, IEEE Trans. Image Process.*, Vol. 10, no. 2, pp. 266–277.

Chen Y, Tagare HD, Thiruvenkadam S, Huang F, Wilson D, Gopinath KS, Briggs RW and Geiser EA (2002). *Using prior shapes in geometric active contours in a variational framework, Int. J. Comp. Vis.*, Vol. 50, no. 3, pp. 315–328.

Chipot M (2009). *Elliptic Equations: An Introductory Course,* Bilkhäuser *Advanced texts,* Bilkhäuser Verlag, Berlin.

Cormack AM (1963). *Representation of a function by its line integrals, with some radiological applications,* J. Appl. Phys., Vol. 34, pp. 2722–2727.

Cormack AM (1992). *75 years of radon transform,* J. Comput. Assist. Tomogr., Vol. 16, p. 673.

Damadian RV (1971). *Tumor detection by nuclear magnetic resonance,* Science, Vol. 171, pp. 1151–1153.

Donoho DL (2006). *Compressed sensing,* IEEE Trans. Inform. Theory, Vol. 52, no. 4, pp. 1289–1306.

Donoho DL and Elad M (2003). *Optimally sparse representation in general (non-orthogonal) dictionaries via ℓ_1 minimization,* Proc. Natl Acad. Sci. USA, Vol. 100, pp. 2197–2202.

Donoho DL and Huo X (1999). *Uncertainty principles and ideal atomic decomposition,* IEEE Trans. Inform. Theory, Vol. 47, pp. 2845–2862.

Duan Q, Angelini ED, Herz SL, Ingrassia CM, Costa KD, Holmes JW, Homma S and Laine AF (2009). *Region-based endocardium tracking on real-time three-dimensional ultrasound,* Ultrasound Med. Biol., Vol. 35, no. 2, pp. 256–265.

Engl HW, Hanke M and Neubauer A (1996). *Regularization of Inverse Problems (Mathematics and its Applications),* Kluwer Academic Publishers, Dordrecht.

Evans LC (2010). *Partial differential equations, graduate studies in mathematics,* Vol. 19, American Mathematical Society, Providence, RI.

Faridani A (2003). *Introduction to the mathematics of computed tomography: Inside out: inverse problems and applications,* Cambridge Univ. Press, Math. Sci. Res. Inst. Publ., Vol. 47, pp. 1–46.

Feldkamp LA, Davis LC and Kress JW (1984). *Practical cone-beam algorithm,* J. Opt. Soc. Am. A, Vol. 1, no. 6, pp. 612–619.

Feldman J and Uhlmann G (2003). *Inverse Problems, Lecture Note.*

Filler AG (2010). *The history, development, and impact of computed imaging in neurological diagnosis and neurosurgery: CT, MRI, DTI,* Internet Journal of Neurosurgery, Vol. 7, no. 1, DOI: 10.5580/23c6.

Folland G (1976). *Introduction to Partial Differential Equations,* Princeton University Press, Princeton, NJ.

Gabriel C, Gabriel S and Corthout E (1996a). *The dielectric properties of biological tissues: I. Literature survey,* Phys. Med. Biol., Vol. 41, pp. 2231–2249.

Gabriel S, Lau RW and Gabriel C (1996b). *The dielectric properties of biological tissues: II. Measurements in the frequency range 10Hz to 20GHz,* Phys. Med. Biol., Vol. 41, pp. 2251–2269.

Geddes LA and Baker LE (1967). *The specific resistance of biological material: a compendium of data for the biomedical engineer and physiologist,* Med. Biol. Eng., Vol. 5, pp. 271–293.

Giaquinta M (1983). *Multiple Integrals in the Calculus of Variations and Nonlinear Elliptic Systems,* Princeton University Press, Princeton, NJ.

Gilbarg D and Trudinger N (2001). *Elliptic Partial Differential Equations of Second Order,* Springer Verlag, Berlin.

Goldenberg R, Kimmel R, Rivlin E and Rudzsky M (2001). *Fast geodesic active contours*, IEEE Trans. Image Process., Vol. 10, no. 10, pp. 1467–1475.

Grimnes S and Martinsen OG (2008). *Bioimpedance and Bioelectricity Basics*, Second edition, Academic Press, Oxford.

Grisvard P (1985). *Elliptic problems in nonsmooth domains*, Pitman, Marshfield, MA.

Griswold MA, Jakob PM, Heidemann RM, Nittka M, Jellus V, Wang J, Kiefer B and Haase A (2002). *Generalized autocalibrating partially parallel acquisitions (GRAPPA)*, Magn. Reson. Med., Vol. 47, pp. 1202–1210.

Haacke E, Brown R, Thompson M and Venkatesan R (1999). *Magnetic resonance imaging Physical Principles and Sequence Design*, Wiley, Hoboken, NJ.

Hadamard J (1902). *Sur les problémes aux dérivées partielles et leur signification physique*, Princeton University Bulletin, Vol. 13, pp. 49–52.

Heidemann RM, Griswold MA, Haase A and Jakob PM (2001). *VD-AUTO-SMASH imaging*, Magn. Reson. Med., Vol. 45, pp. 1066–1074.

Holder D (ed.) (2005). *Electrical Impedance Tomography: Methods, History and Applications*, IOP Publishing, Bristol.

Horn B and Schunk B (1981). *Determining optical flow*, Artif. Intell., Vol. 17, no. 2, pp. 185–203.

Hoult DI (2000). *The principle of reciprocity in signal strength calculations–a mathematical guide*, Concepts Magn. Reson., Vol. 12, pp. 173–187.

Hoult DI and Richards RE (1976). *The signal-to-noise ratio of the nuclear magnetic resonance experiment*, J. Magn. Reson., Vol. 24, pp. 71–85.

Hounsfield GN (1973). *Computerized transverse axial scanning (tomography): I. Description of system Br.*, J. Radiol., Vol. 46, pp. 1016–1022.

Jakob PM, Griswold MA, Edelman RR and Sodickson DK (1998). *AUTO-SMASH: a self-calibrating technique for SMASH imaging*, Magnetic Resonance Materials in Physics, Biology and Medicine, Vol. 7, pp. 42–54.

John F (1982). *Partial differential equations*, App. Math. Sciences, Vol. 1.

Kak AC and Slaney M (1988). *Principles of Computerized Tomographic Imaging*, IEEE Press, New York, NY.

Kalender WA, Hebel R and Ebersberger J (1987). *Reduction of ct artifacts caused by metallic implants*, Radiology, Vol. 164, no. 2, pp. 576–577.

Kalender WA (2006). *X-ray computed tomography*, Phys. Med. Biol., Vol. 51, pp. R29–R43.

Kass M, Witkin A and Terzopoulos D (1987). *Snake: active contour models*, Int. J. Comp. Vis., Vol. 1, pp. 321–331.

Kellogg OD (1953).*Foundations of Potential Theory*, Dover, New York, NY.

Kichenassamy S (1997). *The Perona–Malik paradox*, SIAM Journal on Applied Mathematics, Vol. 57, no. 5, pp. 1328–1342.

Kichenassamy S, Kumar A, Olver P, Tannenbaum A and Yezzi A (1995). *Gradient flows and geometric active contour models*, Proc. ICCV'95, pp. 810–815.

Kyriakos WE, Panych LP, Kacher DF, Westin CF, Bao SM, Mulkern RV and Jolesz FA (2000). *Sensitivity profiles from an array of coils for encoding* and reconstruction in parallel (SPACE RIP), Magn. Reson. Med., Vol. 44, pp. 301–308.

Lambert JH (1760). *Photometria sive de mensura et gradibus luminis, colorum et umbrae, Augsburg ("Augusta Vindelicorum")*, Eberhardt Klett, Berlin.

Landau LD and Lifshitz EM (1960). *Electrodynamics of Continuous Media*, First edition, Pergamon Press, Oxford.

Larkman DJ and Nunes RG (2001). *Parallel magnetic resonance imaging, Phys. Med. Biol.*, Vol. 52, p. R15.

Lauterbur PC (1973). *Image formation by induced local interactions: examples of employing nuclear magnetic resonance, Nature*, Vol. 242, (5394), pp. 190–191.

Lauterbur PC (1974). *Magnetic resonance zeugmatography, Pure Appl. Chem.*, Vol. 40, pp. 149–157.

Leventon M, Faugeras O, Grimson E and Wells W (2000). *Level set based segmentation with intensity and curvature priors, Prc. Math. Meth. Biomed. Image Anal.*, MMBIA 2000, pp. 4–11.

Lieb EH and Loss M (2001). *Analysis: Second Edition*, Graduate Studies in Mathematics, Vol. 14, American Mathematical Society, Providence, RI.

Linguraru MG, Vasilyev NV, Marx GR, Tworetzky W, Nido PJD and Howe RD (2008). *Fast block flow tracking of atrial septal defects in 4D echocardiography, Med. Image Anal.*, Vol. 12, no. 4, pp. 397–412.

Lustig M, Donoho DL and Pauly JM (2007). *Sparse MRI: the application of compressed sensing for rapid MR imaging, Magn. Reson. Med.*, Vol. 58, pp. 1182–1195.

Malladi R, Sethian JA and Vemuri BC (1995). *Shape modeling with front propagation: a level set approach, IEEE Trans. Pattern Anal.*, Vol. 17, no. 2, pp. 158–175.

Marsden JE (1974). *Elementary Classical Analysis*, WH. Freeman and Company, London.

Meyer Y (2002). *Oscillating patterns in image processing and nonlinear evolution equations*, University Lecture Series, Vol. 22, American Mathematical Society, Providence, RI.

Meyer E, Raupach R, Lell M, Schmidt B and Kachelrie M (2010). *Normalized metal artifact reduction (NMAR) in computed tomography, Med. Phys.*, Vol. 37, pp. 5482–5493.

Mumford D and Shah J (1989). *Optimal approximation by piecewise smooth functions and associated variational problems, Commun. Pure Appl. Math.*, Vol. 42, pp. 577–685.

Natterer F (2008). *X-ray tomography, Inverse problems and imaging, Lect. Notes Math.*, Vol. 1943, pp. 17–34.

Nehrke K and Börnert P (2012). *DREAM — a novel approach for robust, ultrafast, multislice B(1) mapping, Magn. Reson. Med.*, Vol. 68, pp. 1517–1526.

Osher S and Fedkiw R (2002). *Level Set Methods and Dynamic Implicit Surfaces*, Springer Verlag, Berlin.

Osher S, Solé A and Vese L (2002). *Image decomposition and restoration using total variation minimization and the H^{-1} Norm, SIAM Multiscale Model. Simul.*, Vol. 1, no. 3, pp. 349–370.

Osher S, Burger M, Goldfarb D, Xu J and Yin W (2005). *An iterative regularization method for total variation-based image restoration*, *SIAM Multiscale Model. Simul.*, Vol. 4, no. 2, pp. 460–489.

Paragios N and Deriche R (1998). *A PDE-based level set approach for detection and tracking of moving objects*, *IEEE Int. Conf. Comp. Vis. (ICCV)*, pp. 1139–1145.

Perona P and Malik J (1990). *Scale space and edge detection using anisotropic diffusion*, *IEEE Trans. Pattern Anal.*, Vol. 12, pp. 629–639.

Pruessmann KP, Weiger M, Scheidegger MB and Boesiger P (1999). *SENSE: sensitivity encoding for fast MRI*, *Magn. Reson. Med.*, Vol. 42, pp. 952–962.

Pruessmann KP, Weiger M, Bornert P and Boesiger P (2001). *Advances in sensitivity encoding with arbitrary k-space trajectories*, *Magn. Reson. Med.*, Vol. 46, pp. 638–651.

Radon JH (1917). *Über die Bestimmung von Funktionen durch ihre Integralwerte längs gewisser Mannigfaltig*, *Ber. vor Sächs. Akad. Wiss.*, Vol. 69, pp. 262–277.

Reed M and Simon B (1980). *Functional Analysis (Methods of Modern Mathematical Physics I)*, Academic Press, Oxford.

Rudin L, Osher SJ and Fatemi E (1992). *Nonlinear total variation-based noise removal algorithms*, *Physica D*, Vol. 60, pp. 259–268.

Rudin W (1970). *Real and Complex Analysis*, McGraw-Hill, London.

Rudin W (1973). *Functional Analysis*, McGraw-Hill, London.

Sacolick LI, Wiesinger F, Hancu I and Vogel MW (2010). *B1 mapping by Bloch-Siegert shift*, *Magn. Reson. Med.*, Vol. 63, pp. 1315–1322.

Scott GC (1993). *NMR Imaging of Current Density and Magnetic Fields*, PhD thesis, University of Toronto, Canada.

Scott GC, Joy M, Armstrong RL and Henkelman MR (1995). *Rotating frame RF current density imaging*, *Magn. Reson. Med.*, Vol. 33, no. 3, pp. 355–369.

Seo JK and Woo EJ (2011). *Magnetic Resonance Electrical Impedance Tomography(MREIT)*, *SIAM Review*, Vol. 53, Issue 1, pp. 40–68.

Seo JK and Woo EJ (2012). *Nonlinear Inverse Problems in Imaging*, Wiley, New York.

Seo JK, Kim DH, Lee J, Kwon OI, Sajib SZK and Woo EJ (2012). *Electrical tissue property imaging using MRI at dc and Larmor frequency*, *Inverse Prob.*, Vol. 28, 084002.

Seo JK, Bera TK, Kwon H and Sadleir R (2013) *Effective admittivity of biological tissues as a coefficient of elliptic PDE*, *Comput. Math. Method. M.*, 2013.

Sodickson DK, Griswold MA, Jakob PM, Edelman RR and Manning WJ (1999). *Signal-to-noise ratio and signal to-noise efficiency in SMASH imaging*, *Magn. Reson. Med.*, Vol. 41, pp. 1009–1022.

Sodickson DK and Manning WJ (1997). *Simultaneous acquisition of spatial harmonics (SMASH): fast imaging with radiofrequency coil arrays*, *Magn. Reson. Med.*, Vol. 38, pp. 591–603.

Stollberger R and Wach P (1996). *Imaging of the active B1 field in vivo* , *Magn. Reson. Med.* , Vol. 35, pp. 246–251.

Strauss W A (1992). *Partial Differential Equations, An Introduction*, (Wiley, New York, NY).

Van de Moortele PF, Akgun C, Adriany G, Moeller S, Ritter J, Collins CM, Smith MB, Vaughan JT and Ugurbil K (2005). *B(1) destructive interferences and spatial phase patterns at 7 T with a head transceiver array coil, Magn. Reson. Med.*, Vol. 54, pp. 1503–1518.

Vese L and Osher S (2002). *Modeling Textures with Total Variation Minimization and Oscillating Patterns in Image Processing, J. Sci. Comput.*, Vol. 19, pp. 553–572.

Wang J, Qiu M, Yang QX, Smith MB and Constable RT (2005). *Measurement and Correction of Transmitter and Receiver Induced Nonuniformities In Vivo, Magn. Reson. Med.*, Vol. 53, pp. 408–417.

Wang Y (2012). *Principles of Magnetic Resonance Imaging*, Cornell University Press, Ithaca, NY.

Weickert J (1997). *A review of nonlinear diffusion filtering, B. t.H. Romeny, L. Florack, J. Koenderink and M. Viergever, eds., Scale-Space Theory in Computer Vision, Lecture Notes in Computer Science*, Vol. 1252, pp. 3–28.

Wheeden RL and Zygmund A (1977). *Measure and integral: An introduction to real analysis, Monographis and textbooks in pure and applied mathematics*, Vol. 43, Marcel Dekker, New York, NY.

Yarnykh VL (2007). *Actual flip-angle imaging in the pulsed steady state: a method for rapid three-dimensional mapping of the transmitted radiofrequency field, Magn. Reson. Med.*, Vol. 57, pp.192–200.

Yezzi A, Tsai A and Willsky A (1999). *Binary and Ternary Flows for Image Segmentation, 6th IEEE International Conference on Image Processing*, Vol. 2, pp. 1–5.

You Y, Xu W, Tannenbaum A and Kaveh M (1996). *Behavioral analysis of anisotropic diffusion in image processing, IEEE Trans. Image Process.*, Vol. 5, pp. 15–53.

Zeidler E (1989). *Nonlinear Functional Analysis and Its Applications*, Springer Verlag, Berlin.

Zhao HK, Chan T, Merriman B and Osher S (1996). *A variational level set approach to multiphase motion, J. Comput. Phys.*, Vol. 127, pp. 179–195.

Chapter 3

Magnetic Resonance Electrical Impedance Tomography

Magnetic resonance electrical impedance tomography (MREIT) is a technique of mapping conductivity distribution at dc or frequency below 1 kHz. See Figure 3.1 for its schematic diagram. The corresponding inverse problem can be described roughly as follows.

- **Input data:** Inject almost dc current (at frequency below 1 kHz) using a pair of surface electrodes that are attached on the boundary of an imaging object. The externally injected current generates the fields $\mathbf{E}, \mathbf{J}, \mathbf{B}$ inside the imaging object. They are approximately governed by

$$\mathbf{J} = \sigma \mathbf{E}, \quad \nabla \times \mathbf{E} = 0, \quad \mathbf{J} = \frac{1}{\mu_0} \nabla \times \mathbf{B}. \tag{3.1}$$

- **Output data:** Measure B_z, the z-component of $\mathbf{B}$, using a magnetic resonance imaging (MRI) scanner. Here, z-axis is the direction of the main magnetic field of the scanner.
- **Inverse problem:** Reconstruct σ from measured data B_z.

Throughout this chapter, we assume that σ is an isotropic, and $\mathbf{B} = \mu_0 \mathbf{H}$ where $\mu_0 = 4\pi \times 10^{-7}$ is the magnetic permeability of the free space. We begin with an overview and brief history of MREIT.

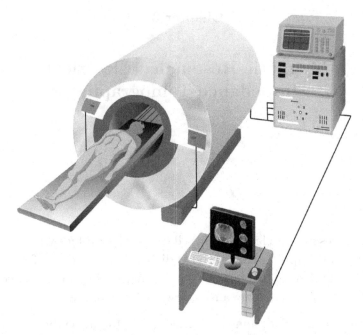

Fig. 3.1.   Diagram of an MREIT system. An imaging object is placed inside the bore of an MRI scanner with two pairs of electrodes attached on its surface. Currents are injected into the object between a chosen pair of electrodes. We obtain the induced B_z data to reconstruct cross-sectional conductivity images of the object.

3.1 Overview and History of MREIT

The motivation for MREIT was from electrical impedance tomography (EIT) and magnetic resonance current density imaging (MRCDI). Electric impedance tomography is an imaging technique that provides tomographic images of a conductivity distribution inside the human body from boundary current-voltage data.

Magnetic resonance current density imaging aims to provide non-invasive visualization of a current density distribution $\mathbf{J} = \nabla \times \mathbf{H}$ inside the human body by externally injecting dc current using a pair of surface electrodes and measuring the induced magnetic field using an MRI scanner.

Henderson and Webster first proposed EIT in 1978 and its mathematical formulation was given by Calderón (1980). Most EIT

Electrodes
(recessed/hyrdogel)

Imaging object
(Phantom/Animal)

Imaging object
inside RF coil

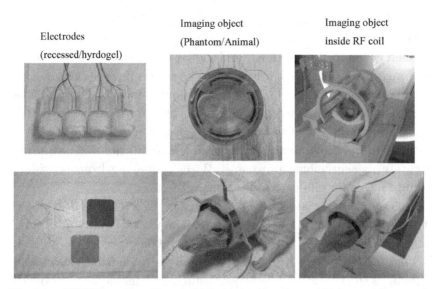

Fig. 3.2. MREIT system. Recessed electrodes have been widely used in experimental studies, and flexible carbon-hydrogel electrodes with conductive adhesive are being used in *in vivo* animal and human experiments.

systems are equipped with multiple current sources and voltmeters so that they can inject currents and measure voltages through multiple surface electrodes. The success of X-ray CT[1] influenced EIT. An EIT version of the CT back-projection algorithm[2] was developed by [Barber and Brown (1984)]. It can be viewed as a reproduction of the CT method with a deep understanding of Maxwell's equations in the context of EIT.

The CT back-projection method is based on the projection property of X-ray data being the line integral of the image data along the straight line with a given projection direction. Unlike X-ray CT,

---

[1]X-ray computed tomography (CT) is one of the most widely used tomographic imaging techniques, which uses X-rays passing through the body at different angles. It visualizes internal structure of the human body by assigning an X-ray attenuation coefficient at each pixel that characterizes how easily a medium can be penetrated by an X-ray beam. The idea was to visualize the imaging object in a slice by taking X-ray data at all angles around the object.

[2]The back-projection method in X-ray CT reconstructs cross-sectional images by reversing the process of projection data measurements.

static EIT has fundamental difficulties in controlling the pathway of the internal current $\mathbf{J}$ since $\mathbf{J}$ depends strongly on the boundary geometry, electrode positions, and global conductivity distribution. The measured boundary voltage data as a non-linear function of σ is very sensitive to small errors in the boundary geometry and the electrode positions, whereas it is insensitive to a local perturbation of σ away from the measuring electrodes. These fundamental ill-posed structures combined with technical limitations in acquiring accurate measurements prevent static EIT imaging from providing useful images for clinical applications.

In contrast to static EIT, difference EIT has better posed structures [Metherall *et al.* (1996); Cheney *et al.* (1999); Holder (2005); Rahman *et al.* (2008); Seo *et al.* (2008); Lee *et al.* (2011)]. It takes advantage of a data subtraction method which effectively eliminates the technical difficulties of static EIT including the boundary geometry errors and electrode position uncertainties. Although difference EIT cannot provide images of absolute conductivity values with a high spatial resolution, its potential in clinical applications has been shown where portability and continuous monitoring capability with a high temporal resolution are needed [Metherall *et al.* (1996); Cheney *et al.* (1999)]. Existing EIT algorithms include the back-projection [Barber and Brown (1984); Brown *et al.* (1985); Santosa and Vogelius (1990)], one-step Newton [Cheney *et al.* (1990)], D-bar [Mueller *et al.* (2009)], factorization [Hanke and Brühl (2003); Harrach *et al.* (2010)] and so on. They are usually combined with a regularization method [Engl *et al.* (1996)] to handle the ill-conditioning problems. Here, EIT reconstruction algorithms using any kind of current-voltage data corresponding to a background conductivity σ_0 are regarded as methods for difference EIT. Since such a background current-voltage data is not available in static EIT, these existing EIT algorithms have not been successfully applied to static EIT imaging.

Numerous endeavors to static EIT during the last three decades have led us to admit methodological limitations in handling forward modeling errors involving the boundary geometry and electrode positions uncertainties. Most theoretical results concerning reconstruction of σ neglect or underestimate the forward modeling errors.

For novel theoretical results guaranteeing a unique identification of σ, we refer to [Kohn and Vogelius (1984); Sylvester and Uhlmann (1986, 1987, 1988); Nachman (1988, 1996); Brown and Uhlmann (1997); Astala and Päivärinta (2006); Kenig *et al.* (2007)] and references contained therein. Considering the methodological limitations of static EIT, the boundary current-voltage data available in EIT may not be sufficient to achieve robust reconstructions of static conductivity images in remote areas away from the measuring electrodes. It seems that robust conductivity image reconstructions demand some kind of internal data probing the conductivity distribution.

Due to its underlying electro-magnetic principles, MRI would be a top candidate to measure internal data for conductivity imaging. In 1989, [Joy *et al.* (1989)] developed a technique to measure the z-component of $\mathbf{H}$ where $\mathbf{H}$ is the internal magnetic field induced by an externally injected current through surface electrodes and z-axis is the direction of the main magnetic field of an MRI scanner. This measurement technique was designed for MRCDI which provides images of an internal current density distribution [Scott *et al.* (1991, 1992)]. Since only H_z is measurable using MRI, computation of $\mathbf{J} = \nabla \times \mathbf{H}$ requires mechanical rotations of the imaging object inside the MRI scanner to measure all three components of $\mathbf{H}$.

In the early 1990s, MREIT was first proposed to overcome the fundamental limitations of the static EIT methods by using the internal current density data $\mathbf{J}$ that is obtained from the MRCDI method. Three different initial trials [Zhang (1992); Woo *et al.* (1994); Birgul and Ider (1995, 1996)] were independently attempted, but none of them could produce high-quality conductivity images in actual imaging experiments. However, these early ideas changed the way we investigate the conductivity imaging problem by suggesting the supplemental use of internal data as well as boundary measurements.

In 1999, [Kwon *et al.* (2002)] proposed the $\mathbf{J}$-substitution algorithm based on the following non-linear partial differential equation (PDE):

$$\nabla \cdot \left(\frac{|\mathbf{J}|}{|\nabla u|} \nabla u \right) = 0 \quad \text{inside the imaging object.} \quad (3.2)$$

This new approach using the non-linear PDE could produce high-resolution conductivity images by displaying $\sigma = \frac{|\mathbf{J}|}{|\nabla u|}$ [Khang *et al.* (2002)]. [Joy *et al.* (2004)] and [Lee (2004)] independently found other direct (non-iterative) reconstruction methods for visualizing $\nabla \ln \sigma$ at each point inside an imaging region. The method, called current density impedance imaging (CDII), was experimentally verified in [Hasanov *et al.* (2008)]. Recently, CDII using a single current density $|\mathbf{J}|$ has been carefully studied in [Nachman *et al.* (2007b, 2009, 2010)]. All of these methods using the full components of $\mathbf{H} = (H_x, H_y, H_z)$, however, suffer from the practical technical difficulties of rotating the imaging object inside the MRI scanner.

We should avoid adopting the object rotation process inside an MRI scanner to give up measuring all three components of $\mathbf{H}$, if we wish to make the MREIT technique applicable to clinical situations. Without rotating the imaging object, only H_z is a measurable quantity, and therefore the inverse problem of reconstructing σ from only H_z is the major issue in MREIT.

In 2001, [Seo *et al.* (2003a)] invented the first constructive H_z-based MREIT algorithm, called the harmonic B_z algorithm, which reconstructs an image of σ from $B_z = \mu_0 H_z$. This method removed the rotation process and has been widely used in subsequent experimental studies. They carefully investigated the non-linear relationship between the conductivity σ and the measured data H_z via the Biot–Savart law, making key observations that the Laplacian of H_z probes $[\hat{\mathbf{z}} \times (\nabla \times \mathbf{H})] \cdot \nabla(\ln \sigma)$ and two linearly independent currents should be injected to reconstruct the transversal change of σ. Based on these key observations, they derived a representation formula of σ which could lead to the development of constructive irrotational MREIT algorithms including the harmonic B_z algorithm. Though this representation formula exists in an implicit form due to the non-linear relationship between the conductivity and the measured data, it was designed to use a fixed point theory. In other words, the formula has a contraction mapping property such that an iterative method can be used. The major drawback of EIT related with its ill-posedness is mainly due to the fact that the overall flow of the current density is insensitive to local perturbations of the conductivity distribution. It is interesting to see that the harmonic B_z method in MREIT could take advantage of this fact to make the algorithm work.

After the invention of the harmonic B_z algorithm [Seo *et al.* (2003a); Oh *et al.* (2003)], imaging techniques in MREIT have advanced rapidly and now can perform state-of-the-art conductivity imaging of animal and human subjects [Woo and Seo (2008); Seo and Woo (2011)]. Future studies of MREIT should overcome a few technical barriers to advance the method to the stage of routine clinical uses. The biggest hurdle at present is the amount of injection currents that may stimulate muscle and nerve. Reducing it down to a level that does not produce undesirable side effects is the key to the success of this new bio-imaging modality. We expect MREIT to be a new clinically useful bio-imaging modality which manifests structural, functional, and pathological conditions of the biological tissues and organs providing valuable diagnostic information.

3.2 Overall Structure of MREIT

The MREIT system comprises an MRI scanner, constant current source and conductivity image reconstruction software. Let the object to be imaged occupy a three-dimensional bounded domain $\Omega \subset \mathbb{R}^3$ with a smooth boundary $\partial\Omega$. We attach a pair of surface electrodes $\mathcal{E}^+$ and $\mathcal{E}^-$ on the boundary $\partial\Omega$. Both electrodes $\mathcal{E}^+$ and $\mathcal{E}^-$ are recessed from the surface of the object $\partial\Omega$ as shown in Figure 3.3. We may regard Ω as the assembly of Ω and the recessed electrodes.

We inject a current of I in mA at a fixed low angular frequency ω ranging over $0 < \frac{\omega}{2\pi} < 500$ Hz. Then, the time-harmonic current density $\mathbf{J}$, electric field intensity $\mathbf{E}$, and magnetic flux density $\mathbf{B}$ due to the injection current approximately satisfy the following relations:

$$\nabla \cdot \mathbf{J} = 0 = \nabla \cdot \mathbf{B}, \quad \mathbf{J} = \frac{1}{\mu_0} \nabla \times \mathbf{B} \quad \text{in } \Omega \qquad (3.3)$$

$$\mathbf{J} = \sigma \mathbf{E}, \quad \nabla \times \mathbf{E} = 0 \quad \text{in } \Omega \qquad (3.4)$$

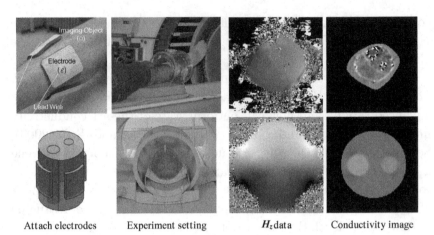

Attach electrodes   Experiment setting H_z data   Conductivity image

Fig. 3.3. MREIT phantom and human leg experiments using four recessed electrodes. Conductivity images were obtained by using the harmonic B_z-algorithm.

$$I = -\int_{\mathcal{E}^+} \mathbf{J} \cdot \mathbf{n} \, ds = \int_{\mathcal{E}^-} \mathbf{J} \cdot \mathbf{n} \, ds \qquad (3.5)$$

$$\mathbf{J} \cdot \mathbf{n} = 0 \text{ on } \partial\Omega \backslash \overline{\mathcal{E}^+ \cup \mathcal{E}^-}, \quad \mathbf{J} \times \mathbf{n} = 0 \text{ on } \mathcal{E}^+ \cup \mathcal{E}^-. \qquad (3.6)$$

The injection current I during the MR data collection process produces extra phase shift in the MR phase image in such a way that its accumulation is proportional to B_z. An MR spectrometer provides complex k-space data including information of B_z data on each slice $\Omega_{z_0} = \Omega \cap \{z = z_0\}$:

$$S(k_x, k_y) = \iint_{\Omega_{z_0}} \mathcal{M}(x, y, z_0) \, e^{i(xk_x + yk_y)} dx dy,$$

$$\mathcal{M}(x, y, z_0) := M(x, y, z_0) \, e^{i(\gamma B_z(x,y,z_0)T_c + \delta(x,y,z_0))} \qquad (3.7)$$

where M is a conventional MR magnitude image, δ any systematic phase artifact, $\gamma = 26.75 \times 10^7 \text{rad/T} \cdot \text{s}$ the gyromagnetic ratio of hydrogen and T_c the current pulse width in seconds. [Haacke *et al.* (1999)] and [Bernstein *et al.* (2004)] explain numerous MR imaging parameters affecting M and δ. The B_z in (3.7) is the major data for the reconstruction of σ in MREIT.

The inverse problem of MREIT is to recover σ from the measured data B_z, where the relation between B_z and σ is determined by the

z-component of the Biot−Savart law:

$$B_z(\mathbf{r}) = \frac{\mu_0}{4\pi} \int_\Omega \frac{\langle \mathbf{r} - \mathbf{r}', \sigma(\mathbf{r}')\mathbf{E}(\mathbf{r}') \times \hat{\mathbf{z}} \rangle}{|\mathbf{r} - \mathbf{r}'|^3} \, d\mathbf{r}' + \mathcal{H}(\mathbf{r}) \quad \text{for } \mathbf{r} \in \Omega,$$

(3.8)

where $\mathcal{H}(\mathbf{r})$ is a harmonic function in Ω representing a magnetic flux density generated by currents flowing through external lead wires.

In the following sections, we give detailed explanations from the data acquisition system to the image reconstruction software.

3.3 Measurement of Internal Data B_z

One of the key issues in MREIT is to minimize the noise level in measured B_z data as well as the data acquisition time for a given amount of injection current; the amount should be within a level that a human subject can tolerate. Hence, numerous advanced MR imaging techniques should be adopted in MREIT to make it applicable for various areas in biomedicine. In this section, we present a typical setup for MREIT imaging experiments as shown in Figure 3.1.

Figure 3.4 shows a basic spin echo pulse sequence commonly used in MREIT experiments. The current source is usually located outside the bore and coaxial cables are used for the connection to the surface electrodes on an imaging object placed inside the bore. Through a pair of electrodes, current is injected in a form of pulses whose timing is synchronized with the MR pulse sequence. The current source is controlled by a microprocessor and includes circuits for waveform generation, current output, switching, discharge and auxiliary voltage measurement. Carbon cables could be advantageous when a high-field MRI scanner is used. Cabling must be done carefully using appropriate filters to reject interferences.

We sequentially inject positive and negative currents, I^+ and I^- to get the following complex k-space data $\mathcal{S}^\pm$ shown in Figure 3.5 corresponding to I^+ and I^-, respectively:

$$S_{I^\pm}(k_x, k_y) = \iint_{\Omega_{z_0}} \mathcal{M}_{I^\pm}(x, y, z_0) \, e^{i(xk_x + yk_y)} dxdy$$

(3.9)

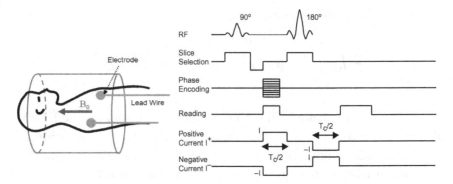

Fig. 3.4.   Typical spin echo pulse sequence for MREIT.

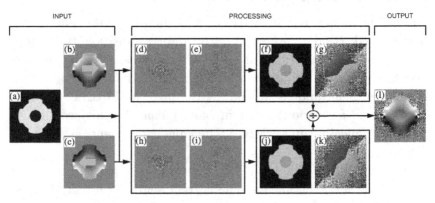

Fig. 3.5.   MREIT k-space data. (a) Cross-section of a cylindrical phantom. (b) Positive current using south and east electrodes. (c) Negative current. (d)−(e) and (h)−(i) Real and imaginary part of $S_{I\pm}$. (f) & (j) MR and phase of $\mathcal{M}_{I\pm}$. (l) B_z.

where

$$\mathcal{M}_{I\pm}(x, y, z_0) := M(x, y, z_0)\, e^{\pm i\gamma B_z(x,y,z_0)T_c}\, e^{i\delta(x,y,z_0)}. \qquad (3.10)$$

Collecting k-space data, we reconstruct multi-slice MR magnitude and phase images. Magnitude images allow us to obtain boundary geometry and electrode positions. Phase images provide B_z data.

Taking two-dimensional discrete Fourier transformations to the k-space MR signal $S_{I\pm}$, we obtain the complex MR images $\mathcal{M}_{I\pm}$ shown in Figure 3.5. We should note that $|\mathcal{M}^+| = |\mathcal{M}^-| = M$ is proportional to the size (volume) of voxels. If $M(x, y, z_0) \neq 0$, dividing $\mathcal{M}_{I+}(x, y, z_0)$ by $\mathcal{M}_{I-}(x, y, z_0)$ extracts a wrapped B_z, denoted by $B_z^\natural$:

$$B_z^\natural(x, y, z_0) = \frac{1}{2\gamma T_c} \Im \left\{ \ln \left(\frac{\mathcal{M}_{I+}(x, y, z_0)}{\mathcal{M}_{I-}(x, y, z_0)} \right) \right\}. \qquad (3.11)$$

Note that injection of positive and negative currents eliminates any systematic phase artifact δ in (3.7) and doubles the phase change.

The $B_z^\natural$ is wrapped by

$$\frac{-\pi}{2\gamma T_c} < B_z^\natural \leq \frac{\pi}{2\gamma T_c}$$

and therefore the function given by

$$\eta(x, y, z_0) := 2\gamma T_c [B_z(x, y, z_0) - B_z^\natural(x, y, z_0)]$$

is a piecewise constant function whose value is an integer multiple of 2π. Hence, we must unwrap $B_z^\natural$ to obtain B_z. Using the fact that B_z is continuous, we can unwrap $B_z^\natural$ in (3.11) to restore B_z:

$$B_z(x, y, z_0) = B_z^\natural(x, y, z_0) + \frac{1}{2\gamma T_c} \eta(x, y, z_0). \qquad (3.12)$$

Figure 3.6(a) shows an MR magnitude image M of a cylindrical saline phantom including an agar object whose conductivity was different from that of the saline. Injection current from the top to the bottom electrodes produced the wrapped phase image in (b). Such

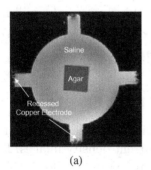
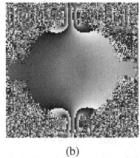
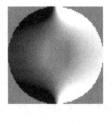

(a)   (b)   (c)

Fig. 3.6.   (a) MR magnitude image M of a cylindrical saline phantom including an agar object. Conductivity values of the saline and agar were different. (b) Wrapped phase image subject to an injection current from the top to the bottom electrodes. (c) Corresponding image of induced B_z after applying a phase-unwrapping algorithm.

phase wrapping may not occur when the amplitude of the injection current is small. Figure 3.6(c) is the B_z image after applying a phase-unwrapping algorithm. We can observe the deflection of B_z across the boundary of the agar object where conductivity contrast exists.

Remark 3.1. After collecting multiple sets of k-space data in (3.7), we perform several data processing tasks. First, we compute the discrete inverse Fourier transformation to get the complex MR image in (3.10). Though this step is straightforward, the second step of computing the incremental phase change $B_z^\natural$ in (3.11) needs a careful numerical implementation of a phase-unwrapping algorithm. Special care must be given to regions near current-injection electrodes where phase changes are very rapid. [Ghiglia and Pritt (1998)] explain details of numerous phase-unwrapping algorithms and one may find a suitable algorithm for obtained MR signals. There exist numerous sources of phase artifacts in an MRI system and current injection may introduce additional phase artifacts. Since MREIT relies on an MR phase image, phase artifacts must be minimized to improve the quality of a reconstructed conductivity image.

Remark 3.2. There are internal regions where the MR signal is weak due to a low proton density. This MR signal void phenomenon usually occurs in lungs, outer layers of bones, and gas-filled organs. Inside such a region, $M \approx 0$ in (3.10). Since this causes $\frac{\mathcal{M}_{I+}}{\mathcal{M}_{I-}} \approx \frac{0}{0}$ in (3.11), the measured B_z data contains an excessive amount of noise even though the B_z signal itself may not be small there.

3.3.1 *Noise analysis*

The B_z data is contaminated with noise, which ultimately limits the quality of reconstructed conductivity and current density images. In this section, we describe the noise analysis based on [Sadleir *et al.* (2005)]. For simplicity of notation, we let $\mathcal{M}^\pm(x,y) := \mathcal{M}_{I\pm}(x,y,z_0)$ with z_0 being fixed.

The measured $\mathcal{M}^\pm$ contain independent and identically distributed complex Gaussian random noise $\mathcal{Z}^\pm$, respectively. That is,

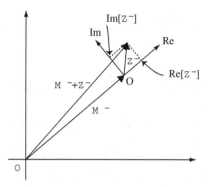

Fig. 3.7.   An example of $\mathcal{M}^-$ and $\mathcal{Z}^-$. Note the definition of the local axis for $\mathcal{Z}^-$.

measured signals may be described by

$$\mathcal{M}^\pm + \mathcal{Z}^\pm \quad \text{where } \mathcal{Z}^\pm = \mathcal{Z}^\pm_{re} + i\mathcal{Z}^\pm_{im} \tag{3.13}$$

and $\mathcal{Z}^\pm_{re}$ and $\mathcal{Z}^\pm_{im}$ are identically distributed Gaussian random variables with zero mean and a variance of s^2. Figure 3.7 shows an example of $\mathcal{M}^-$ and $\mathcal{Z}^-$. Without loss of generality, we may set the local coordinate of $\mathcal{Z}^-$ with its real axis parallel to the direction of $\mathcal{M}^-$. Then, the noise $\mathcal{Z}^-$ can be understood as a vector located at the local origin O, having a random magnitude and direction.

[Scott *et al.* (1992)] defined the SNR (signal-to-noise ratio) in a noisy magnitude image $|\mathcal{M}^- + \mathcal{Z}^-|$ as

$$SNR = \frac{\text{mean}(|\mathcal{M}^- + \mathcal{Z}^-|)}{\text{sd}(\mathcal{M}^- + \mathcal{Z}^-)} = \frac{|\mathcal{M}^-|}{\text{sd}(\mathcal{Z}^-)} = \frac{M}{\sqrt{2}s} \tag{3.14}$$

where mean($\cdot$) and sd($\cdot$) denote the mean and standard deviation, respectively. [Scott *et al.*] derived an expression for the standard deviation in measured B_z data as

$$\text{sd}(B_z) = \frac{1}{2\gamma T_c \, SNR}. \tag{3.15}$$

However, as shown below, we found that it is more convenient to define the SNR_M of the magnitude image as

$$SNR_M = \frac{\text{mean}(|\mathcal{M}^- + \mathcal{Z}^-|)}{\text{sd}(|\mathcal{M}^- + \mathcal{Z}^-|)} = \frac{M}{\text{sd}(|\mathcal{M}^- + \mathcal{Z}^-|)} = \frac{M}{s}. \tag{3.16}$$

Including noise in (3.11), we now have B_z signals proportional to

$$\arg\left(\frac{\mathcal{M}^+ + \mathcal{Z}^+}{\mathcal{M}^- + \mathcal{Z}^-}\right) = \arg\left(\frac{\mathcal{M}^+\left(1 + \frac{\mathcal{Z}^+}{\mathcal{M}^+}\right)}{\mathcal{M}^-\left(1 + \frac{\mathcal{Z}^-}{\mathcal{M}^-}\right)}\right)$$

$$= \arg\left(\frac{\mathcal{M}^+}{\mathcal{M}^-}\right) + \arg\left(1 + \frac{\mathcal{Z}^+}{\mathcal{M}^+}\right) \quad (3.17)$$

$$- \arg\left(1 + \frac{\mathcal{Z}^-}{\mathcal{M}^-}\right).$$

Assuming that $|\mathcal{M}^{\pm}| \gg |\mathcal{Z}^{\pm}|$, we have $\arg(1 + \frac{\mathcal{Z}^{\pm}}{\mathcal{M}^{\pm}}) \approx \text{Im}(\frac{\mathcal{Z}^{\pm}}{\mathcal{M}^{\pm}})$. This can also be understood from Figure 3.7, since the imaginary part of $\mathcal{Z}^-$ perturbs the argument of $\mathcal{M}^-$. Now, the standard deviation of the argument in (3.17) is

$$\text{sd}\left[\arg\left(\frac{\mathcal{M}^+ + \mathcal{Z}^+}{\mathcal{M}^- + \mathcal{Z}^-}\right)\right] \approx \text{sd}\left[\text{Im}\left(\frac{\mathcal{Z}^+}{\mathcal{M}^+}\right) - \text{Im}\left(\frac{\mathcal{Z}^-}{\mathcal{M}^-}\right)\right]$$

$$= \sqrt{2}\text{sd}\left[\text{Im}\left(\frac{\mathcal{Z}^-}{\mathcal{M}^-}\right)\right]$$

$$= \frac{\sqrt{2}}{|\mathcal{M}^-|}\text{sd}\left[\text{Im}\left(\mathcal{Z}^-\right)\right] \quad (3.18)$$

$$= \frac{\sqrt{2}}{|\mathcal{M}^-|\sqrt{2}}\text{sd}(\mathcal{Z}^-) = \frac{1}{M}\text{sd}(\mathcal{Z}^-).$$

We now estimate the standard deviation of the magnitude image, $|\mathcal{M}^- + \mathcal{Z}^-|$. As shown in Figure 3.7, the real part of the complex Gaussian random noise $\mathcal{Z}^-$ mainly perturbs the magnitude of $\mathcal{M}^-$. Assuming $|\mathcal{Z}^-| \ll |\mathcal{M}^-|$, we have

$$\text{sd}(|\mathcal{M}^- + \mathcal{Z}^-|) \approx \text{sd}\left(\text{Re}[\mathcal{Z}^-]\right) = \frac{1}{\sqrt{2}}\text{sd}\left(\mathcal{Z}^-\right). \quad (3.19)$$

The above estimate is based on the approximation $|(1 + a) + ib| = \sqrt{(1+a)^2 + b^2} \approx 1 + a$ for $a, b \ll 1$.

Hence, the standard deviation in measured magnetic flux density B_z can be expressed as

$$\text{sd}(B_z) = \frac{1}{2\gamma T_c |\mathcal{M}^-|}\text{sd}(\mathcal{Z}^-) = \frac{\sqrt{2}}{2\gamma T_c M}\text{sd}(|\mathcal{M}^- + \mathcal{Z}^-|). \qquad (3.20)$$

With the definition of SNR, SNR_M from (3.16), we conclude that

$$\text{sd}(B_z) = \frac{1}{\sqrt{2}\gamma T_c \, SNR_M}. \qquad (3.21)$$

Note that the expression in (3.21) is different from the expression in (3.15) by a factor of $\sqrt{2}$ because of the different definitions of SNR in magnitude images.

We now describe how to estimate SNR_M in (3.16) from the magnitude image of $|\mathcal{M}^- + \mathcal{Z}^-|$. Ideally, in a noise-free magnitude image $|\mathcal{M}^-|$ of a homogeneous object, we should obtain one value everywhere inside the object and zero outside. However, due to factors such as main magnetic field inhomogeneity, gradient non-linearity and non-uniform radio frequency (RF) coil sensitivity, we observe a non-uniform intensity profile inside the object. Outside the object, we have Rayleigh distributed noise $|\mathcal{Z}^-| = \sqrt{(\mathcal{Z}_{re}^-)^2 + (\mathcal{Z}_{im}^-)^2}$ with a standard deviation of about $0.655s$ where s is the standard deviation of identically distributed zero-mean Gaussian random variables $\mathcal{Z}_{re}^-$ and $\mathcal{Z}_{im}^-$ [Haacke *et al.* (1999)]. To evaluate SNR_M, we select a region inside the object that appears the most uniform and compute the average value of all pixels within it. We select a region outside the object and compute the standard deviation of all pixels there. Then, SNR_M is evaluated as the average value times 0.655 divided by the standard deviation. Alternatively, we may compute both the average value and standard deviation in the region chosen inside the object. Then, SNR_M is simply the ratio of the average value over the standard deviation.

3.3.2 *Pulse sequence*

The basic spin echo pulse sequence in Figure 3.4 has been widely used in MREIT since it is most robust to many kinds of undesirable perturbations to the phase image. A prolonged current pulse width (i.e. larger T_c) reduces the noise level in measured B_z data. [Park *et al.* (2006)] proposed a new MREIT pulse sequence called injection current non-linear encoding (ICNE) where the duration of the injection current pulse is extended until the end of the reading gradient. Since the current injection during the reading gradient disturbs the gradient linearity, they developed an algorithm to extract B_z data from the acquired MR signal using the ICNE pulse sequence. They could reduce the noise level by about 25%. For a chosen pulse sequence, [Lee *et al.* (2006)] and [Kwon *et al.* (2007)] analyzed the associated noise level and provided a way to optimize the pulse sequence to minimize it. The ICNE method has been advantageous for obtaining magnetic flux density data, B_z, with better SNR. However, if the ICNE method uses a long data acquisition window, it may result in undesirable side artifacts such as blurring and chemical shift and phase artifacts. To overcome these difficulties, the ICNE method can be extended to a multi-echo train pulse sequence in order to provide multiple k-space lines during a single RF pulse period. By determining a weighting factor for each echo train B_z data, an optimized inversion formula for the magnetic flux density data is proposed for the ICNE multi-echo sequence. Using the ICNE multi-echo method [Nam and Kwon (2010)], the quality of the measured magnetic flux density is considerably increased by injection of multiple currents with a longer effective pulse width and also by optimization of the pixel-by-pixel noise level in the B_z value.

3.4   Forward Model

To facilitate MREIT research, we need a numerical simulator which is useful for algorithm development and validation of experimental processes. An MREIT simulator may include geometry modeling, meshing, finite element modeling and numerical computations of magnetic flux density **B**, current density **J**, and k-space MR data. Given an imaging object with a presumed σ and electrode configuration, we can generate a finite element model of the object to compute **J** and **B** as shown in Figure 3.9, and they are validated by checking

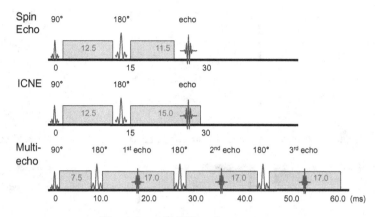

Fig. 3.8. MREIT pulse sequence.

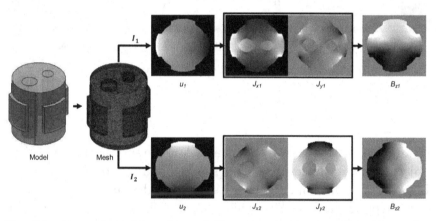

Fig. 3.9. Forward model: u_j ($j = 1, 2$) represents the potential due to the injection current I_j. $\mathbf{J}_j = (J_{xj}, J_{yj}, J_{zj}) = -\sigma \nabla u_j$, and B_{zj} is the z-component of the corresponding magnetic field.

the compatibility condition:

$$\mathbf{J}(\mathbf{r}) = \frac{1}{\mu_0} \nabla \times \mathbf{B}(\mathbf{r}) \quad \text{in } \Omega. \tag{3.22}$$

3.4.1 *Boundary value problem in MREIT*

For electrodes, we may use nonmagnetic conductive materials such as copper, silver, carbon or others. Artifact occurs when a highly

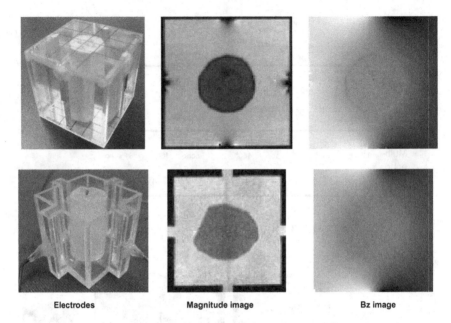

Electrodes   Magnitude image   Bz image

Fig. 3.10.   Electrode artifact problem. Artifact occurs near electrodes.

conductive electrode is directly attached on the surface of the imaging object since it shields RF signals; see Figure 3.10. As shown in Figure 3.1, bulky and rigid recessed electrodes have been used in early experimental studies, while thin and flexible carbon-hydrogel electrodes with conductive adhesive are being used in recent *in vivo* animal and human experiments [Jeong *et al.* (2008); Minhas *et al.* (2008); Kim *et al.* (2008a)]. This kind of recessed electrode with proper materials is desirable to produce artifact-free MR images of an object including its boundary.

To inject two linearly independent currents into the body Ω, we attach two pairs of flexible carbon-hydrogel electrodes, denoted as $\mathcal{E}_1^\pm, \mathcal{E}_2^\pm$, as shown in Figure 3.11. For simplicity of notation, we may regard Ω as the assembly of Ω and the electrodes. Through the pair of electrodes $\mathcal{E}^+$ and $\mathcal{E}^-$ on $\partial\Omega$, we inject current, and let $\mathcal{E}^+ \cup \mathcal{E}^-$ be the portion of the surface $\partial\Omega$ where electrodes are attached.

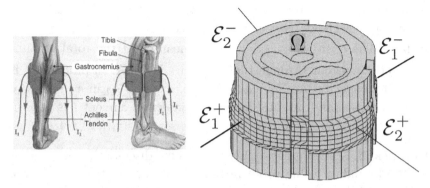

Fig. 3.11. The imaging domain Ω is a part of a knee where two pairs of flexible carbon-hydrogel electrodes are placed.

The injection current I produces an internal current density $\mathbf{J}_j = (J_{xj}, J_{yj}, J_{zj})$ inside the subject Ω satisfying the following problem:

$$
\begin{cases}
\nabla \cdot \mathbf{J}_j = 0 \quad \text{in } \Omega \\[2mm]
I = -\displaystyle\int_{\mathcal{E}_j^+} \mathbf{J}_j \cdot \mathbf{n} ds = \int_{\mathcal{E}_j^-} \mathbf{J}_j \cdot \mathbf{n} ds \\[2mm]
0 = -\displaystyle\int_{\mathcal{E}_k^+} \mathbf{J}_j \cdot \mathbf{n} ds = \int_{\mathcal{E}_k^-} \mathbf{J}_j \cdot \mathbf{n} ds \quad \text{for } k \neq j \\[2mm]
\mathbf{J}_j \times \mathbf{n} = 0 \quad \text{on } \mathcal{E}, \quad \mathbf{J}_j \cdot \mathbf{n} = 0 \quad \text{on } \partial\Omega \backslash \mathcal{E},
\end{cases}
\tag{3.23}
$$

where $\mathcal{E} = \mathcal{E}_1^+ \cup \mathcal{E}_1^- \cup \mathcal{E}_2^+ \cup \mathcal{E}_2^-$. Since $\mathbf{J}_j$ is expressed as $\mathbf{J}_j = -\sigma \nabla u_j$ where u_j is the corresponding electrical potential, (3.23) can be converted to

$$
\begin{cases}
\nabla \cdot (\sigma \nabla u_j) = 0 \quad \text{in } \Omega \\[2mm]
I = \displaystyle\int_{\mathcal{E}_j^+} \sigma \frac{\partial u_j}{\partial \mathbf{n}} ds = -\int_{\mathcal{E}_j^-} \sigma \frac{\partial u_j}{\partial \mathbf{n}} ds \\[2mm]
0 = \displaystyle\int_{\mathcal{E}_k^+} \sigma \frac{\partial u_j}{\partial \mathbf{n}} ds = \int_{\mathcal{E}_k^-} \sigma \frac{\partial u_j}{\partial \mathbf{n}} ds \quad \text{for } k \neq j \\[2mm]
\nabla u_j \times \mathbf{n} = 0 \quad \text{on } \mathcal{E}, \quad \sigma \frac{\partial u_j}{\partial \mathbf{n}} = 0 \quad \text{on } \partial\Omega \backslash \mathcal{E}.
\end{cases}
\tag{3.24}
$$

The above non-standard boundary value problem (3.24) is well posed and has a unique solution in $H^1(\Omega)$ up to a constant.

Remark 3.3. The boundary condition $\nabla u_j \times \mathbf{n}|_{\mathcal{E}} = 0$ ensures that u_j on each electrode is a constant, since ∇u is normal to its level surface. The term $\pm I = \int_{\mathcal{E}_j^\pm} \sigma \frac{\partial u_j}{\partial \mathbf{n}} ds$ means that the total amount of injection current through the electrodes is I mA. In practice, it is difficult to specify the Neumann data $g := -\sigma \frac{\partial u}{\partial \mathbf{n}}|_{\partial \Omega}$ in a point-wise sense because only the total amount of injection current I is known. Note that the Neumann data g is in the set $H^{-1/2}(\partial \Omega) \backslash L^2(\partial \Omega)$.

Remark 3.4. [Uniqueness] Let us briefly discuss the uniqueness for the boundary value problem (3.24). Assume that u_j and $\tilde{u}_j$ are solutions of the boundary value problem (3.24). Denote $w_j = u_j - \tilde{u}_j$. Then, w_j satisfies

$$
\begin{cases}
\nabla \cdot (\sigma \nabla w_j) = 0 \quad \text{in } \Omega \\
0 = \int_{\mathcal{E}_j^+} \sigma \frac{\partial w_j}{\partial \mathbf{n}} ds = -\int_{\mathcal{E}_j^-} \sigma \frac{\partial w_j}{\partial \mathbf{n}} ds \\
0 = \int_{\mathcal{E}_k^+} \sigma \frac{\partial w_j}{\partial \mathbf{n}} ds = \int_{\mathcal{E}_k^-} \sigma \frac{\partial w_j}{\partial \mathbf{n}} ds \quad \text{for } k \neq j \\
\nabla w_j \times \mathbf{n} = 0 \quad \text{on } \mathcal{E}, \quad \sigma \frac{\partial w_j}{\partial \mathbf{n}} = 0 \quad \text{on } \partial \Omega \backslash \mathcal{E}.
\end{cases}
\tag{3.25}
$$

From the boundary conditions in (3.25), we have

$$
\int_\Omega \sigma \nabla w_j \cdot \nabla w_j d\mathbf{r}
$$

$$
= \int_{\mathcal{E}} w_j \sigma \frac{\partial w_j}{\partial \mathbf{n}} ds
$$

$$
= \sum_{k=1}^{2} \left(\underbrace{w_j|_{\mathcal{E}_k^+}}_{constant} \underbrace{\int_{\mathcal{E}_k^+} \sigma \frac{\partial w_j}{\partial \mathbf{n}} ds}_{0} + \underbrace{w_j|_{\mathcal{E}_k^-}}_{constant} \underbrace{\int_{\mathcal{E}_k^-} \sigma \frac{\partial w_j}{\partial \mathbf{n}} ds}_{0} \right)
$$

$$
= 0.
$$

Hence, $\nabla w_j = 0$, which leads to the uniqueness up to a constant.

To numerically compute u_j, we may use the finite element method with meshes with either all hexagonal or all tetrahedral elements.

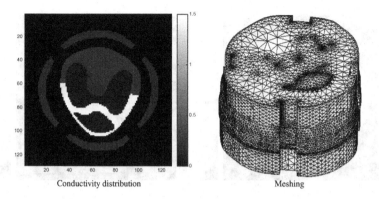

Conductivity distribution   Meshing

Fig. 3.12.   Mesh of the forward model.

Figure 3.12 shows tetrahedral finite element meshes; the domain Ω is subdivided into subdomains $K_1, K_2, \ldots, K_M$. The corresponding approximate domain, denoted by Ω_h, is the domain such that

the closure of Ω_h = the closure of $K_1 \cup K_2 \cup \cdots \cup K_M$.

Let $\mathcal{Q}_1$ be the trilinear (or linear) elements and define the finite element space $\mathcal{V}_h$ as follows:

$$\mathcal{V}_h := \{v \in H^1(\Omega) : v|_K \in \mathcal{Q}_1 \text{ for each } K \in \Omega_h\}.$$

For the approximation of the conductivity, σ belongs to the set of piecewise constant functions:

$$\Sigma_h := \{\sigma : \sigma \text{ is positive constant for each } T \in \Omega_h,$$
$$\sigma = \sigma^* \text{ for } T \in \Omega_h^*\}$$

where Ω_h^* is the set of elements containing the point (x_0, y_0, z_0) at which the conductivity is predetermined as σ^*.

We will only explain the basis (shape) functions of the trilinear element space $\mathcal{V}_h$. Take the following form for the standard element $[-1, 1]^3$:

$$\psi_i = \frac{1}{8}(1 + xx_i)(1 + yy_i)(1 + zz_i), \quad i = 1, \ldots, 8,$$

where x_i, y_i and z_i are the local coordinates of the ith point. Shape functions should satisfy the boundary condition. On the elements

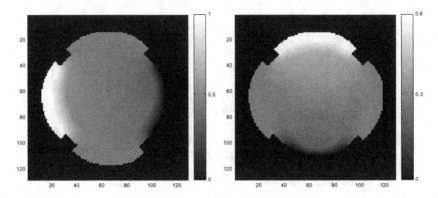

Fig. 3.13.   Cross-sectional images of potentials (left) u_1, (right) u_2.

sharing the boundary surfaces of $\partial\Omega$, basis functions take one of the following forms:

$$\frac{1}{8}(1 + xx_i)(1 + yy_i)(1 \pm z), \quad \frac{1}{8}(1 \pm x)(1 + yy_i)(1 + zz_i)$$

$$\frac{1}{8}(1 + xx_i)(1 \pm y)(1 + zz_i).$$

On the corner and edge elements, basis functions can be defined similarly. Then, we can compute the solutions $u_1, u_2 \in \mathcal{V}_h$ using the variational formulation and the boundary conditions.

Figure 3.13 shows the images of u_1 and u_2. Here, u_1 is the potential due to the injection current using the pair of electrodes along the horizontal direction, and u_2 is the potential induced by the pair of electrodes along the vertical direction.

3.4.2   *Computation of B_z*

For simplicity of notation, let u be either u_1 or u_2. Similarly, $\mathcal{E}^\pm$ denotes either $\mathcal{E}_1^\pm$ or $\mathcal{E}_2^\pm$. The current density $\mathbf{J}$ in Ω can be computed directly by $\mathbf{J} = -\sigma\nabla u$. Figure 3.14 shows the current density $\mathbf{J}$.

The induced magnetic flux density $\mathbf{B}$ can be decomposed into three components:

$$\mathbf{B}(\mathbf{r}) = \mathbf{B}^\Omega(\mathbf{r}) + \mathbf{B}^\mathcal{E}(\mathbf{r}) + \mathbf{B}^\mathcal{L}(\mathbf{r}) \quad \text{in } \Omega \qquad (3.26)$$

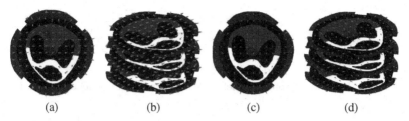

Fig. 3.14. (a)–(b) The current density $\mathbf{J}_1$ generated by the pair of electrodes $\mathcal{E}_1^{\pm}$. (c)–(d) $\mathbf{J}_2$ generated by $\mathcal{E}_2^{\pm}$.

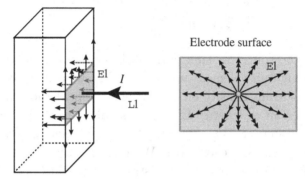

Fig. 3.15. (left) Out-of-plane source and sink currents on the electrode $\mathcal{E}^{+}$ and (right) surface current density within the electrode.

where $\mathbf{B}^{\Omega}$, $\mathbf{B}^{\mathcal{E}}$ and $\mathbf{B}^{\mathcal{L}}$ are magnetic flux densities due to $\mathbf{J}$ in Ω, $\mathcal{E}$ and I in the lead wires $\mathcal{L}$, respectively. From the Biot–Savart law, we have

$$\mathbf{B}^{\Omega}(\mathbf{r}) = \frac{\mu_0}{4\pi} \int_{\Omega} \mathbf{J}(\mathbf{r}') \times \frac{\mathbf{r} - \mathbf{r}'}{|\mathbf{r} - \mathbf{r}'|^3} d\mathbf{r}'$$

$$\mathbf{B}^{\mathcal{E}}(\mathbf{r}) = \frac{\mu_0}{4\pi} \int_{\mathcal{E}} \mathbf{J}(\mathbf{r}') \times \frac{\mathbf{r} - \mathbf{r}'}{|\mathbf{r} - \mathbf{r}'|^3} dS \qquad (3.27)$$

$$\mathbf{B}^{\mathcal{L}}(\mathbf{r}) = \frac{\mu_0 I}{4\pi} \int_{\mathcal{L}} \mathbf{a}(\mathbf{r}') \times \frac{\mathbf{r} - \mathbf{r}'}{|\mathbf{r} - \mathbf{r}'|^3} d\mathbf{l}$$

where $\mathbf{a}(\mathbf{r}')$ is the unit vector in the direction of the current flow at $\mathbf{r}' \in \mathcal{L}$.

The current density $\mathbf{J}$ in the second identity in (3.27) is the surface current. To calculate the surface current density shown in Figure 3.15, we solve the following two-dimensional boundary value

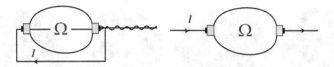

Fig. 3.16.   Lead wire geometry; (left) twisted wires and (right) straight wires.

problem in $\mathcal{E}^+$:

$$\begin{cases} \nabla^2_{x,y} V(x,y) = \eta(x,y) & \text{in } \mathcal{E}^+ \\ \nabla_{x,y} V \cdot \mathbf{n} = 0 & \text{on } \partial\mathcal{E}^+ \end{cases} \tag{3.28}$$

where η is the source or sink current. From the numerical solution of (3.28) using finite element method (FEM), we can easily compute the surface current density on $\mathcal{E}^+$. After we repeat the computation for $\mathcal{E}^-$, we can calculate $\mathbf{B}_{\mathcal{E}}$ in a similar way. We note that the computation of $\mathbf{B}^{\mathcal{L}}$ requires the information on the actual geometrical shape of lead wires. We consider two cases shown in Figure 3.16 (left) together. For the straight wires in Figure 3.16, the lead wires run straight in one direction within a certain range. Note that the current I in a portion of lead wires far away from Ω has a negligible effect on the magnetic flux density in Ω. In either case, we can numerically compute by discretizing the lead wires into many small line segments. For the straight lead wire shown in Figure 3.16 (right), one might use an analytic solution for $\mathbf{B}^{\mathcal{L}}$. Long and straight lead wires in the z-direction may be desirable for measuring B_z in $\partial\Omega$ since only the currents in the x and y-direction determine B_z. Figure 3.17 shows images of B_z.

From the expression in (3.27), $\mathbf{B}^{\mathcal{E}}$ and $\mathbf{B}^{\mathcal{L}}$ are harmonic in Ω. This means that $\nabla^2\mathbf{B}$ in Ω is independent to the geometry of lead wires.

Theorem 3.1. *The $\nabla^2\mathbf{B}$ in Ω is independent to $\mathbf{B}^{\mathcal{E}}$ and $\mathbf{B}^{\mathcal{L}}$, and*

$$\frac{1}{\mu_0}\nabla \times (\mathbf{B}^{\mathcal{E}}(\mathbf{r}) + \mathbf{B}^{\mathcal{L}}(\mathbf{r})) = \nabla \int_{\partial\Omega} \frac{-\mathbf{J}(\mathbf{r}') \cdot \mathbf{n}(\mathbf{r}')}{4\pi|\mathbf{r} - \mathbf{r}'|} dS, \quad \forall \mathbf{r} \in \Omega.$$
$$\tag{3.29}$$

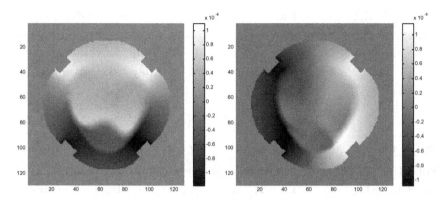

Fig. 3.17. (left) B_{z1} due to $\mathcal{E}_1^{\pm}$ and (right) B_{z2} due to $\mathcal{E}_2^{\pm}$.

Proof. Since $\nabla \cdot \mathbf{J} = 0$, we have

$$\frac{1}{\mu_0}\nabla \times \mathbf{B}^{\Omega}(\mathbf{r}) = \nabla \times \nabla \times \int_{\Omega} \frac{-\mathbf{J}(\mathbf{r}')}{4\pi|\mathbf{r} - \mathbf{r}'|}d\mathbf{r}'$$

$$= (-\nabla^2 + \nabla\nabla\cdot)\int_{\Omega} \frac{-\mathbf{J}(\mathbf{r}')}{4\pi|\mathbf{r} - \mathbf{r}'|}d\mathbf{r}'$$

$$= \mathbf{J}(\mathbf{r}) + \nabla\nabla \cdot \int_{\Omega} \frac{-\mathbf{J}(\mathbf{r}')}{4\pi|\mathbf{r} - \mathbf{r}'|}d\mathbf{r}' \qquad (3.30)$$

$$= \mathbf{J}(\mathbf{r}) - \nabla\int_{\Omega} \nabla_{\mathbf{r}'} \cdot \left(\frac{-\mathbf{J}(\mathbf{r}')}{4\pi|\mathbf{r} - \mathbf{r}'|}\right)d\mathbf{r}'$$

$$= \mathbf{J}(\mathbf{r}) - \nabla\int_{\partial\Omega} \frac{-\mathbf{J}(\mathbf{r}') \cdot \mathbf{n}(\mathbf{r}')}{4\pi|\mathbf{r} - \mathbf{r}'|}dS$$

for all $\mathbf{r}$ in Ω. Since $\mathbf{J} = \nabla \times \mathbf{B}$ in Ω, (3.29) follows from (3.26), (3.27) and (3.30).

Hence, the influences of $\mathbf{B}^{\mathcal{E}}$ and $\mathbf{B}^{\mathcal{L}}$ to $\mathbf{J}$ inside Ω can be reflected to the boundary condition $\mathbf{J} \cdot \mathbf{n}|_{\partial\Omega}$. Moreover, the identity (3.29) leads to

$$\nabla^2(\mathbf{B}^{\mathcal{E}}(\mathbf{r}) + \mathbf{B}^{\mathcal{L}}(\mathbf{r})) = 0 \quad (\forall\, \mathbf{r} \in \Omega) \qquad (3.31)$$

since $\nabla^2\frac{1}{|\mathbf{r}-\mathbf{r}'|} = 0$ when $\mathbf{r} \neq \mathbf{r}'$. Hence, the quantity $\nabla^2\mathbf{B}$ in Ω is independent to $\mathbf{B}^{\mathcal{E}}$ and $\mathbf{B}^{\mathcal{L}}$. □

Remark 3.5. Numerical calculation of the magnetic flux density **B** using the Biot–Savart law requires a large amount of computation time since it is in the form of three-dimensional convolution as in (3.27). For a faster method using FEM, we may take advantage of the identity

$$\nabla^2 \mathbf{B}(\mathbf{r}) = -\mu_0 \nabla \times \mathbf{J}(\mathbf{r}) \quad \text{in } \Omega. \tag{3.32}$$

Since **J** is available, we can solve (3.32) for **B** using FEM if boundary conditions of **B** are known on $\partial\Omega$. We therefore need to compute $\mathbf{B} = \mathbf{B}_\Omega + \mathbf{B}_\mathcal{E} + \mathbf{B}_\mathcal{L}$ only for $\mathbf{r} \in \partial\Omega$. Then, we have the Dirichlet boundary condition on $\partial\Omega$ and can numerically solve (3.32) for **B** using FEM. Please note that it is important to compute all three terms of **B** on $\partial\Omega$ to find the appropriate Dirichlet boundary condition of **B** in (3.32). We can also compute (3.32) in any three-dimensional subdomain of Ω as long as we correctly calculate its boundary condition.

3.5   Uniform Current Density Electrodes

When a highly conducting electrode makes direct contact with biological tissues, the induced current density has strong singularity along the periphery of the electrode, which may cause painful sensation. In MREIT, we should avoid such singularity since more uniform current density underneath a current-injection electrode is desirable. This section presents an optimal geometry of a recessed electrode to produce a well-distributed current density on the contact area under the electrode. The goal is to find the optimal geometry of the electrode surface to minimize the edge singularity and produce nearly uniform current density on the contact area.

Various designs for uniform current density electrodes are suggested to improve the uniformity of current density by altering either the electrode geometry or material property based primarily on numerical simulations. These include a resistive or capacitive coating of a metal electrode to reduce the current density concentration along the perimeter [Wiley and Webster (1982a,b)]; a non-uniform resistive coating of a fixed thickness using materials of different conductivity values [Geuze (1983); Langberg (1993)]; non-uniformly recessed surface electrode making the gap between the electrode surface and the skin [Ksienski (1992); Rubinstein *et al.* (1987); Suesserman *et al.* (1991); Tungjitkusolmun *et al.* (2000)].

In [Song *et al.* (2011)], a special design of a uniform current density electrode was proposed by analyzing the singularity of the current density along the electrode perimeter using the layer potential technique. They investigated the geometry of the electrode surface to minimize the edge singularity on the contact area, and proposed a mathematical framework for the uniform current density electrode and its optimal geometry. This result is given in this section and the design will include a hydrogel layer with varying thickness between the electrode and the skin. In order to keep good contact with the skin, the skin contact surface of the hydrogel layer will be flat while the side making contact with a thin carbon electrode will be curved. The goal is to find an optimal shape of the hydrogel layer which determines a shape of the contact surface in such a way that the induced current density is well distributed on the skin contact surface.

To be precise, let $\mathcal{D}_\pm$ represent hydrogel layers and $\mathcal{E}_\pm$ denote the contact surface of the electrodes. For notational convenience, we denote $\widetilde{\Omega} = \Omega \cup \mathcal{D}_+ \cup \mathcal{D}_-$. $\Gamma_\pm$ denote the contact surfaces between the hydrogel layer and the boundary of the domain Ω. Let u denote the induced electrical potential due to injection current I through $\mathcal{E}_\pm$.

The regularity of the solution is closely related with the domain $\widetilde{\Omega}$ (see, e.g., [Grisvard (1985)]). Near the edge, the current density, $-\sigma \nabla u$, behaves $|\sigma \nabla u| \to \infty$. For a fixed domain Ω, the edge singularity mainly depends on the geometry of the electrodes. For example, on the skin contact area near the periphery of the electrodes, we may experience a strong edge singularity for the case when the electrode is directly attached on the skin. The hydrogel layer between the electrode and the skin weakens the singularity.

The goal is to find an optimal shape of the hydrogel layer $\mathcal{D}_\pm$ which determines a shape of the contact surface $\mathcal{E}_\pm$ in such a way that the induced current density is well distributed on the skin contact surface $\Gamma_\pm$. It would be ideal that $\sigma \frac{\partial u}{\partial \mathbf{n}}$ is constant along $\Gamma_\pm$. Thus we look for a shape of $\mathcal{D}_\pm$ which makes $\sigma \frac{\partial u}{\partial \mathbf{n}}$ on $\Gamma_\pm$ constant. Mathematically, we may express this as a problem to find a geometry of $\mathcal{D}_{\pm}$ which minimizes the following energy functional:

$$\Phi(\mathcal{D}_{\pm}) = \int_{\Gamma_+} \left| \sigma \frac{\partial u}{\partial \mathbf{n}} - \alpha_+ \right|^p dS + \int_{\Gamma_-} \left| \sigma \frac{\partial u}{\partial \mathbf{n}} - \alpha_- \right|^p dS, \qquad (3.33)$$

where $\alpha_{\pm} = \frac{1}{|\Gamma_{\pm}|} \int_{\Gamma_{\pm}} \sigma \frac{\partial u}{\partial \mathbf{n}} dS$, $\mathbf{n}$ represents the outward unit normal vector to $\Gamma_{\pm}$, dS is the surface element of $\Gamma_{\pm}$ and $1 \leq p \leq 2$.

Unfortunately, analyzing the optimization problem (3.33) is a formidable task, because the electrical potential u is a highly non-linear function depending on $\mathcal{D}_{\pm}$. In order to simplify the underlying problem, we assume Ω to be a half space which is reasonable when the electrodes are relatively small compared with the human body.

3.5.1   *Mathematical model for uniform current electrode in half space*

To simplify the underlying uniform current electrode model, we consider the half space. Throughout this subsection, we assume the following:

- $\Omega = \mathbb{R}^3_-$ is the half space. The skin contact surface $\Gamma \subset \partial\Omega$ is convex and symmetric with respect to the origin with its smooth boundary $\partial\Gamma$.
- $\mathcal{D}$ represents the hydrogel layer corresponding to $\mathcal{D}_+$, and the other electrode $\mathcal{D}_-$ is assumed to be located at ∞.
- The shape of the electrode contact surface is expressed by a function ϕ on the subarea $\Gamma_0 \subset \Gamma$ which describes

$$\mathcal{E} = \{\mathbf{r} = (x, y, z) : z = \phi(x, y), \ (x, y, 0) \in \Gamma_0\}.$$

Then, $\mathcal{D}$ can be expressed as

$$\mathcal{D} = \{(x, y, z) : 0 \leq z < \phi(x, y), \ (x, y, 0) \in \Gamma_0\}$$
$$\cup \{(x, y, z) : 0 \leq z < \eta(x, y), \ (x, y, 0) \in \Gamma \backslash \Gamma_0\}$$

where η is a function defined on $\Gamma \backslash \Gamma_0$.
- The conductivity $\sigma = 1$ in both Ω and $\mathcal{D}$.

With the above assumptions, the induced potential, denoted by u, is a solution of

$$\begin{cases} -\nabla^2 u = 0 \quad \text{in } \tilde{\Omega} = \Omega \cup \mathcal{D} \\ \int_{\mathcal{E}} \dfrac{\partial u}{\partial \mathbf{n}} dS = I, \quad \mathbf{n} \times \nabla u|_{\mathcal{E}} = 0 \\ \dfrac{\partial u}{\partial \mathbf{n}} = 0 \quad \text{on } \partial \tilde{\Omega} \backslash \mathcal{E} \\ \lim_{|\mathbf{r}| \to \infty} u(\mathbf{r}) = 0 \end{cases} \tag{3.34}$$

In (3.34), we do not adopt the complete electrode model including the contact impedance [Somersalo et al. (1992)] because we design the uniform current density electrode only for current injection not for voltage measurement. We must consider the contact impedance when we measure a voltage on a current-carrying electrode since the contact impedance induces a voltage drop across it. In MREIT, we do not need to measure voltages on a current-carrying electrode. Instead, we just wish to have a more uniform current density distribution underneath it. For low-frequency injection currents through electrodes with a large surface area of $100 \, \text{cm}^2$, for example, the contact impedance is mostly resistive and small. Including such a contact impedance in the mathematical model of the uniform current density electrode will make the mathematical analysis too complicated with little benefit in practice.

The goal is to get uniform current along the contact surface Γ, that is,

to find optimal $\mathcal{D}$ and $\mathcal{E}$ which minimize $\int_{\Gamma} \left| \dfrac{\partial u}{\partial \mathbf{n}} - \alpha \right|^2 dS, \quad$ (3.35)

where u is a solution of (3.34) and $\alpha = \frac{1}{|\Gamma|} \int_{\Gamma} \frac{\partial u}{\partial \mathbf{n}} dS$ is the average. Note that u is a highly non-linear function of $\mathcal{D}$ and $\mathcal{E}$.

3.5.2 *Optimal geometry of non-uniform recessed electrodes*

Due to the high non-linearity of the problem (3.35), it is very difficult to find its minimizer using a conventional approach such as FEM, finite difference method (FDM), boundary element method (BEM) and domain derivative method.

In order to bypass the difficulty of finding the minimizer of (3.35), we adopt a direct approach using the following special function:

$$\tilde{u}(\mathbf{r}) := \begin{cases} \int_\Gamma \dfrac{1}{4\pi|\mathbf{r} - \mathbf{r}'|}\,dS & \text{in } \Omega \\[4mm] z + \int_\Gamma \dfrac{1}{4\pi|\mathbf{r} - \mathbf{r}'|}\,dS & \text{in } \mathbb{R}^3_+ \cup \Gamma \end{cases} \tag{3.36}$$

where $\mathbb{R}^3_+ = \{\mathbf{r} \in \mathbb{R}^3 : z > 0\}$.

Lemma 3.1. *The potential $\tilde{u}$ satisfies*

$$\nabla^2 \tilde{u} = 0 \quad \text{in } \mathbb{R}^3 \backslash (\partial\Omega \backslash \Gamma)$$
$$\frac{\partial}{\partial z}\tilde{u} = \frac{1}{2} \quad \text{in } \Gamma. \tag{3.37}$$

Proof. It follows from the trace formula of the single layer potential that

$$\nabla^2 \int_\Gamma \frac{1}{4\pi|\mathbf{r} - \mathbf{r}'|}\,dS = 0 \qquad \text{for } \mathbf{r} \in \mathbb{R}^3\backslash\Gamma$$

$$\frac{\partial}{\partial z} \int_\Gamma \frac{1}{4\pi|\mathbf{r} - \mathbf{r}'|}\,dS = 0 \qquad \text{for } \mathbf{r} \in \partial\Omega\backslash\Gamma$$

$$\lim_{z\to 0^\pm} \frac{\partial}{\partial z} \int_\Gamma \frac{1}{4\pi|\mathbf{r} + z\hat{\mathbf{z}} - \mathbf{r}'|}\,dS = \mp\frac{1}{2} \quad \text{for } \mathbf{r} \in \Gamma.$$

The term z in (3.36) plays a crucial role to cancel out the jump of the single layer potential across Γ, so that we have

$$\lim_{z\to 0^+} \frac{\partial\tilde{u}}{\partial z}(\mathbf{r}) = \frac{1}{2} = \lim_{z\to 0^-} \frac{\partial\tilde{u}}{\partial z}(\mathbf{r}) \quad \text{for } \mathbf{r} \in \Gamma.$$

Since normal directional derivatives of $\tilde{u}$ are continuous across Γ, $\nabla^2 \tilde{u} = 0$ in $\mathbb{R}^3\backslash(\partial\Omega\backslash\Gamma)$. $\square$

Now, we define $\mathcal{D}_0$ by

$$\mathcal{D}_0 = \{\mathbf{r} \in \mathbb{R}^3_+ : 0 < \tilde{u}(x, y, z) < \tilde{u}(0) \ \& \ (x, y, 0) \in \Gamma\}.$$

According to the implicit function theorem, there exists φ such that

$$\tilde{u}(x, y, \varphi(x, y)) = \tilde{u}(0),$$

which is equivalent to

$$\varphi(x, y) + \int_\Gamma \frac{1}{4\pi \sqrt{(x - x')^2 + (y - y')^2 + \varphi(x, y)^2}} dS = \int_\Gamma \frac{1}{4\pi |\mathbf{r}'|} dS.$$

$$(3.38)$$

We will choose $\mathcal{D}$ and $\mathcal{E}$ in such a way that

$$\mathcal{D} \subset \mathcal{D}_0 := \{\mathbf{r} \in \mathbb{R}^3_+ : 0 < z < \varphi(x, y), \ (x, y, 0) \in \Gamma\}$$
$$\mathcal{E} \subset \{\mathbf{r} \in \mathbb{R}^3_+ : z = \varphi(x, y), \ (x, y, 0) \in \Gamma\}.$$

$$(3.39)$$

The lateral side of $\mathcal{D}_0$ will be trimmed in the following way: the normal direction of the lateral side becomes pointwisely parallel to the tangential direction of the equipotential surface of $\tilde{u}$, that is,

$$\frac{\partial \tilde{u}}{\partial \mathbf{n}} = 0 \quad \text{on the trimed lateral surface of } \mathcal{D}_0.$$

$$(3.40)$$

To derive a trimmed version of $\mathcal{D}_0$, we compute the trajectory of the lateral surface starting from each point of the bottom Γ by solving the following dynamic system: for each point $\mathbf{p} \in \Gamma$,

$$\begin{cases} T'_p(t) = \nabla \tilde{u}(T_p(t)) / |\nabla \tilde{u}(T_p(t))|, & t > 0 \\ T_p(0) = \mathbf{p}. \end{cases}$$

$$(3.41)$$

See Figure 3.18.

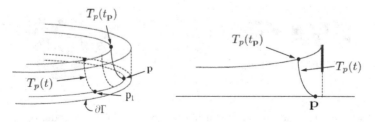

Fig. 3.18. Configuration of the boundary of painless electrode.

From a direct computation, we have

$$(x, y) \cdot \left(\frac{\partial \tilde{u}}{\partial x}(\mathbf{r}), \frac{\partial \tilde{u}}{\partial y}(\mathbf{r}) \right) < 0 \ \& \ \frac{\partial \tilde{u}(\mathbf{r})}{\partial z}(\mathbf{r}) > 0 \quad \text{for all } \mathbf{r} = \in \Gamma \backslash \{0\}.$$

$$(3.42)$$

Due to the properties (3.42), for each $\mathbf{p} \in \Gamma$, there exists a unique $t_{\mathbf{p}} > 0$ such that

$$T_p(t_{\mathbf{p}}) \in \{\mathbf{r} \in \mathbb{R}_+^3 : z = \varphi(x, y) \ \& \ (x, y, 0) \in \Gamma\}.$$

Theorem 3.2. *Let* $\mathcal{E} := \{T_p(t_{\mathbf{p}}) : \mathbf{p} \in \Gamma\}$ *and*

$$\mathcal{D} := \{T_p(t) : 0 < t < t_{\mathbf{p}}, \ \mathbf{p} \in \Gamma\}. \qquad (3.43)$$

If u is a solution of (3.34) with the above $\mathcal{E}$ and $\mathcal{D}$, then

$$\mathbf{n} \cdot \mathbf{J} = -\frac{\partial u}{\partial \mathbf{n}} = constant \quad on \ \Gamma. \qquad (3.44)$$

For the proof of the above theorem, please refer to [Song *et al.* (2011)].

Figure 3.20 shows vector plots of $J_z = -\frac{\partial}{\partial z} u$ along Γ for the two cases (a) the standard electrode and (b) the optimal electrode whose shape is shown in (c).

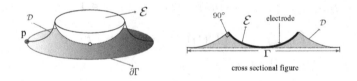

Fig. 3.19.　Configuration of the painless electrode.

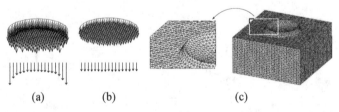

Fig. 3.20.　Current density images using (a) the standard electrode; (b) painless electrode. (c) Finite element structure with painless electrode.

Based on the rigorous mathematical analysis with Theorem 3.2, the uniform current density electrode is designed, and its shape is quite different from the conventional electrode shape. This model may be useful in MREIT where the amount of injection current directly affects the quality of reconstructed conductivity images since the SNR is proportional to the current amplitude. This electrode helps us to inject more current by spreading the current uniformly underneath the electrode to prevent unpleasant sensations usually originated from concentrated current density at its edge.

3.6 Mathematical Model of MREIT for Stable Reconstruction

3.6.1 *Map from σ to B_z data*

The inverse problem in MREIT is to recover the conductivity distribution σ using the knowledge of the measured data $B_{z,1}, B_{z,2}$, geometry of $\partial\Omega$, positions of electrodes $\mathcal{E}_j^\pm$, and the relationship:

$$B_{z,j}(\mathbf{r}) = \underbrace{-\frac{\mu_0}{4\pi} \int_\Omega \frac{\langle \mathbf{r} - \mathbf{r}', \mathbf{J}_j(\mathbf{r}') \times \hat{\mathbf{z}} \rangle}{|\mathbf{r} - \mathbf{r}'|^3} \, d\mathbf{r}'}_{B_{z,j}^\Omega} + \mathcal{H}_j(\mathbf{r}) \quad \text{for } \mathbf{r} \in \Omega,$$

(3.45)

where $\mathbf{J}_j = -\sigma \nabla u_j$ is the current density described in the previous section and $\mathcal{H}_j$ is the z-component of $\mathbf{B}_j^\mathcal{E} + \mathbf{B}_j^\mathcal{L}$.

For setting up a mathematical model of MREIT bearing in mind uniqueness and stability, we need to simplify the problem to identify its key structure. We assume that the conductivity distribution in Ω, denoted by σ, is isotropic and $\sigma \in \mathcal{A} := \{\sigma \in C^1(\bar{\Omega}) : 0 < \sigma < \infty \text{ in } \Omega\}$. These smoothness conditions are only for simplicity of the analysis and can be relaxed considerably.

Remark 3.6 (About the smoothness assumption of σ). The question is whether any practically available B_z data can distinguish true conductivity from its smooth approximation. Suppose that $\tilde{\sigma}$ is a C^1-approximation of the true σ. An MRI scanner provides B_z data as a two-dimensional array of B_z intensities inside voxels within a given field of view, and each intensity is affected by the number of protons in the voxel and an adopted pulse sequence. Hence, B_z data is always a blurred version. Admitting the obvious fact that an achievable spatial resolution of a reconstructed conductivity image cannot be better than the determined voxel size, it may not be possible to distinguish $\tilde{\sigma}$ and σ.

We can define the map $\Upsilon : \mathcal{A} \rightarrow [H^1(\Omega)]^2$ from σ to data $(B_{z,1}^\Omega, B_{z,2}^\Omega)$:

$$\Upsilon : \sigma \rightarrow (\Upsilon_1[\sigma], \Upsilon_2[\sigma])$$

$$\Upsilon_j[\sigma](\mathbf{r}) := \underbrace{\frac{\mu_0}{4\pi} \int_\Omega \frac{\langle \mathbf{r} - \mathbf{r}', \sigma(\mathbf{r}') \nabla u_j[\sigma](\mathbf{r}') \times \hat{\mathbf{z}} \rangle}{|\mathbf{r} - \mathbf{r}'|^3} \, d\mathbf{r}'}_{B_{z,j}^\Omega(\mathbf{r})} \qquad (3.46)$$

where $u_j[\sigma]$ is the solution of (3.24). Since σ is unknown, the solution u_j of (3.24) should be expressed as a function of σ.

When we set up a mathematical model of MREIT or develop reconstruction algorithms, it is necessary to deal with the issue on the uniqueness of a reconstructed resistivity image in MREIT. Is the B_z data enough to provide a stable reconstruction of σ? We need to check whether the map $\Upsilon : \mathcal{A} \rightarrow [H^1(\Omega)]^2$ is invertible. If the map is not so, we should find a proper supplemental measurement to develop an invertible map.

3.6.2   *Toward uniqueness of an MREIT problem*

In summary, the requirements in data collection methods for the uniqueness of a reconstructed conductivity image include the following:

- At least one non-zero boundary voltage measurement or predetermined conductivity value at least at one point in the imaging slice.
- At least two injection currents satisfying $\mathbf{J}_1 \times \mathbf{J}_2 \neq 0$ in Ω. This requirement means that $\mathbf{J}_1$ and $\mathbf{J}_2$ are not collinear in Ω.

3.6.2.1 *Scaling uncertainty of* σ

There exists a scaling uncertainty of σ due to the fact that if σ is a solution of (3.45), so is a scaled conductivity $\alpha\sigma$ for any scaling factor $\alpha > 0$.

Proposition 3.1. *Let* $\alpha > 0$. *If* $u_j[\alpha\sigma]$ *is a solution of* (3.24) *with* σ *replaced by* $\alpha\sigma$, *then*

$$u_j[\alpha\sigma] = \frac{1}{\alpha} u_j[\sigma] + constant. \tag{3.47}$$

Proof. Note that $u_j[\alpha\sigma]$ is a solution of

$$
\begin{cases}
\nabla \cdot (\alpha\sigma\nabla u_j[\alpha\sigma]) = 0 \quad \text{in } \Omega \\[2mm]
I = \int_{\mathcal{E}_j^+} \alpha\sigma \frac{\partial}{\partial \mathbf{n}} u_j[\alpha\sigma] \, ds = -\int_{\mathcal{E}_j^-} \alpha\sigma \frac{\partial}{\partial \mathbf{n}} u_j[\alpha\sigma] ds \\[2mm]
0 = \int_{\mathcal{E}_k^+} \alpha\sigma \frac{\partial}{\partial \mathbf{n}} u_j[\alpha\sigma] \, ds = \int_{\mathcal{E}_k^-} \alpha\sigma \frac{\partial}{\partial \mathbf{n}} u_j[\alpha\sigma] ds \quad \text{for } k \neq j \\[2mm]
\nabla u_j[\alpha\sigma] \times \mathbf{n} = 0 \text{ on } \mathcal{E}, \quad \alpha\sigma \frac{\partial}{\partial \mathbf{n}} u_j[\alpha\sigma] = 0 \text{ on } \partial\Omega\backslash\mathcal{E}.
\end{cases}
$$

It is easy to check that $\frac{1}{\alpha} u_j[\sigma]$ is a solution of the above boundary value problem. The result (3.47) follows from the uniqueness result in Remark 3.4. $\qquad\square$

Proposition 3.2. *For* $j = 1, 2$, *we have*

$$\Upsilon_j[\alpha\sigma] = \Upsilon_j[\sigma] \quad \text{for any constant } \alpha > 0. \tag{3.48}$$

Proof. According to the representation (3.46) and (3.47),

$$\underbrace{\frac{\mu_0}{4\pi} \int_\Omega \frac{\alpha\sigma(\mathbf{r}')[(x - x')\frac{1}{\alpha}\frac{\partial}{\partial y} u_j[\sigma](\mathbf{r}') - (y - y')\frac{1}{\alpha}\frac{\partial}{\partial x} u_j[\sigma](\mathbf{r}')]}{|\mathbf{r} - \mathbf{r}'|^3} \, d\mathbf{r}'}_{\Upsilon_j[\alpha\sigma](\mathbf{r})}$$

$$= \underbrace{\frac{\mu_0}{4\pi} \int_\Omega \frac{\sigma(\mathbf{r}') \, [(x - x')\frac{\partial}{\partial y} u_j[\sigma](\mathbf{r}') - (y - y')\frac{\partial}{\partial x} u_j[\sigma](\mathbf{r}')]}{|\mathbf{r} - \mathbf{r}'|^3} \, d\mathbf{r}'}_{\Upsilon_j[\sigma](\mathbf{r})} \qquad\square$$

The scaling uncertainty of σ can be fixed by measuring a voltage difference at any two fixed boundary points or by including a piece of electrically conducting material with a known conductivity value as a part of the imaging object.

3.6.2.2 *Two linearly independent currents for uniqueness*

In this subsection, we will explain why we need at least two linearly independent injection currents to reconstruct σ uniquely. For simplicity of notation, we will denote $u[\sigma] = u_1[\sigma]$, $B_z = B_{z,1}$, $\mathbf{J} = \mathbf{J}_1$ throughout this subsection.

It is important to observe that B_z data cannot probe *any change* of σ in the direction of $(J_x, J_y, 0)$. Indeed, for a given injection current, there are infinitely many different conductivities that produce the same $\mathbf{J}$. This means that, for a given B_z data, there are infinitely many conductivity distributions which satisfy (3.46) and (3.24).

Theorem 3.3. *Let $\sigma \in \mathcal{A}$. Assume that a function $\varphi : \mathbb{R} \to \mathbb{R}$ is strictly increasing and continuously differentiable. Then $\varphi(u[\sigma])$ is a solution of (3.24) with σ replaced by $\frac{\sigma}{\varphi'(u[\sigma])}$. Moreover,*

$$\sigma(\mathbf{r})\nabla u[\sigma](\mathbf{r}) = \frac{\sigma(\mathbf{r})}{\varphi'(u[\sigma](\mathbf{r}))}\nabla\varphi(u[\sigma](\mathbf{r})), \quad \mathbf{r} \in \Omega. \qquad (3.49)$$

Proof. The identity (3.49) follows from the chain rule. Hence,

$$\underbrace{\nabla \cdot \left(\frac{\sigma(\mathbf{r})}{\varphi'(u[\sigma](\mathbf{r}))}\nabla\varphi(u[\sigma](\mathbf{r})) \right)}_{\nabla \cdot (\sigma(\mathbf{r})\nabla u[\sigma](\mathbf{r}))} = 0, \quad \mathbf{r} \in \Omega.$$

Due to (3.49), $\varphi(u[\sigma])$ has the same boundary conditions as u. This completes the proof. $\qquad \square$

Proposition 3.3. *The $\Upsilon_1[\sigma]$ can be expressed as*

$$\Upsilon_1[\sigma] = \frac{\mu_0}{4\pi}\int_\Omega \frac{-1}{|\mathbf{r}-\mathbf{r}'|} \begin{vmatrix} \dfrac{\partial\sigma}{\partial x} & \dfrac{\partial\sigma}{\partial y} \\[2mm] \dfrac{\partial}{\partial x}u[\sigma] & \dfrac{\partial}{\partial y}u[\sigma] \end{vmatrix} d\mathbf{r}' + \frac{\mu_0}{4\pi}\int_{\partial\Omega} \frac{1}{|\mathbf{r}-\mathbf{r}'|}\mathbf{n}$$

$$\cdot (\sigma\nabla u[\sigma] \times \hat{\mathbf{z}})ds. \qquad (3.50)$$

If $\varphi: \mathbb{R} \to \mathbb{R}$ is strictly increasing and continuously differentiable, then $\tilde{\sigma} := \frac{\sigma}{\varphi'(u)}$ satisfies

$$\begin{vmatrix} \dfrac{\partial \sigma}{\partial x} & \dfrac{\partial \sigma}{\partial y} \\[2mm] \dfrac{\partial}{\partial x} u[\sigma] & \dfrac{\partial}{\partial y} u[\sigma] \end{vmatrix} = \begin{vmatrix} \dfrac{\partial \sigma}{\partial x} & \dfrac{\partial \tilde{\sigma}}{\partial y} \\[2mm] \dfrac{\partial}{\partial x} u[\tilde{\sigma}] & \dfrac{\partial}{\partial y} u[\tilde{\sigma}] \end{vmatrix} \quad in \ \Omega \qquad (3.51)$$

and

$$\Upsilon_1[\sigma] = \Upsilon_1[\tilde{\sigma}.]. \qquad (3.52)$$

Proof. Integrating by parts yields

$$\Upsilon_1[\sigma] = \frac{\mu_0}{4\pi} \int_\Omega \nabla_{\mathbf{r}'} \frac{1}{|\mathbf{r} - \mathbf{r}'|} \cdot (\sigma(\mathbf{r}') \nabla u[\sigma](\mathbf{r}') \times \hat{\mathbf{z}}) \, d\mathbf{r}'$$

$$= \frac{\mu_0}{4\pi} \int_\Omega \frac{-1}{|\mathbf{r} - \mathbf{r}'|} \nabla \cdot (\sigma \nabla u[\sigma] \times \hat{\mathbf{z}}) d\mathbf{r}'$$

$$+ \frac{\mu_0}{4\pi} \int_{\partial\Omega} \frac{1}{|\mathbf{r} - \mathbf{r}'|} \mathbf{n} \cdot (\sigma \nabla u[\sigma] \times \hat{\mathbf{z}}) \, ds.$$

Then (3.50) follows from

$$\nabla \cdot (\sigma \nabla u[\sigma] \times \hat{\mathbf{z}}) = \hat{\mathbf{z}} \cdot [\nabla \sigma \times \nabla u[\sigma]] = \begin{vmatrix} \dfrac{\partial \sigma}{\partial x} & \dfrac{\partial \sigma}{\partial y} \\[2mm] \dfrac{\partial}{\partial x} u[\sigma] & \dfrac{\partial}{\partial y} u[\sigma] \end{vmatrix}.$$

From Theorem 3.3, we have

$$\nabla \times (\tilde{\sigma} \nabla u[\tilde{\sigma}]) = \nabla \times (\sigma \nabla u[\sigma])$$

which leads to (3.51). Then, (3.52) follows from (3.51) and (3.50). $\square$

According to Proposition 3.3, it is easy to see that B_z data is blind to the change of σ in the direction of $(J_x, J_y, 0)$. Therefore, we need at least two injection currents that produce $\mathbf{J}_1$ and $\mathbf{J}_2$ satisfying $(\mathbf{J}_1 \times \mathbf{J}_2) \cdot \hat{\mathbf{z}} \neq 0$ in order to remove the blind side from each current.

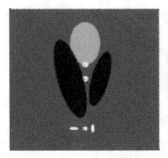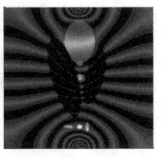

Fig. 3.21.   Shown (left) and (right) are two different conductivity distributions that produce the same B_z data subject to a Neumann data $g(x,y) = \delta((x,y) - (0,1)) - \delta((x,y) - (0,-1))$, $x \in \partial\Omega$ where $\Omega = (-1,1) \times (-1,1)$.

3.7   MREIT with Object Rotations

In early MREIT systems, all three components of $\mathbf{B} = (B_x, B_y, B_z)$ have been utilized as measured data and this requires mechanical rotations of the imaging object within the MRI scanner [Khang *et al.* (2002); Kwon *et al.* (2002a); Lee *et al.* (2003); Birgul *et al.* (2003); Onart *et al.* (2003)]. Assuming the knowledge of the full components of $\mathbf{B}$, we can directly compute the current density $\mathbf{J} = \frac{1}{\mu_0}\nabla \times \mathbf{B}$ and reconstruct σ using an image reconstruction algorithm such as the J-substitution algorithm [Kwon *et al.* (2002a); Khang *et al.* (2002); Lee *et al.* (2003)], current constrained voltage scaled reconstruction (CCVSR) algorithm [Birgul *et al.* (2003)] and equipotential line methods [Kwon *et al.* (2002b); Onart *et al.* (2003)]. Lately, a new non-iterative conductivity image reconstruction method called CDII has been suggested and experimentally verified [Hasanov *et al.* (2008)]. Recently, CDII using a single current density $|\mathbf{J}|$ has been carefully studied in [Nachman *et al.* (2007b, 2009, 2010)]. These methods using $\mathbf{B} = (B_x, B_y, B_z)$ suffer from technical difficulties related with object rotations within the main magnet of the MRI scanner.

This section focuses on the J-substitution algorithm [Kwon *et al.* (2002a)] which is based on the following non-linear PDE:

$$\nabla \cdot \left(\frac{|\mathbf{J}|}{|\nabla u|} \nabla u \right) = 0 \quad \text{inside the imaging object.} \qquad (3.53)$$

The **J**-based MREIT can provide high-resolution conductivity images by displaying $\sigma = \frac{|\mathbf{J}|}{|\nabla u|}$ [Khang *et al.* (2002)].

3.7.1 *Current density imaging*

Throughout this subsection, we will denote $u = u[\sigma] = u_1[\sigma], B_z = B_{z,1}, \mathbf{J} = \mathbf{J}_1$. In 1988, Joy *et al.* at the University of Toronto [Joy *et al.* (1989); Scott *et al.* (1991, 1992)] developed MRCDI to obtain an image of the current density $\mathbf{J} = \nabla \times \mathbf{H}$. The aim of MRCDI is to provide an image of $\mathbf{J}$ in Ω by measuring all three components of $\mathbf{B} = (B_x, B_y, B_z)$ due to an injection current I. However, the existing MRI scanners can measure only one component of $\mathbf{B}$ that is parallel to the direction of the main magnetic field of the machine. More precisely, if we let z be the label of an axis that is parallel to the direction of the main magnetic field, then we can measure only B_z. Hence, measuring all of the three components of $\mathbf{B} = (B_x, B_y, B_z)$ necessitates mechanical rotations of the subject within the MRI machine [Scott *et al.* (1991); Eyuboglu *et al.* (1998); Gamba and Delfy (1998)]. To obtain B_x and B_y, we must rotate the subject as shown in Figure 3.23. Figure 3.23(a) is the initial setup to measure B_z. In Figure 3.23(b), we rotate the subject so that the x-direction becomes parallel to the direction of the main magnetic field. This enables us to obtain B_x by repeating the procedure in Section 3.3 with the same injection current I. With another rotation shown in Figure 3.23(c), we can get B_y.

Once we have measured all three components of $\mathbf{B}$, we can obtain a current density image (CDI) $\mathbf{J}$ in the subject Ω. From $\mathbf{J} = \nabla \times \mathbf{B}/\mu_0$, we compute $\mathbf{J} = (J_x, J_y, J_z)$ as

$$J_x = \frac{1}{\mu_0}\left(\frac{\partial B_z}{\partial y} - \frac{\partial B_y}{\partial z}\right), \quad J_y = \frac{1}{\mu_0}\left(\frac{\partial B_x}{\partial z} - \frac{\partial B_z}{\partial x}\right)$$

and

$$J_z = \frac{1}{\mu_0}\left(\frac{\partial B_y}{\partial x} - \frac{\partial B_x}{\partial y}\right). \tag{3.54}$$

Since we should differentiate B_z with respect to x and y, it is enough to acquire one phase image for B_z from the center slice S_c

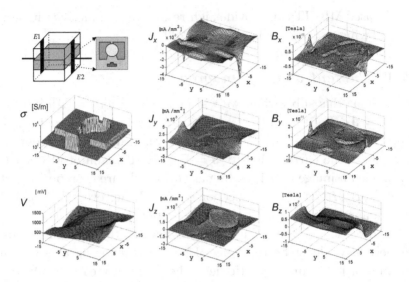

Fig. 3.22.   Images of $u, \mathbf{B}, \mathbf{J}$.

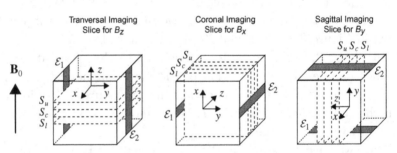

Fig. 3.23.   Subject rotations to measure all three components of $\mathbf{B} = (B_x, B_y, B_z)$.

in Figure 3.23(a). We must differentiate B_x and B_y with respect to z as well as y and x, respectively. This requires us to obtain three magnetic flux density images from three slices of S_u, S_c and S_l for each of B_x and B_y in Figure 3.23(b) and (c), respectively. Therefore, we need to acquire seven magnetic flux density images from three slices to compute $\mathbf{J} = (J_x, J_y, J_z)$ in (3.54).

3.7.1.1 *Recovering a transversal current density* $\mathbf{J}$ *having* $J_z = 0$ *using* B_z

This subsection presents a method of recovering a transversal current density $\mathbf{J}$ having $J_z = 0$ within a thin slice to be imaged from the measured B_z data.

Let Ω_s denote a cut of the subject Ω by an xy-plane $\{z = s\}$. A thin slice $\tilde{\Omega}$ to be imaged could be $\tilde{\Omega} = \cup_{-a<s<a}\Omega_s$ for some small $s > 0$. If the conductivity of the subject Ω does not change much in z-direction, we could produce approximately a transversal internal current density $\mathbf{J}$, that is, $\mathbf{J} \approx (J_x, J_y, 0)$ in the cylindrical chop $\tilde{\Omega}$ using long longitudinal electrodes.

We can express B_z as

$$B_z(\mathbf{r}) = \underbrace{-\frac{\mu_0}{4\pi} \int_{\tilde{\Omega}} \frac{\langle \mathbf{r} - \mathbf{r}', \mathbf{J}(\mathbf{r}') \times \hat{\mathbf{z}} \rangle}{|\mathbf{r} - \mathbf{r}'|^3} \, d\mathbf{r}'}_{B_z^{\tilde{\Omega}}} + G(\mathbf{r}) \quad \text{for } \mathbf{r} \in \Omega,$$

(3.55)

where

$$G(\mathbf{r}) = B_z^{\Omega \setminus \tilde{\Omega}} + B_z^{\mathcal{E}} + B_z^{\mathcal{L}}.$$

See (3.27) for the notation of B_z^{Region}.

Proposition 3.4. *If* $\mathbf{J} \cdot \hat{\mathbf{z}} = 0$ *in* $\tilde{\Omega}$, *then there exists a scalar function* w *such that*

$$\mathbf{J} = \left(\frac{\partial w}{\partial y}, -\frac{\partial w}{\partial x}, 0 \right) \quad \text{and} \quad \nabla^2 \left(w - \frac{1}{\mu_0} B_z \right) = 0 \quad \text{in } \tilde{\Omega}.$$

(3.56)

Proof. Since $\nabla \cdot \mathbf{J} = 0$ in Ω, we have

$$\nabla \times (\mathbf{J} \times \hat{\mathbf{z}}) = 0 \quad \text{in } \tilde{\Omega}.$$

From the Holmholtz decomposition, there is a function w in $\tilde{\Omega}$ such that

$$-\nabla w(\mathbf{r}) = \mathbf{J} \times \hat{\mathbf{z}}, \quad \text{in } \tilde{\Omega}.$$

Substituting $-\nabla w(\mathbf{r}) = \mathbf{J} \times \hat{\mathbf{z}}$ into (3.55) yields

$$B_z(\mathbf{r}) = \frac{\mu_0}{4\pi} \int_{\tilde{\Omega}} \frac{(\mathbf{r} - \mathbf{r}') \cdot \nabla w(\mathbf{r}')}{|\mathbf{r} - \mathbf{r}'|^3} d\mathbf{r}' + G(\mathbf{r}). \qquad (3.57)$$

Using the fact that $-\nabla^2(\frac{1}{4\pi|\mathbf{r}-\mathbf{r}'|}) = \delta(\mathbf{r} - \mathbf{r}')$, integrating by part yields

$$B_z(\mathbf{r}) = \mu_0 w(\mathbf{r}) - \frac{\mu_0}{4\pi} \int_{\partial\tilde{\Omega}} \frac{(\mathbf{r} - \mathbf{r}') \cdot \mathbf{n}(\mathbf{r}')}{|\mathbf{r} - \mathbf{r}'|^3} \mathbf{w}(\mathbf{r}') dS\mathbf{r}' + G(\mathbf{r})$$

$$(3.58)$$

for $\mathbf{r} \in \tilde{\Omega}$. It is easy to see that G and the boundary integral in the right side of the above equality are harmonic in $\tilde{\Omega}$ because $\nabla^2(|\mathbf{r} - \mathbf{r}'|^{-1}) = 0$ for $\mathbf{r} \in \tilde{\Omega}$ and $\mathbf{r}' \in \mathbb{R}^3 \backslash \tilde{\Omega}$. Therefore, $B_z - \mu_0 w$ is harmonic in $\tilde{\Omega}$. □

According to Proposition 3.4, the transversal current $\mathbf{J}$ can be expressed by

$$\mathbf{J} \times \hat{\mathbf{z}} = \frac{-1}{\mu_0}\nabla B_z + \text{Harmonic} \quad \text{in } \tilde{\Omega}.$$

Since a harmonic function is determined by its boundary conditions, we can compute $\mathbf{J}$ as

$$J_x = -\frac{1}{\mu_0}\frac{\partial}{\partial y}B_z + \frac{\partial\eta}{\partial y}, \quad J_x = \frac{1}{\mu_0}\frac{\partial}{\partial y}B_z - \frac{\partial\eta}{\partial x} \qquad (3.59)$$

where η is a harmonic function in $\tilde{\Omega}$ with its Neumann boundary condition $\mathbf{n} \cdot (\mathbf{J} \times \hat{\mathbf{z}} = \frac{1}{\mu_0}\nabla B_z)$.

The CDI method in (3.59) is based on the assumption that a two-dimensional current is produced in a thin imaging slice by an appropriate external injection current and electrodes. Hence, the presence of out-of-plane current in the imaging slice deteriorates the accuracy of the reconstructed image and several numerical experiments can manifest this effect. The injection current provided by long longitudinal electrodes may produce an internal current density $\mathbf{J}$ such that its longitudinal component J_z within a thin transversal slice near the middle of the electrodes is negligible. In such a case, (3.59) provides current density. However, out-of-plane current J_z increases as the longitudinal length of the electrodes decreases and also as the conductivity distribution changes significantly along z-direction. For subjects like human limbs with long electrodes, we can safely assume that $J_z \approx 0$ where z is the longitudinal direction of each limb.

3.7.2 *Early MREIT algorithms*

The first conductivity image reconstruction algorithm in MREIT was based on the line integral technique. [Zhang (1992)] proposed a conductivity image reconstruction algorithm utilizing the measurement of internal $\mathbf{J}$ and many boundary voltages. The method is based on the relationship, $V_{1,2} = \int_C \frac{1}{\sigma} \mathbf{J} \cdot \mathbf{dl}$ where $V_{1,2}$ is the voltage difference between two locations 1 and 2 at the boundary; C is an interior line integral path connecting 1 and 2. After discretization of an imaging slice into M pixels, we can construct a linear system of equation $\mathbf{V}_{N \times 1} = \mathbf{G}_{N \times M} \mathbf{S}_{M \times 1}$ where $\mathbf{V}$ is a vector of N boundary voltage measurements, $\mathbf{S}$ a vector of conductivity values from M pixels and $\mathbf{N}$ a noise vector in measured voltages. Assuming that we have obtained current density at every pixel, the matrix $\mathbf{G}$ contains internal current density data and we can reconstruct the conductivity image $\mathbf{S}$ by solving the linear system of equations. A drawback of this method is the requirement of many boundary voltage measurements to improve the accuracy and spatial resolution of the conductivity image.

[Woo *et al.* (1994)] proposed a different method where the error between the measured and computed current density is minimized as a function of σ of a finite element model of the imaging object. They used a sensitivity matrix relating the measured current density to changes in conductivity values. [Ider and Birgul (1998)] suggested a method based on a sensitivity matrix between the magnetic flux density and conductivity. They used the singular value decomposition to reconstruct conductivity images. [Eyuboglu *et al.* (2001)] used an FEM with measured boundary voltages and injection current as boundary conditions. Their method is iterative assuming an initial guess on the conductivity distribution. For a given conductivity distribution of the model, they computed internal current density using FEM and updated the conductivity distribution to minimize the error between this current density and the measured one. These early algorithms initiated the MREIT research to develop more effective and practically applicable new algorithms.

3.7.3 J-substitution algorithm

Assuming that measured data of $\mathbf{J}_1$ and $\mathbf{J}_2$ are available, σ can be expressed as

$$\sigma = \frac{|\mathbf{J}_1|}{|\nabla u_1|} = \frac{|\mathbf{J}_2|}{|\nabla u_2|}$$

where $u_j = u_j[\sigma]$ is a solution of (3.24). The main idea of the J-substitution algorithm is that the potential u_j is viewed as a solution of non-linear PDE [Kwon *et al.* (2002a)]

$$\nabla \cdot \left(\frac{|\mathbf{J}_j|}{|\nabla u_j|} \nabla u_j \right) = 0 \quad \text{in } \Omega \tag{3.60}$$

with the same boundary conditions in (3.24).

Remark 3.7 (Non-uniqueness). We should note that the non-linear PDE (3.60) with a standard boundary condition may have infinite solutions. For example, in the case when $|\mathbf{J}| = 1$ and $\Omega = [0,1] \times [0,1] \times [0,1]$, the following boundary value problem has infinite solutions including $u = x, x^2, x^2, x^4, \ldots$:

$$\begin{cases} \nabla \cdot \left(\dfrac{1}{|\nabla u|} \nabla u \right) = 0 \quad \text{in } \Omega \\[2mm] u(0,y,z) = 0, \quad u(1,y,z) = 1 \quad \text{for } (x,y) \in [0,1] \times [0,1] \\[2mm] \dfrac{\partial u}{\partial \mathbf{n}} = 0 \quad \text{on the other boundaries.} \end{cases}$$

$$\tag{3.61}$$

Remark 3.8 (Non-uniqueness). For any strictly increasing function $\varphi : \mathbb{R} \to \mathbb{R}$, $\nabla \varphi(u_j) = \varphi'(u_j) \nabla u_j$ and $\varphi'(u_j) > 0$. Hence,

$$\nabla \cdot \left(\frac{|\mathbf{J}_j|}{|\nabla \varphi(u_j)|} \nabla \varphi(u_j) \right) = \nabla \cdot \left(\frac{|\mathbf{J}_j|}{|\nabla u_j|} \nabla u_j \right) = 0. \tag{3.62}$$

If u_j is a solution of (3.60), then $\varphi(u_j)$ is also a solution of (3.60). This means that there are infinite conductivities producing the same $\mathbf{J}_1$ as shown in Figure 3.21.

As mentioned in Section 3.6.2.2, the uniqueness of a reconstructed conductivity image requires two injection currents I_1 and I_2. [Kown et al. (2002)] suggested the following coupled system:

$$
\begin{cases}
\nabla \cdot \left(\dfrac{|\mathbf{J}_j|}{|\nabla u_j|} \nabla u_j \right) = 0 & \text{in } \Omega, \quad j = 1, 2 \\[2ex]
\dfrac{|\mathbf{J}_1|}{|\nabla u_1|} = \dfrac{|\mathbf{J}_2|}{|\nabla u_2|} & \text{in } \Omega \\[2ex]
-\dfrac{|\mathbf{J}_j|}{|\nabla u_j|} \nabla u_j \cdot \mathbf{n} = g_j & \text{on } \partial\Omega, \quad j = 1, 2 \\[2ex]
u_j(\mathbf{r}_0) = 0, \quad \dfrac{|\mathbf{J}_j(\mathbf{r}_0)|}{|\nabla u_j(\mathbf{r}_0)|} = 1 &
\end{cases}
\tag{3.63}
$$

where g_j is the corresponding Neumann boundary condition to the injection current I_j and $\mathbf{r}_0$ is a point on $\partial\Omega$.

The second coupling identity connecting u_1 and u_2 in (3.63) stems from the fact that the change of σ due to different injection currents is negligible. The last condition in (3.63) is for fixing the scaling uncertainty that corresponds to the normalization of conductivity values with $\sigma(\mathbf{r}_0) = 1$:

$$
\frac{|\mathbf{J}_j(\mathbf{r}_0)|}{|\nabla u_j(\mathbf{r}_0)|} = 1 \Leftrightarrow \sigma(\mathbf{r}_0) = 1.
$$

In practice, we may attach a small piece of conductive material with a known conductivity value at the point $\mathbf{r}_0$ and image the subject including it. As explained in Section 3.6.2.1, we need to fix the scaling uncertainty by either measuring a voltage difference or specifying conductivity at one point $\mathbf{r}_0 \in \partial\Omega$.

The J-substitution algorithm is a natural iterative scheme of the coupled system (3.63). After [Kwon et al. (2002a)] first introduced the J-substitution algorithm and provided its numerical simulations, [Khang et al. (2002)] and [Lee et al. (2003a)] applied it to reconstruct conductivity images of saline phantoms. The fundamental questions such as the uniqueness of the coupled MREIT system itself and the convergence of the algorithm have been studied by [Kim et al. (2004)].

3.7.3.1 J-*substitution: Uniqueness*

We will discuss the desired uniqueness which implies that the conductivity is uniquely decided by two measurements of $\mathbf{J}_1$ and $\mathbf{J}_2$ for both two- and three-dimensional space. For ease of explanation, let $(u_1, u_2) \in H^1(\Omega) \times H^1(\Omega)$ be the solution of (3.63) and $\mathbf{J}_j = -\sigma \nabla u_j$. We assume that

$$\mathbf{J}_1(\mathbf{r}) \times \mathbf{J}_2(\mathbf{r}) \neq 0 \quad \text{for all } \mathbf{r} \in \Omega. \tag{3.64}$$

This could be possible by a suitable arrangement of electrodes $\mathcal{E}_1^\pm$, $\mathcal{E}_2^\pm$ (or proper Neumann data g_1 and g_2).

Theorem 3.4 (Uniqueness). *Assume that* $(\tilde{u}_1, \tilde{u}_2) \in H^1(\Omega) \times H^1(\Omega)$ *is a pair of solutions of the system* (3.63) *and* $|\nabla \tilde{u}_j(\mathbf{r})| \neq 0$ *for all* $\mathbf{r} \in \Omega$, $j = 1, 2$. *Then*

$$\sigma = \tilde{\sigma}, \quad u_j = \tilde{u}_j \quad in \ \Omega, \quad j = 1, 2. \tag{3.65}$$

Proof. Since u_j and $\tilde{u}_j$ have the same Neumann data g_j, we have

$$\int_\Omega (\sigma \nabla u_j - \tilde{\sigma} \nabla \tilde{u}_j) \cdot \nabla (u_j - \tilde{u}_j) dx = \int_{\partial \Omega} (g_j - g_j)(u_j - \tilde{u}_j) ds = 0.$$

Using $\tilde{\sigma} |\nabla \tilde{u}_j| = \sigma |\nabla u_j|$, the above identity becomes

$$0 = \int_\Omega \sigma |\nabla u_j| (|\nabla u_j| + |\nabla \tilde{u}_j|) \left(1 - \frac{\nabla u_j \cdot \nabla \tilde{u}_j}{|\nabla u_j| |\nabla \tilde{u}_j|} \right) dx.$$

Since each factor of the above integrand is non-negative, the whole integrand should be identically zero. Hence, it must be $\frac{\nabla u_j \cdot \nabla \tilde{u}_j}{|\nabla u_j| |\nabla \tilde{u}_j|} = 1$ which leads to

$$\frac{\nabla u_j}{|\nabla u_j|} = \frac{\nabla \tilde{u}_j}{|\nabla \tilde{u}_j|}. \tag{3.66}$$

Since $\nabla \times \nabla u_j = \mathbf{0}$,

$$\mathbf{0} = \nabla \times \left(\frac{1}{\sigma} \mathbf{J}_j \right) = \frac{1}{\sigma} (-\nabla \log \sigma \times \mathbf{J}_j + \nabla \times \mathbf{J}_j) \quad \text{in } \Omega \tag{3.67}$$

which leads to $\nabla \log \sigma \times \mathbf{J}_j = \nabla \times \mathbf{J}_j$, and similarly we have $\nabla \log \tilde{\sigma} \times \mathbf{J}_j = \nabla \times \mathbf{J}_j$ using the identity $\mathbf{J}_j = \tilde{\mathbf{J}}_j$. By taking the difference of these two identities, we have

$$\nabla\left(\log\frac{\sigma}{\bar{\sigma}}\right)\times \mathbf{J}_j = \mathbf{0} \quad \text{in } \Omega, \quad j = 1, 2. \tag{3.68}$$

Setting $\eta(x) = \log\frac{\sigma(x)}{\bar{\sigma}(x)}$, we will show $\eta = 0$ in Ω. Let $\mathbf{J}_j = (a_1^j, a_2^j, a_3^j)$. The linear independence between $\mathbf{J}^1$ and $\mathbf{J}^2$ leads that for each $\mathbf{r} \in \Omega$ at least one of the following three matrix should be invertible:

$$A_1(\mathbf{r}) := \begin{pmatrix} a_2^1(\mathbf{r}) & a_3^1(\mathbf{r}) \\ a_2^2(\mathbf{r}) & a_3^2(\mathbf{r}) \end{pmatrix}, \quad A_2(\mathbf{r}) := \begin{pmatrix} a_3^1(\mathbf{r}) & a_1^1(\mathbf{r}) \\ a_3^2(\mathbf{r}) & a_1^2(\mathbf{r}) \end{pmatrix},$$

$$A_3(\mathbf{r}) := \begin{pmatrix} a_1^1(\mathbf{r}) & a_2^1(\mathbf{r}) \\ a_1^2(\mathbf{r}) & a_2^2(\mathbf{r}) \end{pmatrix}, \quad \mathbf{r} \in \Omega. \tag{3.69}$$

Moreover, (3.68) implies that

$$A_1(\mathbf{r})\begin{pmatrix} -\dfrac{\partial}{\partial z}\eta(\mathbf{r}) \\ \dfrac{\partial}{\partial y}\eta(\mathbf{r}) \end{pmatrix} = \begin{pmatrix} 0 \\ 0 \end{pmatrix}, \quad A_2(\mathbf{r})\begin{pmatrix} -\dfrac{\partial}{\partial x}\eta(\mathbf{r}) \\ \dfrac{\partial}{\partial z}\eta(\mathbf{r}) \end{pmatrix} = \begin{pmatrix} 0 \\ 0 \end{pmatrix},$$

$$A_3(\mathbf{r})\begin{pmatrix} -\dfrac{\partial}{\partial y}\eta(\mathbf{r}) \\ \dfrac{\partial}{\partial x}\eta(\mathbf{r}) \end{pmatrix} = \begin{pmatrix} 0 \\ 0 \end{pmatrix}, \quad \mathbf{r} \in \Omega. \tag{3.70}$$

Now, we are ready to prove that $\nabla\eta(\mathbf{r}) = \mathbf{0}$ for all $\mathbf{r} \in \Omega$. Since at least one $A_j(\mathbf{r})$ is invertible, without loss of generality we assume that $A_1(\mathbf{r})$ is invertible. According to (3.70), we have

$$\frac{\partial}{\partial y}\eta(\mathbf{r}) = 0 \quad \text{and} \quad \frac{\partial}{\partial z}\eta(\mathbf{r}) = 0$$

and

$$A_2(\mathbf{r})\begin{pmatrix} -\dfrac{\partial}{\partial x}\eta(\mathbf{r}) \\ 0 \end{pmatrix} = \begin{pmatrix} 0 \\ 0 \end{pmatrix} = A_3(\mathbf{r})\begin{pmatrix} 0 \\ \dfrac{\partial}{\partial x}\eta(\mathbf{r}) \end{pmatrix},$$

which is equivalent to

$$A_1(\mathbf{r}) \begin{pmatrix} \dfrac{\partial}{\partial x}\eta(\mathbf{r}) \\ -\dfrac{\partial}{\partial x}\eta(\mathbf{r}) \end{pmatrix} = \begin{pmatrix} 0 \\ 0 \end{pmatrix}.$$

The invertibility of $A_1(\mathbf{r})$ yields $\frac{\partial}{\partial x}\eta(\mathbf{r}) = 0$. Hence, we have $\nabla\eta(\mathbf{r}) = \mathbf{0}$ for all $\mathbf{r} \in \Omega$. Due to $\sigma(\mathbf{r}_0) = 1 = \tilde{\sigma}(\mathbf{r}_0)$, we have $\eta(\mathbf{r}) = 0$ or $\sigma(\mathbf{r}) = \tilde{\sigma}(\mathbf{r})$ for all $\mathbf{r} \in \Omega$.

Since $\sigma = \tilde{\sigma}$, u_j and $\tilde{u}_j$ are solutions of the same elliptic PDE with the same Neumann data and, hence the uniqueness of the Neumann problem implies $u_j = \tilde{u}_j$. This completes the proof. □

3.7.3.2 J-substitution algorithm: Iterative scheme

The **J-substitution** algorithm is a natural iterative scheme of the coupled system (3.63). Using the **J-substitution** MREIT model (3.63), we may design an iterative J-substitution algorithm as follows:

(1) Initial guess $\sigma_0 = 1$.
(2) For each $n = 0, 1, \ldots$, solve

$$\begin{cases} \nabla \cdot (\sigma_n \nabla u_1^n) = 0 & \text{in } \Omega \\ \sigma_n \dfrac{\partial u_1^n}{\partial \nu} = g_1 & \text{on } \partial\Omega, \quad u_1^n(\mathbf{r}_0) = 0. \end{cases}$$

(3) Update the conductivity using

$$\sigma_{n+1/2}(\mathbf{r}) = C_n \frac{|\mathbf{J}_1(\mathbf{r})|}{|\nabla u_1^n(\mathbf{r})|} \quad \text{with } C_n = \frac{|\nabla u_1^n(\mathbf{r}_0)|}{|\mathbf{J}_1(\mathbf{r}_0)|}.$$

(4) Solve

$$\begin{cases} \nabla \cdot (\sigma_{n+1/2} \nabla u_2^{n+1/2}) = 0 & \text{in } \Omega \\ \sigma_{n+1/2} \dfrac{\partial u_2^{n+1/2}}{\partial \nu} = g_2 & \text{on } \partial\Omega, \quad u_2^{n+1/2}(\mathbf{r}_0) = 0. \end{cases}$$

(5) Stop the process if $\||\mathbf{J}_2| - \sigma_{n+1/2}|\nabla u_2^{n+1/2}|\|_{L^2(\Omega)} < \epsilon$ where ϵ is a given tolerance.

(6) Update the conductivity using

$$\sigma_{n+1}(\mathbf{r}) = C_{n+1/2} \frac{|\mathbf{J}_2(\mathbf{r})|}{|\nabla u_2^{n+1/2}(\mathbf{r})|} \quad \text{with } C_{n+1/2} = \frac{|\nabla u_2^{n+1/2}(\mathbf{r}_0)|}{|\mathbf{J}_2(\mathbf{r}_0)|}.$$

In this iterative method, we start with the homogeneous initial guess. We can easily obtain the boundary shape of the subject since MR images are available.

In the $\mathbf{J}$-substitution algorithm, we use only the magnitude of the current density vector for the following reasons. When two pairs of electrodes are used, the magnitude information is sufficient to guarantee the uniqueness of the reconstructed conductivity image as far as $\mathbf{J}_1 \times \mathbf{J}_2 \neq 0$. Thus, for noise-free current density data, the reconstructed image using only the magnitude must be the same as the image using the direction as well. Numerical simulations show convergence characteristics good enough for most highly complicated conductivity distributions that we can face in medical applications. We also observe that any reasonable initial guesses make the algorithm convergent to the degree needed for successful image reconstructions. The $\mathbf{J}$-substitution algorithm does not require a non-linear least squares optimization such as Newton-type algorithms. Since it requires simple substitutions, it only needs a fast-forward solver.

3.8   MREIT Without Subject Rotation

The $\mathbf{J}$-based MREIT has practical difficulties in imaging experiments because the process of rotating the imaging object implies other technical difficulties such as pixel misalignments, movement of internal organs and distortion of boundary geometry in addition to the simple fact that there is no room to rotate a large object inside the MRI scanner. To avoid the rotation process, we should use only B_z data to reconstruct conductivity images.

In order to eliminate the problem related with rotations, we should find a B_z-based MREIT algorithm (conductivity imaging using only B_z data). Until 2000, conductivity imaging using only B_z data seemed impossible. According to Maxwell's equations, the current density is directly related to the three components of the magnetic flux density $\mathbf{B}$ and the conductivity must be computed from the relationship between the current density and the electrical field. Hence, most researchers consider that B_z data is insufficient for conductivity image reconstructions.

In 2001, [Seo *et al.* (2003a)] developed a constructive B_z-based MREIT algorithm called the harmonic B_z algorithm, and its numerical simulations and phantom experiments showed that high-resolution conductivity imaging is possible without rotating the object [Seo *et al.* (2003a); Oh *et al.* (2003, 2004, 2005)]. Since then, imaging techniques in MREIT have been advanced rapidly and now reached the stage of *in vivo* animal and human imaging experiments [Park *et al.* (2004a, b); Seo *et al.* (2004); Kwon *et al.* (2005); Oh *et al.* (2005); Liu *et al.* (2006, 2007)]. This section discusses the harmonic B_z algorithm and its variations based on two review papers [Woo and Seo (2008); Seo and Woo (2011)].

3.8.1 *Harmonic B_z algorithm*

The harmonic B_z algorithm [Seo *et al.* (2003a)] is based on the following key observations:

- The Laplacian of B_z data probes changes in the logarithm of the conductivity distribution along any equipotential curve in each imaging slice.
- With a suitable arrangement of four electrodes $\mathcal{E}_1^{\pm}, \mathcal{E}_2^{\pm}$, there exists an exact representation formula[3] of σ using two data $B_{z,1}$ and $B_{z,2}$.
- The representation formula of σ can be somewhat explicit (to some degree) by taking advantage of the fact that the overall flow of the current density is insensitive to local perturbations in the conductivity distribution, which behaves as a drawback in EIT.

From Ampère's law $\mathbf{J}_j = \frac{1}{\mu_0} \nabla \times \mathbf{B}_j$,

$$\mu_0 \nabla \times \mathbf{J}_j = \nabla \times \nabla \times \mathbf{B}_j = -\nabla^2 \mathbf{B}_j + \nabla \underbrace{\nabla \cdot \mathbf{B}_j}_{=0} = -\nabla^2 \mathbf{B}. \qquad (3.71)$$

---

[3]The representation formula of σ in terms of $B_{z,1}$ and $B_{z,2}$ exists in an implicit form due to the non-linear relationship between the conductivity and the measured data.

On the other hand, $\nabla \times \mathbf{J}_j$ can be expressed as

$$\nabla \times \mathbf{J}_j = -\nabla \times [\sigma \nabla u_j] = -\nabla \sigma \times \nabla u_j - \underbrace{\sigma \nabla \times \nabla u}_{=0}. \tag{3.72}$$

Combining (3.71) and (3.72), we have

$$\frac{1}{\mu_0} \nabla^2 B_{z,j} = \hat{\mathbf{z}} \cdot \nabla \sigma \times \nabla u_j = \mathbf{d} \cdot \nabla \sigma \quad (\mathbf{d}(\mathbf{r}) := \hat{\mathbf{z}} \times \nabla u_j(\mathbf{r})).$$
$$\tag{3.73}$$

The above formula provides how the distribution of $\nabla^2 B_z$ traces a change of σ:

- If $B_{z,j}$ is convex at $\mathbf{r}$, then $\sigma(\mathbf{r}) \nearrow$ in $\mathbf{d}(\mathbf{r})$-direction.
- If $B_{z,j}$ is concave at $\mathbf{r}$, then $\sigma(\mathbf{r}) \searrow$ in $\mathbf{d}(\mathbf{r})$-direction.
- If $\nabla^2 B_{z,j}(\mathbf{r}) = 0$, then $\sigma(\mathbf{r})$ does not change in $\mathbf{d}(\mathbf{r})$-direction.

To be precise, let $\boldsymbol{\zeta} : (0,1) \to \Omega$ be a vector-valued function such that

$$\frac{d}{dt} \boldsymbol{\zeta}(t) = \mathbf{J}_j(\boldsymbol{\zeta}(t)) \times \hat{\mathbf{z}}.$$

Then, the identity $\nabla^2 B_{z,j} = \nabla \ln \sigma \cdot (\mathbf{J}_j \times \hat{\mathbf{z}})$ is equivalent to

$$\frac{d}{dt} \ln \sigma(\boldsymbol{\zeta}(t)) = \nabla^2 B_{z,j}(\boldsymbol{\zeta}(t)) \quad (\forall\, t \in (0,1)). \tag{3.74}$$

The vector field $\sigma \nabla u_j \times \hat{\mathbf{z}}$ is a non-linear function of the unknown conductivity σ, and hence its estimation without knowledge of σ is necessary. Fortunately, numerous experiences show that the overall vector flow of the current density $\mathbf{J}_j = -\sigma \nabla u_j$ is mostly dictated by given positions of electrodes $\mathcal{E}_j^{\pm}$, amount of injection current I, and geometry of the boundary $\partial \Omega$, while the influence of changes in σ on $\mathbf{J}_j$ is relatively small. This is one of the major drawbacks of EIT. However, the harmonic B_z method takes advantage of this fact to make the algorithm work.

Based on the observations above, two data $B_{z,1}$ and $B_{z,2}$ probe a change of σ on the slice Ω_{z_0} in both directions of $\mathbf{J}_1$ and $\mathbf{J}_2$. If $(\mathbf{J}_1 \times \mathbf{J}_2) \cdot \hat{\mathbf{z}} \neq 0$ in Ω_{z_0}, we can perceive a transversal change of σ on the slice Ω_{z_0}. It is desirable to attach four surface electrodes so that, in the imaging region, the area of parallelogram made by two vectors

$\mathbf{J}_1 \times \hat{\mathbf{z}}$ and $\mathbf{J}_2 \times \hat{\mathbf{z}}$ is as large as possible. This is the main reason why we usually use two pairs of surface electrodes $\mathcal{E}_1^{\pm}$ and $\mathcal{E}_2^{\pm}$.

3.8.1.1 *Mathematical model and corresponding inverse problem*

We define a map $\Lambda : \mathcal{A} \to H^1(\Omega) \times H^1(\Omega) \times \mathbb{R}$ by

$$\Lambda[\sigma](\mathbf{r}) = \begin{pmatrix} \dfrac{\mu_0}{4\pi} \displaystyle\int_\Omega \dfrac{\langle \mathbf{r} - \mathbf{r}', \sigma \nabla u_1[\sigma](\mathbf{r}') \times \hat{\mathbf{z}} \rangle}{|\mathbf{r} - \mathbf{r}'|^3} \, d\mathbf{r}' \\[2ex] \dfrac{\mu_0}{4\pi} \displaystyle\int_\Omega \dfrac{\langle \mathbf{r} - \mathbf{r}', \sigma \nabla u_2[\sigma](\mathbf{r}') \times \hat{\mathbf{z}} \rangle}{|\mathbf{r} - \mathbf{r}'|^3} \, d\mathbf{r}' \\[2ex] u_1[\sigma]\big|_{\mathcal{E}_2^+} - u_1[\sigma]\big|_{\mathcal{E}_2^-} \end{pmatrix}, \quad \mathbf{r} \in \Omega. \tag{3.75}$$

We should note that, according to (3.46),

$$\Lambda[\sigma](\mathbf{r}) = (B_{z,1}^\Omega(\mathbf{r}),\ B_{z,2}^\Omega(\mathbf{r}),\ V_{12}^{\pm}) \quad (\forall\,\mathbf{r} \in \Omega) \tag{3.76}$$

where $V_{12}^{\pm}$ is the voltage difference $u_1[\sigma]$ between the electrodes $\mathcal{E}_2^+$ and $\mathcal{E}_2^-$, that is, $V_{12}^{\pm} = u_1[\sigma]\big|_{\mathcal{E}_2^+} - u_1[\sigma]\big|_{\mathcal{E}_2^-}$. Since $B_{z,j}^\Omega = B_{z,j} + harmonic$, the first two components of $\Lambda[\sigma]$ are available up to harmonic factors. Recall that the harmonic term $B_{z,j} - \Lambda[\sigma]$ depends only on configuration of lead wires and electrodes and does not depend on $\nabla \sigma$ inside Ω. Since computation of $B_{z,j} - \Lambda_j[\sigma]$ is quite difficult, it would be desirable to eliminate the harmonic terms in any image reconstruction algorithm. Recall that if $\nabla^2 B_{z,j} = 0$ in Ω, σ does not change in the direction $\hat{\mathbf{z}} \times \mathbf{J}_j$. If $\nabla^2 B_{z,1} = 0$, $\nabla^2 B_{z,2} = 0$, and $(\mathbf{J}_1 \times \mathbf{J}_2) \cdot \hat{\mathbf{z}} \neq 0$ in Ω, then σ is constant on each slice Ω_{z_0}. Therefore, the harmonic terms are not an important issue in reconstructing the conductivity image. This means that the Laplacian $\nabla^2 \Lambda_j[\sigma] = \nabla^2 B_{z,j}$ $(j = 1, 2)$ conveys the same information on σ (up to constants) as the data $B_{z,j}$ $(j = 1, 2)$.

The inverse problem of MREIT is to invert the map $\Lambda : \sigma \to (B_{z,1}^\Omega, B_{z,2}^\Omega, V_{12}^{\pm})$. The uniqueness is a very important issue even in a practical sense because in the absence of the uniqueness we never know whether the reconstructed solution is close to the true one or not. The uniqueness of the conductivity can be obtained by showing that $\Lambda[\sigma] = \Lambda[\tilde{\sigma}]$ implies $\sigma = \tilde{\sigma}$.

Since $\nabla^2 B_{z,j}$ probes the change of σ in the direction $\hat{\mathbf{z}} \times \mathbf{J}_j$, the following condition is essential for the uniqueness:

$$|(\mathbf{J}_1(\mathbf{r}) \times \mathbf{J}_2(\mathbf{r})) \cdot \hat{\mathbf{z}}| > 0 \quad \text{for } \mathbf{r} \in \Omega. \tag{3.77}$$

However, this issue related to (3.77) in the third dimension is wide open, while there are some two-dimensional results based on the geometric index theory [Alessandrini and Magnanini (1992); Bauman *et al.* (2000); Seo (1996)]. In this section, we briefly explain the two-dimensional uniqueness.

3.8.1.2 *Two-dimensional MREIT model*

Two-dimensional MREIT models occur when the imaging object is locally cylindrical and $\frac{\partial \sigma}{\partial z} \approx 0$. For such an object, we may produce a transversally dominating current density $\mathbf{J}$ inside a truncated cylindrical region by using longitudinal electrodes. This two-dimensional problem has some practical meaning because many parts of the human body are locally cylindrical in their shape.

By the two-dimensional MREIT model, we mean the following:

(1) The subject to be imaged is a cylinder described by the set $\{(x, y, z) : (x, y) \in \Omega, -a < z < a\}$ where Ω is a two-dimensional domain occupying the cross-section of the cylinder.
(2) $\frac{\partial \sigma}{\partial z} = 0$ in the cylindrical subject.
(3) Using longitudinal electrodes $\mathcal{E}_1^{\pm}$ and $\mathcal{E}_2^{\pm}$, the corresponding voltages $u_1[\sigma]$ and $u_2[\sigma]$ in (3.24) are independent to z.

Theorem 3.5 (Uniqueness). *Under the assumption of the two-dimensional MREIT model, the map* $\Lambda : \mathcal{A} \to H^1(\Omega) \times H^1(\Omega) \times \mathbb{R}$ *in* (3.75) *is one-to-one.*

Proof. It suffices to prove that $\Lambda[\sigma] = \Lambda[\tilde{\sigma}]$ implies $\sigma = \tilde{\sigma}$. By taking the Laplacian of $\Lambda_j[\sigma] = \Lambda_j[\tilde{\sigma}], j = 1, 2$, we have

$$\mu_0 \nabla \cdot [\sigma \nabla u_j \times \hat{\mathbf{z}}] = \nabla^2 \Lambda_j[\sigma] = \nabla^2 \Lambda_j[\tilde{\sigma}] = \mu_0 \nabla \cdot [\tilde{\sigma} \nabla \tilde{u}_j \times \hat{\mathbf{z}}] \quad \text{in } \Omega$$

where $u_j = u_j[\sigma]$ and $\tilde{u}_j = u_j[\tilde{\sigma}]$.

The above identity leads to $\nabla \cdot [\sigma \nabla u_j \times \hat{\mathbf{z}} - \tilde{\sigma} \nabla \tilde{u}_j \times \hat{\mathbf{z}}] = 0$ which can be rewritten as

$$0 = \nabla_{xy} \times \left(\sigma \frac{\partial u_j}{\partial x} - \tilde{\sigma} \frac{\partial \tilde{u}_j}{\partial x}, \, \sigma \frac{\partial u_j}{\partial y} - \tilde{\sigma} \frac{\partial \tilde{u}_j}{\partial y} \right)$$

where $\nabla_{xy} = (\frac{\partial}{\partial x}, \frac{\partial}{\partial y})$ is the two-dimensional gradient. Hence, there exists a scalar function $\phi_j(\mathbf{r})$ such that

$$\nabla_{xy} \phi_j := \left(\sigma \frac{\partial u_j}{\partial x} - \tilde{\sigma} \frac{\partial \tilde{u}_j}{\partial x}, \, \sigma \frac{\partial u_j}{\partial y} - \tilde{\sigma} \frac{\partial \tilde{u}_j}{\partial y} \right) \quad \text{in } \Omega. \tag{3.78}$$

Then, ϕ_j satisfies the two-dimensional Laplace equation $\nabla_{xy}^2 \phi_j = 0$ in Ω with zero Neumann data, and hence ϕ_j is a constant function. Using $\sigma \nabla_{xy} u_j - \tilde{\sigma} \nabla_{xy} \tilde{u}_j = \nabla_{x,y} \phi^j = 0$ and (3.78), we can derive

$$\begin{bmatrix} \sigma \dfrac{\partial u_1}{\partial x} & -\sigma \dfrac{\partial u_1}{\partial y} \\[2mm] \sigma \dfrac{\partial u_2}{\partial x} & -\sigma \dfrac{\partial u_2}{\partial y} \end{bmatrix} \begin{bmatrix} \dfrac{\partial}{\partial y} \ln \dfrac{\sigma}{\tilde{\sigma}} \\[2mm] \dfrac{\partial}{\partial x} \ln \dfrac{\sigma}{\tilde{\sigma}} \end{bmatrix} = \begin{bmatrix} 0 \\[2mm] 0 \end{bmatrix} \quad \text{in } \Omega.$$

We can show that

$$A(\mathbf{r}) := \begin{bmatrix} \sigma \dfrac{\partial u_1}{\partial x}(\mathbf{r}) & -\sigma \dfrac{\partial u_1}{\partial y}(\mathbf{r}) \\[2mm] \sigma \dfrac{\partial u_2}{\partial x}(\mathbf{r}) & -\sigma \dfrac{\partial u_2}{\partial y}(\mathbf{r}) \end{bmatrix} \quad \text{is invertible for all } \mathbf{r} \in \Omega.$$

$$\tag{3.79}$$

The proof of (3.79) is based on the geometric theory in [Alessandrini and Magnanini (1992); Alessandrini and Nesi (2001)]. We will defer the proof.

Under the assumption of (3.79), $\ln \frac{\sigma}{\tilde{\sigma}}$ is constant or $\sigma = c\tilde{\sigma}$ for a scaling constant c. From the condition that $u_1|_{\mathcal{E}_2^+} - u_1|_{\mathcal{E}_2^-} = \Lambda_3[\sigma] = \Lambda_3[\tilde{\sigma}] = \tilde{u}_1|_{\mathcal{E}_2^+} - \tilde{u}_1|_{\mathcal{E}_2^-}$, we have $c = 1$ which leads to $\sigma = \tilde{\sigma}$.

It remains to prove (3.79). It suffices to prove that $|\det A(P)| > 0$ for all $P \in \Omega$. To derive a contradiction, we assume that there is a point $P_0 = (x_0, y_0) \in \Omega$ such that $\det(\mathbb{A}[\sigma](P_0)) = 0$. Then $\nabla u_1[\sigma](P_0) \times \nabla u_2[\sigma](P_0) = 0$, and there is a non-zero constant vector (α, β) such that $\alpha \nabla u_1[\sigma](P_0) = \beta \nabla u_2[\sigma](P_0)$. Setting $w = \alpha u_1[\sigma] -$

$\beta u_2[\sigma]$, w satisfies

$$\begin{cases} \nabla \cdot (\sigma \nabla w) = 0 & \text{in } \Omega \\ w|_{\mathcal{E}_1^+} = \alpha, \quad w|_{\mathcal{E}_2^+} = -\beta, \quad w|_{\mathcal{E}_1^- \cup \mathcal{E}_2^-} = 0 \\ \dfrac{\partial w}{\partial \mathbf{n}} = 0 \quad \text{on } \partial\Omega \backslash \overline{\mathcal{E}_1^+ \cup \mathcal{E}_1^- \cup \mathcal{E}_2^+ \cup \mathcal{E}_2^-}. \end{cases} \quad (3.80)$$

Since (α, β) is non-zero, w is not a constant. From the maximum principle and $\nabla w(P_0) = 0$, the level curve $\mathcal{C} := \{(x, y) \in \overline{\Omega} : w(x, y) = w(P_0)\}$ divides Ω into at least four regions. For simplicity, we assume that the level curve $\mathcal{C}$ divides Ω into k pieces $\Omega_1, \Omega_2, \ldots, \Omega_k$ and use the same notation Ω_4 to denote $\Omega_4 := \Omega \backslash \overline{\Omega_1 \cup \Omega_2 \cup \Omega_3}$. It is easy to see that $\partial\Omega_j \cap \overline{\mathcal{E}_1^+ \cup \mathcal{E}_1^- \cup \mathcal{E}_2^+ \cup \mathcal{E}_2^-} \neq \emptyset$, otherwise w is a constant in Ω from the boundary conditions in (3.80) and the unique continuation property. Without loss of generality, we assume that $\Omega_1, \Omega_2, \ldots, \Omega_4$ are ordered counterclockwise with respect to P_0. By Hopf's boundary lemma with the maximum principle, there is at least one point $Q_j \in \partial\Omega \cap \partial\Omega_j$ such that $\frac{\partial w}{\partial n}(Q_j) \neq 0$ for each $j = 1, 2, 3, 4$. Otherwise $w = w(P_0)$ is constant in Ω_k. Without loss of generality, we may assume $\frac{\partial w}{\partial n}(Q_1) > 0$. Then we can choose Q_2, Q_3, Q_4 such that

$$\frac{\partial w}{\partial n}(Q_2) < 0, \quad \frac{\partial w}{\partial n}(Q_3) > 0, \quad \frac{\partial w}{\partial n}(Q_4) < 0. \quad (3.81)$$

(To see this, suppose that we cannot choose Q_2 such that $\frac{\partial w}{\partial n}(Q_2) < 0$. Then $\inf_{\Omega_1 \cup \Omega_2} w = w(P_0)$, and w has a local minimum along an interface curve between Ω_1 and Ω_2 which is not possible from the maximum principle.)

In the case where $\alpha\beta \leq 0$, it follows from the boundary condition (3.80) that w has either the maximum or minimum on $\overline{\mathcal{E}_1^- \cup \mathcal{E}_2^-}$. Since $\mathcal{E}_1^-$ and $\mathcal{E}_2^-$ are adjacent electrodes and $\{Q_1, Q_2, Q_3, Q_4\}$ are ordered in a counterclockwise direction, $\overline{\mathcal{E}_1^+ \cup \mathcal{E}_2^+}$ contains at least three points out of $\{Q_1, Q_2, Q_3, Q_4\}$. Hence one of $\{\overline{\mathcal{E}_1^+}, \overline{\mathcal{E}_2^+}\}$ must have at least two points, say $\{Q_3, Q_4\} \subset \overline{\mathcal{E}_1^+}$. In this case, the level curve Γ hits the curve $\overline{\mathcal{E}_1^+}$ between Q_3 and Q_4 and hence $w = w(P_0)$ in $\Omega_3 \cup \Omega_4$. It follows from the maximum principle and the unique continuation that $\nabla w = 0$ in Ω, a contradiction. For the case where $\alpha\beta > 0$, w has its maximum or minimum on either $\overline{\mathcal{E}_1^+}$ or $\overline{\mathcal{E}_2^+}$. Hence

$\overline{\mathcal{E}_1^+ \cup \mathcal{E}_2^+}$ must be included in the boundary of two pieces, say Ω_1, Ω_2. Then $\overline{\mathcal{E}_1^- \cup \mathcal{E}_2^-} \subset \overline{\Omega_3 \cup \Omega_4}$ and $w = w(P_0)$ in $\Omega_3 \cup \Omega_4$ and $\nabla w = 0$ in Ω, a contradiction. This completes the proof.   □

Although the uniqueness in the third dimension is still an open problem, we can expect the three-dimensional uniqueness by looking at roles of the three components $\Lambda_1[\sigma], \Lambda_2[\sigma]$, and $\Lambda_3[\sigma]$ with appropriate attachments of electrodes. Typical experimental and simulated B_z data sets are shown in Figures 3.24 and 3.25, respectively.

- Comparing Figure 3.24(a) and (c), we can see that the first component $\Lambda_1[\sigma]$ probes the vertical change of $\ln \sigma$ where the current density vector field $\mathbf{J}_1$ flows mostly in the horizontal direction. Figure 3.25(b) shows the simulated $\Lambda_1[\sigma]$ data with a horizontally oriented current. It is clearer that the B_z data subject to the horizontal current flow distinguishes the conductivity contrast along the vertical direction.

- Comparing Figure 3.24(b) and (d), the second component $\Lambda_2[\sigma]$ probes the horizontal change of $\ln \sigma$ where $\mathbf{J}_2$ flows mostly in the vertical direction. Figure 3.25(c) shows the simulated $\Lambda_2[\sigma]$ data with a vertically oriented current. It is clear that the B_z data subject to the vertical current flow distinguishes the conductivity contrast along the horizontal direction.

- The third component $\Lambda_3[\sigma]$ is used to fix the scaling uncertainty mentioned in Section 2.2.

In general, if we could produce two currents such that $\mathbf{J}_1(\mathbf{r}) \times \hat{\mathbf{z}}$ and $\mathbf{J}_2(\mathbf{r}) \times \hat{\mathbf{z}}$ are linearly independent for all $\mathbf{r} \in \Omega$, we can expect the uniqueness roughly by observing the roles of $\Lambda[\sigma]$. Taking account of the uniqueness and stability, we carefully attach two pairs of surface electrodes (which determine the two different Neumann data), as shown in Figure 3.26, so that the area of the parallelogram $|(\mathbf{J}_1 \times \mathbf{J}_2) \cdot \hat{\mathbf{z}}|$ is as large as possible in the truncated cylindrical region. However, the proof of $|(\mathbf{J}_1(\mathbf{r}) \times \mathbf{J}_2(\mathbf{r})) \cdot \hat{\mathbf{z}}| > 0$ for $\mathbf{r} \in \Omega$ would be difficult due to examples in [Briane *et al.* (2004); Laugesen (1996)].

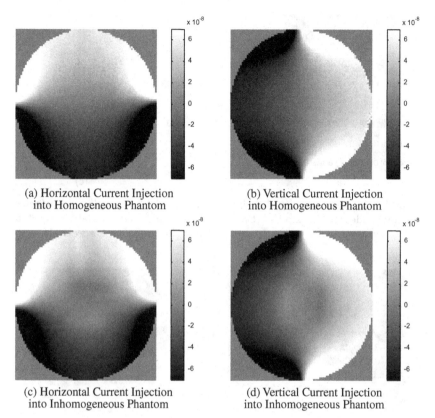

(a) Horizontal Current Injection
into Homogeneous Phantom

(b) Vertical Current Injection
into Homogeneous Phantom

(c) Horizontal Current Injection
into Inhomogeneous Phantom

(d) Vertical Current Injection
into Inhomogeneous Phantom

Fig. 3.24.   Here, (a) and (b) are measured B_z data from a cylindrical homogeneous saline phantom subject to current injections along the horizontal and vertical directions, respectively; (c) and (d) are measured B_z data from the same phantom containing an agar anomaly with a different conductivity value from the background saline.

3.8.1.3 *Representation formula*

The harmonic B_z algorithm is based on the following identity:

$$\mathbb{A}[\sigma](\mathbf{r}) \begin{bmatrix} \dfrac{\partial \ln \sigma}{\partial x}(\mathbf{r}) \\ \dfrac{\partial \ln \sigma}{\partial y}(\mathbf{r}) \end{bmatrix} = \begin{bmatrix} \nabla^2 \Lambda_1[\sigma](\mathbf{r}) \\ \nabla^2 \Lambda_2[\sigma](\mathbf{r}) \end{bmatrix}, \quad \mathbf{r} \in \Omega \qquad (3.82)$$

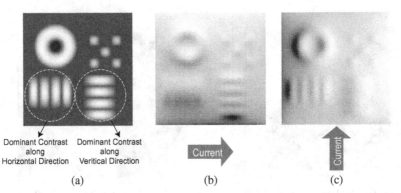

Fig. 3.25. (a) Conductivity distribution of a model. Electrodes are attached along four sides of the model; (b) and (c) are simulated B_z data subject to current injections along the horizontal and vertical directions, respectively.

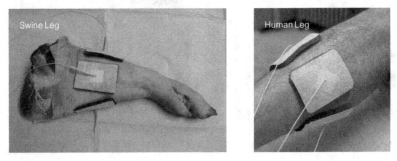

Fig. 3.26. Typical examples of electrode attachment to maximize the area of parallelogram $|(\mathbf{J}_1 \times \mathbf{J}_2) \cdot \hat{\mathbf{z}}|$.

where

$$\mathbb{A}[\sigma](\mathbf{r}) = \mu_0 \begin{bmatrix} \sigma \dfrac{\partial u_1[\sigma]}{\partial y}(\mathbf{r}) & -\sigma \dfrac{\partial u_1[\sigma]}{\partial x}(\mathbf{r}) \\ \sigma \dfrac{\partial u_2[\sigma]}{\partial y}(\mathbf{r}) & -\sigma \dfrac{\partial u_2[\sigma]}{\partial x}(\mathbf{r}) \end{bmatrix}, \quad \mathbf{r} \in \Omega.$$

Noting that $\nabla^2 \Lambda_j[\sigma] = \nabla^2 B_{z,j}$ for $j = 1, 2$ from (3.46), we have

$$\begin{bmatrix} \dfrac{\partial \ln \sigma}{\partial x}(\mathbf{r}) \\ \dfrac{\partial \ln \sigma}{\partial y}(\mathbf{r}) \end{bmatrix} = (\mathbb{A}[\sigma](\mathbf{r}))^{-1} \begin{bmatrix} \nabla^2 B_{z,1}(\mathbf{r}) \\ \nabla^2 B_{z,2}(\mathbf{r}) \end{bmatrix}, \quad \mathbf{r} \in \Omega \qquad (3.83)$$

provided that $\mathbb{A}[\sigma]$ is invertible.

Denoting the cross-sectional slice at $z = z_0$ by $\Omega_{z_0} := \Omega \cap \{z = z_0\}$, the transversal divergence of (3.83) leads to

$$\nabla_{xy} \cdot \nabla_{xy} \ln \sigma(\mathbf{x}, z_0) = \nabla_{xy} \cdot F_\sigma(\mathbf{x}, z_0) \quad \text{for } (\mathbf{x}, z_0) \in \Omega_{z_0} \qquad (3.84)$$

where

$$F_\sigma(\mathbf{r}) := \mathbb{A}[\sigma]^{-1}(\mathbf{r}) \begin{bmatrix} \nabla^2 B_{z,1}(\mathbf{r}) \\ \nabla^2 B_{z,2}(\mathbf{r}) \end{bmatrix}.$$

The above identity (3.84) leads to an implicit representation formula for σ on each slice Ω_{z_0} in terms of the measured data set $(B_{z,1}, B_{z,2}, V_{12}^{\pm})$. Denoting $\mathbf{x} = (x, y)$ and $\mathbf{x}' = (x', y')$, we have

$$\mathcal{L}_{z_0} \ln \sigma(\mathbf{x}) = \frac{1}{2\pi} \int_{\Omega_{z_0}} \frac{\mathbf{x} - \mathbf{x}'}{|\mathbf{x} - \mathbf{x}'|^2}$$

$$\cdot F_\sigma(\mathbf{x}', z_0) \, ds_{\mathbf{x}'} \quad \text{for all } (\mathbf{x}, z_0) \in \Omega_{z_0} \qquad (3.85)$$

where

$$\mathcal{L}_{z_0} \ln \sigma(\mathbf{x}) = \ln \sigma(\mathbf{x}, z_0) + \frac{1}{2\pi} \int_{\partial \Omega_{z_0}} \frac{(\mathbf{x} - \mathbf{x}') \cdot \nu(\mathbf{x}')}{|\mathbf{x} - \mathbf{x}'|^2} \ln \sigma(\mathbf{x}', z_0) d\ell_{\mathbf{x}'}.$$

$$(3.86)$$

Here, ν is the unit outward normal vector to the curve $\partial \Omega_{z_0}$ and $d\ell$ is the line element. From the trace formula for the double layer potential in (3.86), the identity (3.85) on the boundary $\partial \Omega_{z_0}$ can be expressed as

$$\mathcal{T}_{z_0} \ln \sigma(\mathbf{x}) = \frac{1}{2\pi} \int_{\Omega_{z_0}} \frac{\mathbf{x} - \mathbf{x}'}{|\mathbf{x} - \mathbf{x}'|^2} \cdot F_\sigma(\mathbf{x}', z_0) ds_{\mathbf{x}'} \quad \text{for } (\mathbf{x}, z_0) \in \partial \Omega_{z_0}$$

$$(3.87)$$

where

$$\mathcal{T}_{z_0} \ln \sigma(\mathbf{x}) = \frac{\ln \sigma(\mathbf{x}, z_0)}{2} + \frac{1}{2\pi} \int_{\partial \Omega_{z_0}} \frac{(\mathbf{x} - \mathbf{x}') \cdot \nu(\mathbf{x}')}{|\mathbf{x} - \mathbf{x}'|^2} \ln \sigma(\mathbf{x}', z_0) \, d\ell_{\mathbf{x}'}.$$

Noting that the operator $\mathcal{T}_{z_0}$ is invertible on $L_0^2(\partial \Omega_{z_0}) = \{\phi \in L^2(\partial \Omega_{z_0}) : \int_{\partial \Omega_{z_0}} \phi \, d\ell = 0\}$ from the well-known potential theory [Folland (1976)], we may expect that the following iterative algorithm based on the identities (3.85) and (3.87) can determine σ up to a scaling factor:

$$\begin{cases} \nabla^2_{xy} \ln \sigma^{n+1} = \nabla_{xy} \cdot F_{\sigma^n} & \text{in } \Omega_{z_0} \\ \ln \sigma^{n+1} = \mathcal{T}_{z_0}^{-1} \Phi_{z_0}[\sigma^n] & \text{on } \partial\Omega_{z_0} \end{cases} \qquad (3.88)$$

where

$$\Phi_{z_0}[\sigma^n](\mathbf{x}, z_0) = \frac{1}{2\pi} \int_{\Omega_{z_0}} \frac{\mathbf{x} - \mathbf{x}'}{|\mathbf{x} - \mathbf{x}'|^2} \cdot F_\sigma(\mathbf{x}', z_0) \, ds_{\mathbf{x}'} \text{ on } \partial\Omega_{z_0}.$$

From the first step in (3.88), we can update $\nabla_{xy}\sigma^{n+1}$ for all imaging slices of interest within the object as long as the measured data B_z are available for the slices. Next, we obtain $\sigma^{n+1}|_{\partial\Omega}$ by solving the integral equation (3.87) for the given right side of the second step in (3.88). Since $\sigma^{n+1}|_{\partial\Omega_{z_0}}$ is known, we determine the value σ^{n+1} inside Ω_{z_0} by simple substitutions of $\sigma^{n+1}|_{\partial\Omega_{z_0}}$ and $\nabla_{xy}\sigma^{n+1}$ into the corresponding integrals. This harmonic B_z algorithm has shown a remarkable performance in various numerical simulations [Seo *et al.* (2003); Oh *et al.* (2003)] and imaging experiments summarized in Section 3.10.

Early MREIT methods required all three components of the magnetic flux density $\mathbf{B} = (B_x, B_y, B_z)$ using impractical rotations of the imaging object inside the MRI scanner. The invention of the harmonic B_z algorithm using only B_z instead of $\mathbf{B}$ [Seo *et al.* (2003a)] changed the problem of impractical rotations into a mathematical problem (3.84) with achievable data through applications of two linearly independent Neumann data. This harmonic B_z algorithm has been widely used in subsequent experimental studies including the latest *in vivo* animal and human imaging experiments [Kim *et al.* (2007, 2008a, b, c, 2009)].

We should mention the convergence behavior of (3.88). When σ has a low contrast in Ω, the direction of the vector field $\sigma\nabla u_j[\sigma]$ is mostly dictated by the geometry of the boundary $\partial\Omega$ and the electrode positions $\mathcal{E}_j^{\pm}$ (or Neumann boundary data) instead of the distribution of σ. This ill-posedness was the fundamental drawback of the corresponding inverse problem of EIT. But, in MREIT, we take advantage of this insensitivity of EIT. This means that the direction of the vector field $\sigma\nabla u_j[\sigma]$ is similar to that of $\sigma^0\nabla u_j[\sigma^0]$ with $\sigma^0 = 1$, and therefore the data $B_{z,1}$ and $B_{z,2}$ hold the major information of the conductivity contrast. Various numerical simulations show that only one iteration of (3.88) may provide a conductivity image σ^1 which is quite similar to the true conductivity σ. Rigorous mathematical theories regarding its convergence behavior have not been proven yet. In [Liu *et al.* (2007)], there are some convergence results on (3.88) under *a priori* assumption on the target conductivity.

3.8.1.4 *Local reconstruction using harmonic B_z algorithm*

This subsection is based on [Seo *et al.* (2008b)]. When we apply the harmonic B_z algorithm to measured B_z data from animal or human subjects, there occur a few technical difficulties that are mainly related to measurement errors in B_z data, especially in local regions where MR signals are very small. Such local regions may include bones, lungs, and air-filled organs. Therefore, it would be desirable to reconstruct accurate conductivity values in regions away from the problematic ones.

This demands a local image reconstruction algorithm to prevent defective data at one local region from influencing badly on conductivity images of other regions. Let $D \subset \Omega_{z_0}$ be a local area away from such problematic regions. Define

$$\Phi_D[\sigma](\mathbf{x}) := \frac{1}{2\pi} \int_{\Omega_{z_0}} \frac{\mathbf{x} - \mathbf{x}'}{|\mathbf{x} - \mathbf{x}'|^2}$$

$$\cdot \mathbb{A}[\sigma]^{-1} \begin{bmatrix} \nabla^2 B_{1,z}(\mathbf{x}', z_0) \\ \nabla^2 B_{2,z}(\mathbf{x}', z_0) \end{bmatrix} d\mathbf{x}' \qquad (3.89)$$

for $(\mathbf{x}, z_0) = (x, y, z_0) \in D$ and

$$\mathcal{L}_{\partial D}\phi(\mathbf{x}) := -\frac{1}{2\pi} \int_D \frac{(\mathbf{x} - \mathbf{x}') \cdot \nu(\mathbf{x}')}{|\mathbf{x} - \mathbf{x}'|^2} \phi(\mathbf{x}', z_0) \, d\ell_{\mathbf{x}'}. \qquad (3.90)$$

The next theorem explains how to reconstruct σ in a local disk D contained in the slice Ω_{z_0}.

Theorem 3.6. *If D is an arbitrary disk lying on Ω_{z_0}, then, for $(\mathbf{x}, z_0) = (x, y, z_0) \in D$, we have*

$$\ln \sigma(\mathbf{x}, z_0) = \beta_{\partial D} + \Phi_D[\sigma](\mathbf{x})$$
$$- \frac{1}{\pi} \int_{\partial D} \frac{(\mathbf{x} - \mathbf{x}') \cdot \nu(\mathbf{x}')}{|\mathbf{x} - \mathbf{x}'|^2} \Phi_D[\sigma](\mathbf{x}') dl_{\mathbf{x}'} \quad (3.91)$$

where r is the radius of D, $\mathbf{x}_0 = (x_0, y_0)$ the center of D, and $\beta_{\partial D} = \frac{1}{2\pi r} \int_{\partial D} \ln \sigma dl$ the average of σ along the boundary ∂D.

Proof. Based on the idea of the harmonic B_z algorithm, σ in D can be expressed as

$$\ln \sigma(\mathbf{x}, z_0) = \Phi_D[\sigma](\mathbf{x}) + \mathcal{L}_{\partial D} \ln \sigma(\mathbf{x}), \quad (x, y, z_0) \in D. \quad (3.92)$$

According to the trace formula of the double layer potential [Folland (1976); Verchota (1984)], we have

$$\lim_{t \to 0^+} \mathcal{L}_{\partial D} \ln \sigma(\mathbf{x} - t\nu, z_0)$$
$$= \frac{1}{2} \ln \sigma(\mathbf{x}, z_0) - \frac{1}{2\pi} \int_{\partial D} \frac{(\mathbf{x} - \mathbf{x}') \cdot \nu(\mathbf{x}')}{|\mathbf{x} - \mathbf{x}'|^2} \ln \sigma(\mathbf{x}', z_0) dl_{\mathbf{x}'}$$
$$(\mathbf{x}, z_0) \in \partial D.$$
$$(3.93)$$

Since D is the disk with the radius r, a direct computation yields

$$\frac{(\mathbf{x} - \mathbf{x}') \cdot \nu(\mathbf{x}')}{|\mathbf{x} - \mathbf{x}'|^2} = -\frac{1}{2r} \quad \text{for all } \mathbf{x}, \mathbf{x}' \in \partial D.$$

Hence, the trace formula (3.93) becomes

$$\mathcal{L}_{\partial D} \ln \sigma(\mathbf{x}) = \frac{1}{2} \ln \sigma(\mathbf{x}, z_0) + \frac{1}{2} \beta_{\partial D}, \quad \mathbf{x} \in \partial D. \quad (3.94)$$

From (3.92) and (3.94), we have the expression of σ along the boundary:

$$\ln \sigma(\mathbf{x}, z_0) = 2\Phi_D[\sigma](\mathbf{x}) + \beta_{\partial D}, \quad \mathbf{x} \in \partial D. \quad (3.95)$$

Now, we substitute (3.95) into the term involving $\mathcal{L}_{\partial D}$ in (3.92) to get

$$\Phi_D[\sigma](\mathbf{x}) = \ln \sigma + \frac{1}{2\pi} \int_{\partial D} \frac{(\mathbf{x} - \mathbf{x}') \cdot \nu(\mathbf{x}')}{|\mathbf{x} - \mathbf{x}'|^2} [2\Phi_D[\sigma](\mathbf{x}') + \beta_{\partial D}] \, dl_{\mathbf{x}'},$$

$$\mathbf{x} \in D.$$

$$(3.96)$$

Using the fact that $-1 = \frac{1}{2\pi} \int_{\partial D} \frac{(\mathbf{x}-\mathbf{x}')\cdot\nu(\mathbf{x}')}{|\mathbf{x}-\mathbf{x}'|^2} dl_{\mathbf{x}'}$ for all $\mathbf{x} \in D$, the identity (3.96) becomes

$$\Phi_D[\sigma](\mathbf{x}) = \ln \sigma - \beta_{\partial D} + \frac{1}{\pi} \int_{\partial D} \frac{(\mathbf{x} - \mathbf{x}') \cdot \nu(\mathbf{x}')}{|\mathbf{x} - \mathbf{x}'|^2} \Phi_D[\sigma](\mathbf{x}') \, dl_{\mathbf{x}'}.$$

This completes the proof. □

3.8.1.5 *Conductivity reconstructor using harmonic* B_z *algorithm*

The MREIT technique involves (1) current injection into an electrically conducting object through surface electrodes, (2) measurement of induced B_z, and (3) conductivity reconstruction by solving nonlinear boundary value problems with the known injected current and measured magnetic flux density data, employing FEM. Although it looks straightforward to reconstruct conductivity images using the three steps, the computations involve several innovative approaches including preprocessing of the magnetic flux density data, segmentation of MR magnitude images, denoising, missing data recovery, and forward/inverse problem solving.

The image reconstruction procedure using the harmonic B_z algorithm includes three major tasks of preprocessing: model construction, data recovery, and conductivity image reconstruction. We obtain magnetic flux density images $B_{z,1}$ and $B_{z,2}$ corresponding to two injection currents I_1 and I_2, respectively, from the k-space data after applying proper phase unwrapping and unit conversion. To compute $A[\sigma]$, we need the geometrical modeling of the conducting domain which includes identifications of the outermost boundary and electrode locations for imposing boundary conditions. There could be an internal region where MR signal void occurred. In such a

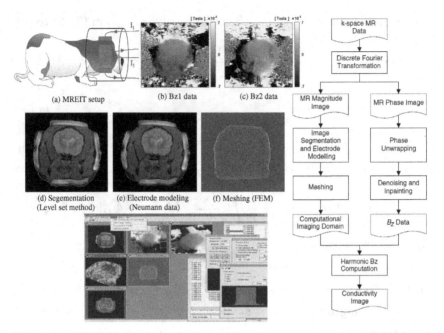

Fig. 3.27.   MREIT software includes preprocessing, segmentation, meshing, and image reconstruction.

problematic region, measured B_z data are defective. We need to segment those defected regions to prevent noise propagation. For conductivity reconstructions, we use the harmonic B_z algorithm as the default algorithm for three-dimensional conductivity image reconstructions. We may apply the local harmonic B_z algorithm [Seo *et al.* (2008b)] for conductivity image reconstructions in chosen regions of interest. Figure 3.27 shows a screen capture of the MREIT software, CoReHA (conductivity reconstructor using harmonic algorithms) [Jeon *et al.* (2009a, b)].

The MREIT image reconstruction procedure is as follows:

Step 1   Attach two pairs of electrodes $\mathcal{E}_1^{\pm}$ and $\mathcal{E}_2^{\pm}$ on the surface of an electrically conducting domain Ω to be imaged.

Step 2   Inject electrical currents I_1 and I_2 through the pairs of electrodes $\mathcal{E}_1^{\pm}$ and $\mathcal{E}_2^{\pm}$, respectively. The injection current produces $\mathbf{E}_j(\mathbf{r}) = -\nabla u_j[\sigma](\mathbf{r})$, $\mathbf{J}_j(\mathbf{r}) = -\sigma \nabla u_j[\sigma](\mathbf{r})$, and $\mathbf{B}_j$ inside Ω.

Step 3 Acquire k-space data from an MRI scanner. The MR spectrometer provides the complex k-space data $\mathcal{S}_j^{\pm}$:

$$\mathcal{S}_j^{\pm}(\mathbf{k_x}, z_0) = \int_{\Omega_{z_0}} \underbrace{M(\mathbf{x}, z_0)e^{i\delta(\mathbf{x}, z_0)}e^{\pm i\gamma B_{z,j}(\mathbf{x}, z_0)T_c}}_{\mathcal{M}_j^{\pm}(\mathbf{x}, z_0)} e^{i\mathbf{x}\cdot\mathbf{k_x}} \, d\mathbf{x}.$$

(3.97)

Hence, we obtain

$$B_{z,j}(\mathbf{x}, z_0) = \text{phase unwrapping of } \underbrace{\frac{1}{2\gamma T_c} \arg\left(\frac{\mathcal{M}_j^+(\mathbf{x}, z_0)}{\mathcal{M}_j^-(\mathbf{x}, z_0)}\right)}_{\Theta_j}.$$

(3.98)

The phase image Θ_j is wrapped in the range of $-\pi$ and π due to the branch cut of the argument operator. Apply a two-dimensional phase-unwrapping operator on each slice to make B_z continuous along xy-direction, and add or subtract integer multiples of π to each slice of wrapped B_z images to make B_z continuous along z-direction (see Figure 3.5.)

Step 3* *Get simulated* $\mathbf{E}_j, \mathbf{J}_j, B_{z,j}$.

— *Geometric modeling of the imaging domain* Ω *and Neumann data* $\mathcal{E}_j^{\pm}$. *We may use the MR magnitude image* $M(\mathbf{r})$ *to segment* $\partial\Omega$ *and* $\mathcal{E}_j^{\pm}$. *One can adopt a segmentation technique such as the snake algorithm, thresholding, or level set method.*

— *Computation of* $\mathbf{E}_j = -\nabla u_j[\sigma]$:

$$\nabla u_j[\sigma](\mathbf{r}) = \beta_j \nabla \tilde{u}_j(\mathbf{r}) \quad (\forall \mathbf{r} \in \Omega)$$

where $\tilde{u}_j$ is the solution of

$$\begin{cases} \nabla \cdot (\sigma\nabla\tilde{u}_j) = 0 & \text{in } \Omega \\ \tilde{u}_j|_{\mathcal{E}_j^{\pm}} = \pm 1, \quad -\sigma\dfrac{\partial\tilde{u}_j}{\partial\mathbf{n}}\bigg|_{\partial\Omega\setminus(\mathcal{E}^+\cup\mathcal{E}^-)} = 0 \end{cases}$$

and $\beta_j = I(\int_{\partial\mathcal{E}_j^+} \sigma\frac{\partial\tilde{u}_j}{\partial\mathbf{n}})^{-1}$.

— *Computation of* $B_{z,j}^{\Omega}$. Compute its Fourier transform

$$\mathcal{F}_3\{B_{z,j}^{\Omega}\}(\mathbf{k}) = \frac{i}{2\pi\mu_0|\mathbf{k}|^2}\hat{\mathbf{z}} \cdot [\mathbf{k} \times \mathcal{F}_3(\sigma\nabla u_j[\sigma])])$$

Recall that the measured data is $B_{z,j} = B_{z,j}^{\Omega} + \mathcal{H}_j$ where $\mathcal{H}_j$ is the effect of the current outside Ω such as lead wires and electrodes.

Step 4 For $\sigma_0 = 1$, compute the $\mathbb{A}[\sigma^0]^{-1}(\mathbf{r})$ for $\mathbf{r} \in \Omega$.

Step 5 Compute

$$F_\sigma(\mathbf{r}) := \mathbb{A}[\sigma_0]^{-1}(\mathbf{r}) \begin{bmatrix} \nabla^2 B_{z,1}(\mathbf{r}) \\ \nabla^2 B_{z,2}(\mathbf{r}) \end{bmatrix} (1 - \chi_{\Omega^\delta}(\mathbf{r}))$$

where Ω^δ is a subdomain of Ω:

$$\Omega^\delta := \{\mathbf{r} \in \Omega : |M(\mathbf{r})| < \delta_M, \ |\det\mathbb{A}[\sigma_0](\mathbf{r})| < \delta_A\}.$$

Here, δ_M and δ_A are small positive numbers depending on the SNR of measured B_z data.

Step 6 For each slice Ω_{z_0}, solve the two-dimensional Poisson equation

$$\begin{cases} \nabla_{xy}^2 \ln\sigma^1(x,y,z_0) & \text{for } (x,y,z_0) \in \Omega_{z_0} \\ \quad = \nabla_{xy} \cdot F_{\sigma^0}(x,y,z_0) & \\ \ln\sigma^1 = 0 & \text{on } \partial\Omega_{z_0}. \end{cases} \tag{3.99}$$

Step 7 Scale σ^1 as

$$\sigma^1 \leftarrow \frac{V_1^+ - V_1^-}{u_1[\sigma^1]|_{\mathcal{E}_2^+} - u_1[\sigma^1]|_{\mathcal{E}_2^-}}\sigma_1$$

where $V_1^+ - V_1^-$ is the measured voltage difference between electrodes $\mathcal{E}_2^+$ and $\mathcal{E}_2^1$ due to the injection current I_1.

Step 8 If necessary, repeat steps 4 to 7, replacing σ^0 by σ^1 and denoting the updated conductivity as σ^2. Repeat the process to improve the quality of the reconstructed conductivity image.

3.8.1.6   *Non-iterative harmonic B_z algorithm with transversally dominant current density*

The harmonic B_z algorithm utilizes an iterative procedure to update conductivity values and in each iteration we need to solve an elliptic boundary value problem with a presumed conductivity distribution. This iteration is often troublesome in practice due to excessive amounts of noise in some local regions where weak MR signals are produced. For certain applications where conductivity contrast information is primarily of concern, it will be better and sufficient to use a non-iterative reconstruction algorithm, which does not depend on a global structure of the conductivity distribution.

Based on [Seo *et al.* (2011)], this subsection presents a non-iterative harmonic B_z algorithm under the assumption that we can produce a transversally dominant current density within a region to be imaged. Assuming that the imaging object is locally cylindrical in its shape, we will adopt thin, flexible, wide, and long electrodes to produce a transversally dominant current density $\mathbf{J} = (J_x, J_y, J_z)$ within multiple slices of the imaging object around the middle of the electrode plane.

Noting that the iteration stems from the non-linear relation of $\sigma \mathbb{A}[\sigma]$ with respect to the unknown σ, we need to maximize the use of measured B_z data to get rid of the iteration. The following observation enables us to eliminate the iteration process in theory.

- **Observation.** We fix an imaging slice Ω_{z_0}. Let Γ_j^+ and Γ_j^- be sub-arcs of the closed curve $\partial\Omega_{z_0}$ such that $\partial\Omega_{z_0}$ is divided into four arcs $\mathcal{E}_j^+ \cap \partial\Omega_{z_0}, \mathcal{E}_j^- \cap \partial\Omega_{z_0}, \Gamma_j^+$ and Γ_j^-. Suppose ϕ_j and Ψ_j are, respectively, solutions of

$$
\begin{cases}
\nabla_{xy}^2 \phi_j(\mathbf{r}) = \dfrac{1}{\mu_0}\nabla^2 B_{z,j}(\mathbf{r}) & \text{for } \mathbf{r} \in \Omega_{z_0} \\[2mm]
\nu \cdot \nabla_{xy}\phi_j = 0 & \text{on } (\mathcal{E}_j^+ \cup \mathcal{E}_j^-) \cap \partial\Omega_{z_0} \\[2mm]
\phi_j = 0 & \text{on } \Gamma_j^+ \cup \Gamma_j^- \\[1mm]
& = \partial\Omega_{z_0}\backslash(\mathcal{E}_j^+ \cup \mathcal{E}_j^-)
\end{cases}
\tag{3.100}
$$

and

$$\begin{cases} \nabla^2_{xy}\Psi_j(\mathbf{r}) = 0 & \text{for } \mathbf{r} \in \Omega_{z_0} \\ \nu \cdot \nabla_{xy}\Psi_j = 0 & \text{on } (\mathcal{E}_j^+ \cup \mathcal{E}_j^-) \cap \partial\Omega_{z_0} \\ \Psi_j|_{\Gamma_j^+} = +1 & \text{and} \quad \Psi_j|_{\Gamma_j^-} = -1 \end{cases} \qquad (3.101)$$

where ∇^2_{xy} is the transversal Laplacian and ν is the outward unit normal vector to the two-dimensional curve $\partial\Omega_{z_0}$. Then, there exists β_j such that

$$\int_{\Omega_{z_0}} |\nabla_{xy}(\beta_j\Psi_j + \phi_j) - \sigma\nabla^\perp_{xy}u_j[\sigma]|^2 \, dS$$

$$\leq C \int_{\Omega_{z_0}} \left| \frac{\partial}{\partial z}\left(\sigma\frac{\partial u_j}{\partial z}\right) \right|^2 \, dS \qquad (3.102)$$

where $\nabla^\perp_{xy} = (\frac{\partial}{\partial y}, -\frac{\partial}{\partial x})$ and C is a positive constant depending only on the geometry of Ω_{z_0}. Hence, if $\frac{\partial}{\partial z}(\sigma\frac{\partial u_j}{\partial z}) \approx 0$ on Ω_{z_0}, we have the following approximation of $\sigma\nabla^\perp_{xy}u$ (i.e., one row of $\sigma\mathbb{A}[\sigma]$):

$$\nabla_{xy}(\beta_j\Psi_j + \phi_j) \approx \sigma\mathbb{L}\nabla_{xy}u_j[\sigma] \quad \text{on } \Omega_{z_0}. \qquad (3.103)$$

Proof. According to the Helmholtz decomposition,

$$(\sigma\nabla^\perp_{xy}u_j) = \nabla_{xy}G_j + \nabla^\perp_{xy}W_j \quad \text{on } \Omega_{z_0}. \qquad (3.104)$$

For the unique determination of $\nabla_{xy}G_j$ and $\nabla^\perp_{xy}W_j$, we impose the following boundary conditions for W_j:

$$\begin{aligned} \nu \cdot \nabla_{xy}W_j(\mathbf{r}) = 0 & \quad \text{for } \mathbf{r} \in \partial\Omega_{z_0}\backslash(\mathcal{E}_j^+ \cup \mathcal{E}_j^-), \\ W_j(\mathbf{r}) = 0 & \quad \text{for } \mathbf{r} \in (\mathcal{E}_j^+ \cup \mathcal{E}_j^-) \cap \partial\Omega_{z_0}. \end{aligned} \qquad (3.105)$$

Note that the z-component of the curl of the Ampère law $\nabla \times \mathbf{J} = \frac{1}{\mu_0}\nabla \times \nabla \times \mathbf{B}$ can be written as

$$\nabla_{xy} \cdot (\sigma\nabla^\perp_{xy}u_j(\mathbf{r})) = \frac{1}{\mu_0}\nabla^2 B_{z,j}(\mathbf{r}). \qquad (3.106)$$

From (3.106), the transversal divergence to (3.104) leads to the identity $\nabla^2_{xy}G_j = \frac{1}{\mu_0}\nabla^2 B_{z,j}$. It follows from the boundary conditions of W_j in (3.105) and u_j that G_j satisfies

$$\begin{cases} \nabla^2_{xy} G_j(\mathbf{r}) = \frac{1}{\mu_0} \nabla^2 B_{z,j}(\mathbf{r}) & \text{in } \Omega_{z0} \\ \nu \cdot \nabla^\perp_{xy} G_j = 0 & \text{on } \partial\Omega_{z0} \backslash (\mathcal{E}^+_j \cup \mathcal{E}^-_j) \\ \nu \cdot \nabla_{xy} G_j = 0 & \text{on } (\mathcal{E}^+_j \cup \mathcal{E}^-_j) \cap \partial\Omega_{z0}. \end{cases} \quad (3.107)$$

Since $\nu \cdot \nabla^\perp_{xy}(G_j - \phi_j) = 0$ on $\Gamma^+_j \cup \Gamma^-_j = \partial\Omega_{z0} \backslash (\mathcal{E}^+_j \cup \mathcal{E}^-_j)$, there exist constants c_+ and c_- such that

$$G_j - \phi_j = c_+ \quad \text{on } \Gamma^+_j \quad \text{and} \quad G_j - \phi_j = c_- \quad \text{on } \Gamma^-_j. \quad (3.108)$$

Let

$$F_j(\mathbf{r}) := G_j(\mathbf{r}) - \phi_j(\mathbf{r}) - \frac{c_+ - c_-}{2} \Psi_j(\mathbf{r}) - \frac{c_+ + c_-}{2} \quad \text{for } \mathbf{r} \in \Omega_{z0}.$$

From (3.100), (3.101), (3.107) and (3.108), F_j satisfies

$$\begin{cases} \nabla^2_{xy} F_j(\mathbf{r}) = 0 & \text{in } \Omega_{z0} \\ F_j = 0 & \text{on } \partial\Omega_{z0} \backslash (\mathcal{E}^+_j \cup \mathcal{E}^-_j) \\ \nu \cdot \nabla_{xy} F_j = 0 & \text{on } (\mathcal{E}^+_j \cup \mathcal{E}^-_j) \cap \partial\Omega_{z0}. \end{cases}$$

Hence, $F_j = 0$ in Ω_{z0} and we can take $\beta_j = \frac{c_+ - c_-}{2}$ in (3.102).

Multiplying $\nabla^\perp_{xy} W_j$ to both sides of (3.104), we have

$$\int_{\Omega_{z0}} |\nabla_{xy} W_j|^2 \, dS = \int_{\Omega_{z0}} \sigma \nabla_{xy} u_j \cdot \nabla_{xy} W_j \, dS$$

$$- \int_{\Omega_{z0}} \nabla_{xy} G_j \cdot \nabla^\perp_{xy} W_j \, dS.$$

Due to the boundary conditions (3.105) and (3.107), we have

$$\int_{\Omega_{z0}} \nabla_{xy} G_j \cdot \nabla^\perp_{xy} W_j \, dS = 0.$$

Thus we have

$$\int_{\Omega_{z0}} |\nabla_{xy} W_j|^2 \, dS$$

$$= \int_{\Omega_{z0}} \sigma \nabla_{xy} u_j \cdot \nabla_{xy} W_j \, dS$$

$$= -\int_{\Omega_{z_0}} \nabla_{xy} \cdot (\sigma \nabla_{xy} u_j) W_j \, dS$$

$$= \int_{\Omega_{z_0}} \frac{\partial}{\partial z} \left(\sigma \frac{\partial u_j}{\partial z} \right) W_j \, dS$$

$$\leq \left(\int_{\Omega_{z_0}} \left| \frac{\partial}{\partial z} \left(\sigma \frac{\partial u_j}{\partial z} \right) \right|^2 dS \right)^{1/2} \left(\int_{\Omega_{z_0}} |W_j|^2 \, dS \right)^{1/2}.$$

The estimate (3.102) follows from the Poincaré inequality with the above estimate. Here, the Poincaré inequality is applicable since $W_j|_{\mathcal{E}_j^\pm} = 0$. This completes the proof of the observation. □

Using the smallness of $\frac{\partial}{\partial z}(\sigma \frac{\partial u_j}{\partial z})$, we can replace the non-linear term $\sigma \mathbb{A}[\sigma]$ by known quantities via the following approximation:

$$\sigma(\mathbf{r})\mathbb{A}[\sigma](\mathbf{r}) \approx \underbrace{\begin{bmatrix} \frac{\partial}{\partial x}(\beta_1 \Psi_1(\mathbf{r}) + \phi_1(\mathbf{r})) & \frac{\partial}{\partial y}(\beta_1 \Psi_1(\mathbf{r}) + \phi_1(\mathbf{r})) \\ \frac{\partial}{\partial x}(\beta_2 \Psi_2(\mathbf{r}) + \phi_2(\mathbf{r})) & \frac{\partial}{\partial y}(\beta_2 \Psi_2(\mathbf{r}) + \phi_2(\mathbf{r})) \end{bmatrix}}_{:= \mathbb{C}(\mathbf{r})}.$$

$$(3.109)$$

In practice, from (3.109), we may choose β_j such that

$$\beta_j = \frac{\left(\int_{\mathcal{E}_j^+ \cap \Omega_{z_0}} \sigma \nabla_{xy} u_j \cdot \nu \, d\ell - \int_{\mathcal{E}_j^+ \cap \partial\Omega_{z_0}} \nabla_{xy} \phi_j \times \nu \, d\ell \right)}{\int_{\mathcal{E}_j^+ \cap \partial\Omega_{z_0}} \nabla_{xy} \Psi_j \times \nu \, d\ell}. \qquad (3.110)$$

Here, the two-dimensional cross product means $(a_1, a_2) \times (b_1, b_2) = a_1 b_2 - a_2 b_1$. It is designed to satisfy

$$\int_{\mathcal{E}_j^+ \cap \Omega_{z_0}} [\nabla_{xy}(\beta \Psi_j + \phi_j) - \sigma \nabla_{xy}^\perp u] \times \nu d\ell = 0.$$

The non-iterative harmonic B_z algorithm is based on the following approximate representation for $\nabla_{xy} \ln \sigma$:

$$\nabla_{xy} \ln \sigma \approx \underbrace{\frac{1}{\mu_0}(\mathbb{C}(\mathbf{r}))^{-1} \begin{bmatrix} \nabla^2 B_{z,1}(\mathbf{r}) \\ \nabla^2 B_{z,2}(\mathbf{r}) \end{bmatrix}}_{:= \Theta(\mathbf{r})}, \quad \text{for } \mathbf{r} \in \Omega_{z_0}. \qquad (3.111)$$

Now, we describe the non-iterative algorithm.

Step 1. Compute Θ in (3.111) and the scaling constant α. The scaling factor α can be obtained by using measured boundary voltage data on the pairs of electrodes.

Step 2. Compute $\tilde{\sigma}$ by solving the problem

$$
\begin{cases}
\left(\dfrac{\partial^2}{\partial x^2} + \dfrac{\partial^2}{\partial y^2} \right) \ln \tilde{\sigma}(\mathbf{r}) = \nabla_{xy} \cdot \Theta(\mathbf{r}) & \text{for } \mathbf{r} \in \Omega_{z_0} \\[2mm]
\nu \cdot \nabla_{xy} \ln \tilde{\sigma}(\mathbf{r}) = \nu \cdot \Theta(\mathbf{r}) & \text{for } \mathbf{r} \in \partial\Omega_{z_0} \\[2mm]
\displaystyle\int_{\Omega_{z_0}} \ln \tilde{\sigma}\, d\mathbf{r} = 0.
\end{cases}
$$

$$(3.112)$$

Step 3. Display $\sigma = \alpha\tilde{\sigma}$.

3.8.1.7 *A posteriori error estimate: two-dimensional MREIT model*

We consider a two-dimensional MREIT model which occurs in the case when the imaging object is locally cylindrical and $\frac{\partial\sigma}{\partial z} = 0$. For such an object, we may produce a transversally dominating current density $-\sigma\nabla u_j[\sigma]$ inside a truncated cylindrical region by using longitudinal electrodes such that $\frac{\partial u_j}{\partial z} = 0$.

We consider the two-dimensional MREIT model and use the same notation Ω for the two-dimensional domain representing the middle slice of a cylindrical subject. For simplicity, we assume $u_j[\sigma]$ in (3.24) is a constant multiple of the solution to

$$
\begin{cases}
\nabla \cdot (\sigma\nabla u_j) = 0 & \text{in } \Omega \\[2mm]
u_j|_{\mathcal{E}_j^+} = 1, \qquad u|_{\mathcal{E}_j^-} = 0 \\[2mm]
\dfrac{\partial u_j}{\partial \mathbf{n}} = 0 & \text{on } \partial\Omega \backslash \overline{\mathcal{E}_j^+ \cup \mathcal{E}_j^-},
\end{cases}
$$

$$(3.113)$$

where $\nabla = (\frac{\partial}{\partial x}, \frac{\partial}{\partial y})$ is the two-dimensional gradient and we denote by $u_j[\sigma]$ the solution of (3.113) instead of (3.24).

We denote by σ^* the true conductivity which is unknown. Let $B_{z,*}^j$ denote the exact magnetic flux density corresponding to σ^* in such a way that it satisfies (3.111). We assume that the boundary value $\sigma^*|_{\partial\Omega}$ is known. If the change of the internal current density $-\sigma\nabla u_j[\sigma]$ due to a perturbation of σ is relatively small, we can reconstruct σ using the following iterative process: for $(x,y) \in \Omega :=$ $\Omega \cap \{z = z_0\}$ and $n = 1, 2, \ldots,$

$$\begin{cases} \nabla \ln \sigma^{n+1}(x,y) := \mathbb{A}[\sigma^n]^{-1} \begin{bmatrix} \nabla^2 B^1_{z,*} \\ \nabla^2 B^2_{z,*} \end{bmatrix}, \\ \ln \sigma^{n+1}(x,y) := \mathcal{L}(\ln \sigma^*) - \frac{1}{2\pi} \int_\Omega \frac{(x-x', y-y')}{|x-x'|^2 + |y-y'|^2} \\ \qquad\qquad \cdot \nabla \ln \sigma^{n+1}(x', y')dx'dy', \end{cases} \qquad (3.114)$$

where

$$\mathcal{L}(\ln \sigma^*) := \frac{1}{2\pi} \int_{\partial\Omega} \frac{(x-x', y-y') \cdot \nu(x', y')}{|x-x'|^2 + |y-y'|^2} \ln \sigma^*(x', y')\, dl.$$

An *a posteriori* error estimate for the two-dimensional MREIT model provides a rigorous estimate of how close the reconstructed σ^n of the iteration scheme in (3.88) is to the unknown true conductivity σ^*. Let $\widetilde{\Omega}$ be a subdomain of Ω with $\widetilde{\Omega} \subset\subset \Omega$. We assume that $\nabla \sigma^*$ is compactly supported in a domain $\widetilde{\Omega}$ with

$$\nabla \sigma^*|_{\Omega \setminus \widetilde{\Omega}} = 0 \quad \text{and} \quad \|\nabla \ln \sigma^*\|_{L^\infty(\Omega)} \le C_0, \qquad (3.115)$$

where C_0 is a positive constant. Notice that the norm $\|\nabla \ln \sigma^*\|_{L^\infty(\Omega)}$ chosen here is natural in the sense that it measures the oscillations on the σ^*. We put a bound C_0 on the oscillation of the target conductivity.

These assumptions with the standard electrode configuration shown in Figure 3.2 provide a positive lower bound for $\det(\mathbb{A}[\sigma^*])$ in $\widetilde{\Omega}$:

$$\inf_{\widetilde{\Omega}} \begin{vmatrix} \dfrac{\partial u_1[\sigma^*]}{\partial y} & -\dfrac{\partial u_1[\sigma^*]}{\partial x} \\ \dfrac{\partial u_2[\sigma^*]}{\partial y} & -\dfrac{\partial u_2[\sigma^*]}{\partial x} \end{vmatrix} > 0. \qquad (3.116)$$

We should note that (3.116) is not true for the entire domain $\overline{\Omega}$ due to the fact that two induced currents satisfy $\nabla u_1[\sigma^*] \times \nabla u_2[\sigma^*] = 0$

on $\partial\Omega \setminus \cup_{j=1,2} \overline{\mathcal{E}_j^+ \cup \mathcal{E}_j^-}$. This means that (3.116) is correct only for the interior region $\tilde{\Omega}$. The above positive lower bound for a three-dimensional domain remains an open problem. In the two-dimensional case, the estimate (3.116) can be proven using the results in [Bauman *et al.* (2000)] when σ^* is smooth. For the case where σ^* is just measurable, the non-vanishing determinant of the Jacobian $\frac{\partial(u_1[\sigma^*], u_2[\sigma^*])}{\partial(x,y)}$ holds in the *a.e.* sense from the results in [Alessandrini and Nesi (2001)]. In the three-dimensional case, there are examples [Briane *et al.* (2004); Laugesen (1996)], which suggest that it may be very difficult to prove (3.116) independently on σ^*, even assuming the smoothness of σ. See [Liu *et al.* (2006)] for details.

Let $\{\sigma^n : n = 1, 2, \ldots\}$ denote the iteration sequence in (3.88) with the exact input data $B_{z,*}^j$ for $j = 1, 2$. Let $\nabla^2 B_{z,n}^j$ for $j = 1, 2$ be solutions of

$$\begin{cases} \nabla^2 B_{z,n}^j = \mu_0 \left[\dfrac{\partial u_j[\sigma^n]}{\partial y}, -\dfrac{\partial u_j[\sigma^n]}{\partial x} \right] \cdot \left[\dfrac{\partial \sigma^n}{\partial x}, \dfrac{\partial \sigma^n}{\partial y} \right] & \text{in } \Omega \\ B_{z,n}^j = B_{z,*}^j \text{ on } \partial\Omega \setminus \mathcal{E}^\pm, \quad \nabla B_{z,n}^j \cdot \mathbf{n} = \nabla B_{z,*}^j \cdot \mathbf{n} \text{ on } \partial\mathcal{E}^\pm. \end{cases}$$

$$(3.117)$$

Note that $B_{z,n}^j$ for $j = 1, 2$ are available quantities by solving the Poisson equation (3.117) and the elliptic equation (3.113) for each σ^n. We are now ready to present an *a posteriori* estimate.

Theorem 3.7. *Assume that $\sigma^* > 0$ satisfies (3.115). The error between the reconstructed conductivity σ^n in (3.88) and the unknown true conductivity σ^* can be estimated by*

$$\| \ln \sigma^n - \ln \sigma^* \|_{L^\infty(\tilde{\Omega})}$$

$$\leq M \left\| (\sigma^n \mathbb{A}[\sigma^n])^{-1} \right\|_{L^{p_2}(\tilde{\Omega})} \sum_{j=1}^{2} \left\| B_{z,*}^j - B_{z,n}^j \right\|_{W^{2,p_3}(\tilde{\Omega})},$$

$$(3.118)$$

where

$$M = \frac{1 + C_0}{2\pi\mu_0(2 - p_1)^{1/p_1}} \left(diam(\Omega) \right)^{\frac{2}{p_1} - 1} \qquad (3.119)$$

and p_1, p_2, p_3 are any positive numbers such that $1 < p_1 < 2$, $\frac{1}{p_1} + \frac{1}{p_2} + \frac{1}{p_3} = 1$.

Proof. According to the Helmholtz decomposition, there exist two scalar functions $\Phi_j(x,y)$ and $\Psi_j(x,y)$ such that

$$\sigma^n \nabla u_j^n - \sigma^* \nabla u_j^* = \nabla \Phi_j + \nabla^\perp \Psi_j, \quad j = 1, 2, \qquad (3.120)$$

where $\nabla^\perp := (\partial_y, -\partial_x)$. Taking divergence to the right side of (3.120) and using $\nabla \cdot \nabla^\perp = 0$, we have

$$\nabla \cdot \nabla \Phi_j + \nabla \cdot \nabla^\perp \Psi_j = \nabla^2 \Phi_j, \quad j = 1, 2.$$

Then (3.120) with the above identity leads to

$$\nabla^2 \Phi_j = \nabla \cdot (\sigma^n \nabla u_j^n - \sigma^* \nabla u_j^*) = 0 \quad \text{in } \Omega. \qquad (3.121)$$

From the boundary condition on u_j^n and u_j^*, we have

$$0 = (\sigma^n \nabla u_j^n - \sigma^* \nabla u_j^*) \cdot \mathbf{n} = \frac{\partial \Phi_j}{\partial \mathbf{n}} + \nabla^\perp \Psi_j \cdot \mathbf{n} \quad \text{in } \partial\Omega \backslash \mathcal{E}^\pm,$$

$$0 = (\sigma^n \nabla u_j^n - \sigma^* \nabla u_j^*) \cdot \mathbf{t} = \frac{\partial \Phi_j}{\partial \mathbf{t}} + \nabla^\perp \Psi_j \cdot \mathbf{t} \quad \text{in } \partial\mathcal{E}^\pm,$$

where $\mathbf{t}$ is the unit tangent vector with $\mathbf{t} \cdot \nabla^\perp = \frac{\partial}{\partial \mathbf{n}}$. In order to determine Φ_j, we fix the boundary condition for Ψ_j by choosing

$$\Psi_j = 0 \quad \text{on } \partial\Omega \backslash \mathcal{E}^\pm, \quad \nabla^\perp \Psi_j \cdot \mathbf{t} = 0 \quad \text{on } \partial\mathcal{E}^\pm. \qquad (3.122)$$

Then Φ_j is a solution of the Laplace equation with the boundary condition

$$\frac{\partial \Phi_j}{\partial \mathbf{n}} = 0 \quad \text{on } \partial\Omega \backslash \mathcal{E}^\pm, \quad \frac{\partial \Phi_j}{\partial \mathbf{t}} = 0 \quad \text{on } \partial\mathcal{E}^\pm. \qquad (3.123)$$

From (3.120) and (3.122), we have

$$\begin{cases} \nabla^\perp \cdot \nabla^\perp \Psi_j = \nabla^\perp \cdot (\sigma^n \nabla u_j^n - \sigma^* \nabla u_j^*) & \text{in } \Omega \\ \Psi_j = 0 \quad \text{on } \partial\Omega \backslash \mathcal{E}^\pm, \quad \nabla \Psi_j \cdot \mathbf{n} = 0 & \text{on } \partial\mathcal{E}^\pm. \end{cases} \qquad (3.124)$$

From (3.117), it is easy to see that

$$\nabla^\perp \cdot (\sigma^n \nabla u_j^n - \sigma^* \nabla u_j^*) = -\nabla \sigma^n \cdot \nabla^\perp u_j^n + \nabla \sigma^* \cdot \nabla^\perp u_j^*$$

$$= \frac{1}{\mu_0}(\nabla^2 B_{z,*}^j - \nabla^2 B_{z,n}^j). \qquad (3.125)$$

Hence Ψ_j satisfies

$$
\begin{cases}
\nabla^2 \Psi_j = \dfrac{1}{\mu_0}(\nabla^2 B_{z,*}^j - \nabla^2 B_{z,n}^j) & \text{in } \Omega \\[2mm]
\Psi_j = 0 \quad \text{on } \partial\Omega \backslash \mathcal{E}^{\pm}, \quad \nabla \Psi_j \cdot \mathbf{n} = 0 \quad \text{on } \partial\mathcal{E}^{\pm}.
\end{cases}
\tag{3.126}
$$

The uniqueness of the problem (3.126) leads to $\Psi_j = \frac{1}{\mu_0}(B_{z,*}^j - B_{z,n}^j)$. Noting that

$$
-\sigma^n \nabla^{\perp} u_j^n + \sigma^* \nabla^{\perp} u_j^* = \nabla \Psi_j = \frac{1}{\mu_0}\nabla(B_{z,*}^j - B_{z,n}^j)
$$

and

$$
\sigma^* \mathbb{A}[\sigma^*]\nabla \ln \sigma^* - \sigma^n \mathbb{A}[\sigma^n]\nabla \ln \sigma^n = \frac{1}{\mu_0}\begin{pmatrix} \nabla^2 B_{z,*}^1 - \nabla^2 B_{z,n}^1 \\ \nabla^2 B_{z,*}^2 - \nabla^2 B_{z,n}^2 \end{pmatrix},
$$

we have

$$
\begin{aligned}
\nabla \ln \frac{\sigma^n}{\sigma^*} = \frac{1}{\mu_0}(\sigma^n \mathbb{A}[\sigma^n])^{-1} & \left[\begin{bmatrix} \nabla(B_{z,*}^1 - B_{z,n}^1) \\ \nabla(B_{z,*}^1 - B_{z,n}^2) \end{bmatrix} \nabla \ln \sigma^* \right. \\
& \left. + \begin{bmatrix} \nabla^2(B_{z,*}^1 - B_{z,n}^1) \\ \nabla^2(B_{z,*}^2 - B_{z,n}^2) \end{bmatrix} \right].
\end{aligned}
\tag{3.127}
$$

In order for the above expression to be meaningful, the matrix $\mathbb{A}[\sigma^n]$ must be invertible. As we mentioned before, the invertibility can be proved based on a very careful use of the results in [Alessandrini and Magnanini (1992)] and [Alessandrini and Nesi (2001)].

We now return to the expression (3.127) which would be uniformly bounded in $\tilde{\Omega}$ due to the boundedness of $\|(\sigma^n \mathbb{A}[\sigma^n])^{-1}\|_{L^{\infty}(\tilde{\Omega})}$. Note that $\nabla \sigma^* = 0$ in $\Omega \backslash \tilde{\Omega}$ implies $\nabla^2 B_{z,*}^j = 0$ in $\Omega \backslash \tilde{\Omega}$ and therefore $\nabla \sigma^n = 0$ in $\Omega \backslash \tilde{\Omega}$ due to the relation (3.88). Since $\nabla \ln \frac{\sigma^n}{\sigma^*} = 0$ in $\Omega \backslash \tilde{\Omega}$, it follows from (3.88) that

$$
(\ln \sigma^n - \ln \sigma^*)(x,y) := -\frac{1}{2\pi}\int_{\tilde{\Omega}} \frac{(x-x', y-y')}{|x-x'|^2 + |y-y'|^2}
$$

$$
\cdot \nabla \ln \frac{\sigma^n}{\sigma^*}(x',y')\, dx' dy'.
\tag{3.128}
$$

From (3.127), (3.128), and the generalized Hölder inequality, we have

$$\left\| \ln \frac{\sigma^n}{\sigma^*} \right\|_{L^\infty(\tilde{\Omega})}$$

$$\leq M \left\| (\sigma^n \mathbb{A}[\sigma^n])^{-1} \right\|_{L^{p_2}(\tilde{\Omega})} \sum_{j=1}^{2} \left\| B_{z,*}^j - B_{z,n}^j \right\|_{W^{2,p_3}(\tilde{\Omega})},$$

$$(3.129)$$

where

$$M = \frac{1}{2\pi\mu_0(2 - p_1)^{1/p_1}} (\text{diam}(\Omega))^{\frac{2}{p_1}-1} (1 + \| \nabla \ln \sigma^* \|_{L^\infty(\tilde{\Omega})})$$

$$(3.130)$$

and p_1, p_2, p_3 are positive numbers such that $1 < p_1 < 2$, $\frac{1}{p_1} + \frac{1}{p_2} + \frac{1}{p_3} = 1$. This completes the proof using the *a priori* information about $\| \nabla \ln \sigma^* \|_{L^\infty(\tilde{\Omega})}$.

3.8.2 *Variational B_z and gradient B_z decomposition algorithm*

Experimental studies in MREIT have demonstrated that conductivity imaging with a spatial resolution comparable to that of MR images is possible as long as we inject enough current into the imaging object to induce B_z signals with enough SNR. However, the performance of the harmonic B_z algorithm is deteriorated when the SNR in measured B_z data is not high enough. The SNR of the signal B_z is proportional to the amplitude of the injection current. To make MREIT easily applicable to clinical situations, however, it is highly desirable to reduce the amount of injection current down to less than 1 mA and not to produce any side effects. To be able to reduce it, we need to minimize the noise level in measured B_z data by improving experimental and data processing techniques.

Since the harmonic B_z algorithm requires twice differentiations of B_z data, which tend to amplify its noise, there has been an effort to improve the harmonic B_z algorithms noise tolerance by reducing the number of differentiations of B_z. They include the gradient

B_z decomposition algorithm [Park *et al.* (2004a)] and variational gradient B_z algorithm [Park *et al.* (2004b)] that need to differentiate B_z only once. They showed a better performance in some numerical simulations. However, in practical environments those algorithms were fruitless and produced some artifacts. Analysis of PDE models often plays an important role in the achievement of major advances in these areas, but it should not be studied in an isolated way. Symbiotic interplay between theoretical mathematics and experiments is crucial to solve these realistic model problems. Although these algorithms [Park *et al.* (2004a, b)] are theoretically interesting, they failed in practice and we discuss them for pedagogical purposes.

For ease of explanation, we assume that $u_j[\sigma]$ is a solution of the following classical boundary value problem:

$$\begin{cases} \nabla \cdot (\sigma \nabla u_j) = 0 & \text{in } \Omega \\ -\sigma \nabla u_j \cdot \mathbf{n} = g_j & \text{on } \partial\Omega \end{cases} \tag{3.131}$$

where g_j is the normal component of the current density $\mathbf{J}_j$ on the boundary. We will denote $u = u_1[\sigma]$, $g = g_1, \mathbf{J} = \mathbf{J}_1$, $\mathbf{B} = \mathbf{B}_1$ throughout this subsection.

3.8.2.1 *Variational B_z algorithm*

The major ingredient in deriving the variational B_z algorithm is the elimination of the two components B_x and B_y from the physical relations

$$\mathbf{J} = \frac{1}{\mu_0} \nabla \times \mathbf{B} \quad \text{and} \quad \mathbf{J} = -\sigma \nabla u. \tag{3.132}$$

This can be achieved by utilizing $\nabla \cdot \mathbf{J} = 0$ and $\nabla \cdot \mathbf{B} = 0$ with a carefully chosen space of test functions.

The identities in (3.132) can be expressed as the following integral form:

$$\int_\Omega \nabla \times \mathbf{B} \cdot \Psi d\mathbf{r} = -\mu_0 \int_\Omega \sigma \nabla u \cdot \Psi d\mathbf{r} \quad \text{for all } \Psi \in [L^2(\Omega)]^3. \tag{3.133}$$

To eliminate the terms B_x and B_y in the integrand in (3.133), we need to force suitable constraints on Ψ by introducing the following class:

$$T := \begin{cases} \psi \in H^1(\Omega): & \text{for } \mathbf{r} \in \partial\Omega, \\ (i)\ \dfrac{\partial\psi}{\partial x}(\mathbf{r}) = 0 = \dfrac{\partial\psi}{\partial y}(\mathbf{r}) & \text{if } \mathbf{n}(\mathbf{r}) \cdot \hat{\mathbf{z}} \neq 0 \\ (ii)\ \dfrac{\partial\psi}{\partial z}(\mathbf{r}) = 0 & \text{if } \mathbf{n}(\mathbf{r}) \times \hat{\mathbf{z}} \neq \vec{0} \end{cases}.$$

This class T plays an important role in eliminating B_x and B_y in (3.133). For the choice of $\Psi = (\frac{\partial\psi}{\partial y}, -\frac{\partial\psi}{\partial x}, 0)$ with $\psi \in T$, the integral identity (3.133) can be written as

$$\int_\Omega \left[\left(\frac{\partial B_z}{\partial y} - \frac{\partial B_y}{\partial z} \right) \frac{\partial\psi}{\partial y} + \left(\frac{\partial B_z}{\partial x} - \frac{\partial B_x}{\partial z} \right) \frac{\partial\psi}{\partial x} \right] d\mathbf{r}$$

$$= \mu_0 \int_\Omega \sigma \left(\frac{\partial u}{\partial y} \frac{\partial\psi}{\partial x} - \frac{\partial u}{\partial x} \frac{\partial\psi}{\partial y} \right) d\mathbf{r}. \qquad (3.134)$$

Taking advantage of the boundary condition on $\psi \in T$ and using integration by parts twice, the left side of (3.134) becomes

$$\int_\Omega \left[\left(\frac{\partial B_z}{\partial y} - \frac{\partial B_y}{\partial z} \right) \frac{\partial\psi}{\partial y} + \left(\frac{\partial B_z}{\partial x} - \frac{\partial B_x}{\partial z} \right) \frac{\partial\psi}{\partial x} \right] d\mathbf{r}$$

$$= \int_\Omega \nabla B_z \cdot \nabla\psi d\mathbf{r}. \qquad (3.135)$$

The identity (3.135) was derived as follows:

$$\int_\Omega \left[\left(\frac{\partial B_z}{\partial y} - \frac{\partial B_y}{\partial z} \right) \frac{\partial\psi}{\partial y} + \left(\frac{\partial B_z}{\partial x} - \frac{\partial B_x}{\partial z} \right) \frac{\partial\psi}{\partial x} \right] d\mathbf{r}$$

$$= \int_\Omega \left[\frac{\partial B_z}{\partial y} \frac{\partial\psi}{\partial y} + \frac{\partial B_z}{\partial x} \frac{\partial\psi}{\partial x} \right] d\mathbf{r} - \int_\Omega \left[\frac{\partial B_y}{\partial z} \frac{\partial\psi}{\partial y} + \frac{\partial B_x}{\partial z} \frac{\partial\psi}{\partial x} \right] d\mathbf{r}$$

$$= \int_\Omega \left[\frac{\partial B_z}{\partial y} \frac{\partial\psi}{\partial y} + \frac{\partial B_z}{\partial x} \frac{\partial\psi}{\partial x} \right] d\mathbf{r} + \int_\Omega \left[B_y \frac{\partial^2\psi}{\partial z \partial y} + B_x \frac{\partial^2\psi}{\partial z \partial x} \right] d\mathbf{r}$$

$$= \int_\Omega \left[\frac{\partial B_z}{\partial y} \frac{\partial\psi}{\partial y} + \frac{\partial B_z}{\partial x} \frac{\partial\psi}{\partial x} \right] d\mathbf{r} - \int_\Omega \left[\frac{\partial B_x}{\partial x} + \frac{\partial B_y}{\partial y} \right] \frac{\partial\psi}{\partial z} d\mathbf{r}$$

$$= \int_\Omega \left[\frac{\partial B_z}{\partial y} \frac{\partial \psi}{\partial y} + \frac{\partial B_z}{\partial x} \frac{\partial \psi}{\partial x} + \frac{\partial B_z}{\partial z} \frac{\partial \psi}{\partial z} \right] d\mathbf{r}$$

$$= \int_\Omega \nabla B_z \cdot \nabla \psi d\mathbf{r}.$$

The first identity follows from rearranging the left side of (3.135). For the second and third, we used integration by parts. The fourth identity follows from $\nabla \cdot \mathbf{B} = 0$.

From (3.134) and (3.135), we arrive at the useful form for MREIT using only B_z data:

$$\int_\Omega \sigma(\nabla u \times \hat{\mathbf{z}}) \cdot \nabla \psi d\mathbf{r} = \frac{1}{\mu_0} \int_\Omega \nabla B_z \cdot \nabla \psi d\mathbf{r}, \quad \forall \psi \in \mathcal{T}. \quad (3.136)$$

Hence, the relation between B_z and the conductivity σ is dictated by the following B_z-based MREIT system:

$$\begin{cases} \nabla \cdot (\sigma \nabla u) = 0 & \text{in } \Omega \\ -\sigma \nabla u \cdot \mathbf{n} = g & \text{on } \partial \Omega \\ \int_\Omega \sigma(\nabla u \times \hat{\mathbf{z}}) \cdot \nabla \psi d\mathbf{r} = \frac{1}{\mu_0} \int_\Omega \nabla B_z \cdot \nabla \psi d\mathbf{r}, & \forall \psi \in \mathcal{T}. \end{cases}$$
$$(3.137)$$

Now, we are ready to state the iterative algorithm as follows.

Step 1. Let $m = 0$ and assume an initial conductivity distribution σ_0.

Step 2. Compute u_m^j by solving the Neumann boundary value problem (3.131) for $j = 1, 2$.

Step 3. Compute σ_{m+1} in each slice by solving

$$\int_\Omega \sigma_{m+1} \begin{bmatrix} (\nabla u_1^m \times \hat{\mathbf{z}}) \cdot \nabla \psi \\ (\nabla u_2^m \times \hat{\mathbf{z}}) \cdot \nabla \psi \end{bmatrix} d\mathbf{r}$$

$$= \begin{bmatrix} \dfrac{1}{\mu_0} \int_\Omega \nabla B_{z,1} \cdot \nabla \psi d\mathbf{r} \\ \dfrac{1}{\mu_0} \int_\Omega \nabla B_{z,2} \cdot \nabla \psi d\mathbf{r} \end{bmatrix}, \quad \forall \psi \in \mathcal{T}. \quad (3.138)$$

Step 4. $\sigma = \lim_{m \to \infty} \sigma_m$.

When the B_z data are contaminated with random noise, the variational B_z algorithm can be worse than the harmonic B_z algorithm due to some undesirable side effects. In order to understand the behavior of the variational B_z algorithm, we define the electrically blind spot as the region inside the subject where the current density is negligibly small. This means that any change of the conductivity value within the blind spot does not produce any noticeable change in the B_z data. This kind of blind spot may occur due to the shape of the subject and also the electrode configuration.

In the harmonic B_z algorithm, the computation of $\nabla^2 B_z$ at one point provides the information on the spatial change of the conductivity there, that is, $\nabla\sigma$. In other words, the harmonic B_z algorithm is a pixel-by-pixel algorithm and any blind spot at a pixel has negligible effect on computing $\nabla\sigma$ at other pixels. Therefore, relatively simple regularization technique can effectively handle blind spots. In the variational B_z algorithm, we end up getting rid of this advantage at the price of reducing the number of differentiations.[4] The matrix associated with (3.138) includes the global structure of the entire subject including all blind spots and blind spots where we can not reconstruct conductivity values accurately, cause the matrix to be ill-conditioned. This explains the reason why errors propagate toward other interior regions in the variational B_z algorithm.

3.8.2.2 *Gradient B_z decomposition algorithm*

The gradient B_z decomposition algorithm deals with a cylindrical domain $\Omega = \{\mathbf{r} = (x, y, z) | (x, y) \in D, -\delta < z < \delta\}$ where D is a two-dimensional, smooth, and simply connected domain. The gradient B_z decomposition algorithm is based on the following implicit reconstruction formula:

$$\sigma = \frac{\left| -\left(\frac{\partial \Upsilon}{\partial y} + \Theta_x[u]\right)\frac{\partial u}{\partial x} + \left(\frac{\partial \Upsilon}{\partial x} + \Theta_y[u]\right)\frac{\partial u}{\partial y} \right|}{\left(\frac{\partial u}{\partial x}\right)^2 + \left(\frac{\partial u}{\partial y}\right)^2} \quad \text{in } \Omega \qquad (3.139)$$

---

[4]This may be somewhat misleading. The harmonic B_z algorithm essentially needs to differentiate B_z only once because it uses twice differentiation of B_z and one integration.

where

$$\Theta_x[u] := \frac{\partial \psi}{\partial y} - \frac{\partial W_z}{\partial x} + \frac{\partial W_x}{\partial z} \quad \text{and}$$

$$\Theta_y[u] := \frac{\partial \psi}{\partial x} + \frac{\partial W_z}{\partial y} - \frac{\partial W_y}{\partial z} \quad \text{in } \Omega$$

and

$$\Upsilon = \phi + \frac{1}{\mu_0} B_z, \quad W(\mathbf{r}) := \int_\Omega \frac{1}{4\pi |\mathbf{r} - \mathbf{r}'|} \frac{\partial (\sigma \nabla u(\mathbf{r}'))}{\partial z} d\mathbf{r}'.$$

Here, ϕ is a solution of

$$\begin{cases} \nabla^2 \phi = 0 & \text{in } \Omega \\ \phi = \tilde{g} - \dfrac{1}{\mu_0} B_z & \text{on } \partial\Omega \backslash \{z = \pm\delta\} \\ \dfrac{\partial \phi}{\partial z} = -\dfrac{1}{\mu_0} \dfrac{\partial B_z}{\partial z} & \text{on } \partial\Omega \cap \{z = \pm\delta\} \end{cases} \tag{3.140}$$

and ψ is a solution of

$$\begin{cases} \nabla^2 \psi = 0 & \text{in } \Omega \\ \nabla \psi \cdot \tau = \nabla \times W \cdot \mathbf{n}^\perp & \text{on } \partial\Omega \backslash \{z = \pm\delta\} \\ \dfrac{\partial \psi}{\partial z} = -\nabla \times W \cdot \hat{\mathbf{z}} & \text{on } \partial\Omega \cap \{z = \pm\delta\} \end{cases} \tag{3.141}$$

where $\mathbf{n}^\perp := (-\mathbf{n} \cdot \hat{\mathbf{y}}, \mathbf{n} \cdot \hat{\mathbf{x}}, 0)$ is the tangent vector on the lateral boundary $\partial\Omega \backslash \{z = \pm\delta\}$. Here, $\tilde{g}$ is

$$\tilde{g}(x(t), y(t), z) := \int_0^t g((x(t), y(t), z)) \sqrt{|x'(t)|^2 + |y'(t)|^2} dt$$

where $\partial D := \{(x(t), y(t)) : 0 \leq t \leq 1\}$.

We may use an iterative reconstruction scheme with multiple Neumann data $g_j, j = 1, 2$ to find σ. Denoting by u_j^m a solution of $\nabla \cdot (\sigma^m \nabla u) = 0$ in Ω with a Neumann data g_j, the reconstructed σ is the limit of a sequence σ^m that is obtained by the following formula:

$$\sigma^{m+1} = \frac{\sum_{i=1}^2 \left| -\left(\frac{\partial \Upsilon_i}{\partial y} + \Theta_x[u_i^m]\right) \frac{\partial u_i^m}{\partial x} + \left(\frac{\partial \Upsilon_i}{\partial x} + \Theta_y[u_i^m]\right) \frac{\partial u_i^m}{\partial y} \right|}{\sum_{i=1}^2 \left[\left(\frac{\partial u_i^m}{\partial x}\right)^2 + \left(\frac{\partial u_i^m}{\partial y}\right)^2\right]}.$$

(3.142)

This method needs to differentiate B_z only once in contrast to the harmonic B_z algorithm where the numerical computation of $\nabla^2 B_z$ is required. It has an advantage of improved noise tolerance and numerical simulations with added random noise of a realistic amount showed its feasibility and robustness against measurement noise. However, in practical environments, it shows poorer performance compared with the harmonic B_z algorithm and may produce some artifacts.

The major reason is that the updated conductivity σ^{m+1} by the iteration process (3.142) is influenced by the global distribution of σ^m. We should note that there always exist some local regions having defected B_z data in human or animal experiments and we always deal with a truncated region of the imaging object which causes geometrical modeling errors. Hence, it would be impossible to reconstruct the conductivity distribution in the entire region of the human or animal subject with a reasonable accuracy and it would be best to achieve robust reconstruction of σ in local regions where measured B_z data are reliable. In order to achieve a stable local reconstruction of conductivity contrast with moderate accuracy, poor conductivity reconstruction at one local region should not influence badly on conductivity reconstructions in other regions. This means that a conductivity image reconstruction algorithm should not depend too much on the global distribution of B_z, global structure of σ, and geometry $\partial \Omega$.

3.9   Anisotropic Conductivity Reconstruction Problem

All of the previous sections in MREIT are limited to the isotropic conductivity imaging problem. Some biological tissues are known to have anisotropic conductivity values and the ratio of anisotropy depends on the type of tissue. For example, the human skeletal muscle shows the anisotropy of up to one to ten between the longitudinal and transversal directions.

The anisotropy appears when we view tissues at a macroscopic scale as packed cells in an extracellular fluid. The anisotropic conductivity $\boldsymbol{\sigma}$ can be viewed as the effective conductivity and can be regarded as a function of tissue composition within a voxel V_{oxel}. It can be determined by Ohm's law:

$$\int_{V_{\text{oxel}}} \mathbf{J}(\mathbf{r})d\mathbf{r} \approx \boldsymbol{\sigma} \int_{V_{\text{oxel}}} \mathbf{E}(\mathbf{r})d\mathbf{r} \tag{3.143}$$

for a time-harmonic electric field $\mathbf{E}$ and the corresponding current density $\mathbf{J} = \sigma\mathbf{E}$. In some very special cases with a periodic structure in the pointwise conductivity distribution, the relation between the pointwise conductivity σ and the effective conductivity $\boldsymbol{\sigma}$ can be described by the well-known concept of the homogenization [Bensoussan *et al.* (1978)]. We begin by describing the precise definition of the effective conductivity $\boldsymbol{\sigma}$ in a given cubic voxel based on [Seo *et al.* (2013)].

3.9.1 *Definition of effective conductivity for a cubic sample*

Let us consider a rectangular tissue sample occupied in the unit cube $\Omega = \{\mathbf{r} : 0 < x, y, z < 1 \text{ cm}\}$ with its three pairs of facing surfaces (Figure 3.28):

$$\mathcal{E}_+^x = \{\mathbf{r} \in \partial\Omega : x = 1\}, \quad \mathcal{E}_-^x = \{\mathbf{r} \in \partial\Omega : x = 0\},$$
$$\mathcal{E}_+^y = \{\mathbf{r} \in \partial\Omega : y = 1\}, \quad \mathcal{E}_-^y = \{\mathbf{r} \in \partial\Omega : y = 0\},$$
$$\mathcal{E}_+^z = \{\mathbf{r} \in \partial\Omega : z = 1\}, \quad \mathcal{E}_-^z = \{\mathbf{r} \in \partial\Omega : z = 0\}.$$

Assume that the pointwise conductivity $\sigma(\mathbf{r})$ is a scalar-valued function depending only on position $\mathbf{r}$. Hence, $\sigma(\mathbf{r})$ is isotropic on a microscopic scale. If we apply a current of $I(t) = I_0 \cos(\omega t)$ at frequencies below 1 kHz through the pair of electrodes attached on $\mathcal{E}_+^a$ and $\mathcal{E}_-^a$, then the resulting time-harmonic potential $u^a(\mathbf{r})$ satisfies the

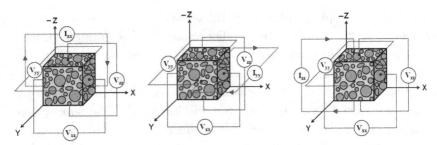

Fig. 3.28. Anisotropic conductivity measurement of a unit cube of anisotropic material by applying three injection currents.

following equation from a suitable arrangement of Maxwell equations:

$$\begin{cases} \nabla \cdot (\sigma(\mathbf{r})\nabla u^a(\mathbf{r})) = 0 & \text{for } \mathbf{r} \in \Omega \\ \mathbf{n} \cdot (\sigma\nabla u^a)|_{\mathcal{E}_+^a} = I_0 = -\mathbf{n} \cdot (\sigma\nabla u^a)|_{\mathcal{E}_-^a} \end{cases} \quad (a \in \{x, y, z\}) \quad (3.144)$$

where $\mathbf{n}$ is the unit outward normal vector on $\partial\Omega$. For each $a, b \in \{x, y, z\}$, we denote the voltage difference $\mathcal{E}_+^b$ by

$$V^{ab} = \int_{\mathcal{E}_+^b} u^a \, dS - \int_{\mathcal{E}_-^b} u^a \, dS. \quad (3.145)$$

Lemma 3.2 (Reciprocity). *For $a, b \in \{x, y, z\}$, we have*

$$V^{ab} = V^{ba}. \quad (3.146)$$

Proof. From the boundary conditions of u^b and divergence theorem, we have

$$V^{ba} = \frac{1}{I_0} \int_{\mathcal{E}_+^b} \mathbf{n} \cdot (\sigma\nabla u^a) u^b \, dS = \frac{1}{I_0} \int_\Omega \sigma\nabla u^a \cdot \nabla u^b \, d\mathbf{r}.$$

Hence, the symmetry (3.146) follows from the reciprocity relation:

$$V^{ab} = \frac{1}{I_0} \int_\Omega \sigma\nabla u^a \cdot \nabla u^b \, d\mathbf{r} = V^{ba} \quad \text{for all } a, b \in \{x, y, z\}. \quad \square$$

If $\nabla\sigma(\mathbf{r}) = 0$ (homogeneous), then $V^{xx} = V^{yy} = V^{zz}$ and $V^{xy} = V^{xz} = V^{yz} = 0$, and σ must be $\sigma = \frac{V^{xx}}{V_0}$. If the effective conductivity

σ is a diagonal matrix satisfying

$$\begin{pmatrix} \sigma_{xx} & 0 & 0 \\ 0 & \sigma_{yy} & 0 \\ 0 & 0 & \sigma_{zz} \end{pmatrix} \int_\Omega \nabla u^a(\mathbf{r})d\mathbf{r} = \int_\Omega \sigma(\mathbf{r})\nabla u^a(\mathbf{r})d\mathbf{r} \quad \forall\, a \in \{x,y,z\},$$

then it must be $\sigma_{xx} = V^{yy}/V_0, \sigma_{yy} = V^{yy}/V_0, \sigma_{zz} = V^{zz}/V_0$.

Now, we are ready to define the effective conductivity tensor σ. For a given unit cubic Ω and each $a, b \in \{x, y, z\}$, let V^{ab} be the potential difference given in (3.145). Then the effective conductivity tensor σ is defined by

$$[\sigma]^{-1} = \begin{pmatrix} \sigma_{xx} & \sigma_{xy} & \sigma_{xz} \\ \sigma_{xy} & \sigma_{yy} & \sigma_{yz} \\ \sigma_{xz} & \sigma_{yz} & \sigma_{zz} \end{pmatrix}^{-1} := \frac{1}{I_0}\begin{pmatrix} V^{xx} & V^{xy} & V^{xz} \\ V^{xy} & V^{yy} & V^{yz} \\ V^{xz} & V^{yz} & V^{zz} \end{pmatrix}. \quad (3.147)$$

The proposed definition may not have a coordinate invariance due to its limitation of the tensor expression. For a proper invariance, we need to compute all the tensor (3.147) by rotating the coordinate system. We may define the effective conductivity tensor as the best fit of a minimization problem related to (3.143).

3.9.2 *Anisotropic conductivity reconstruction in MREIT*

In theory, MREIT technique using internal measurements can provide anisotropic conductivity images unlike EIT using only boundary measurements. [Seo *et al.* (2004)] applied the MREIT technique to anisotropic conductivity image reconstructions. Investigating how an anisotropic conductivity σ affects the internal current density and thereby the magnetic flux density, they understood that at least seven different injection currents are necessary for the anisotropic conductivity image reconstruction algorithm. The algorithm is based on the following two identities:

$$\mathbf{Us} = \mathbf{b} \quad \text{and} \quad \nabla \cdot \left[\underbrace{\begin{pmatrix} \sigma_{11} & \sigma_{12} & \sigma_{13} \\ \sigma_{12} & \sigma_{22} & \sigma_{23} \\ \sigma_{13} & \sigma_{23} & \sigma_{33} \end{pmatrix}}_{\sigma} \nabla u^j \right] = 0 \quad (3.148)$$

where

$$b = \frac{1}{\mu_0} \begin{bmatrix} \nabla^2 B_{z,1} \\ \vdots \\ \nabla^2 B_{z,N} \end{bmatrix}, \quad s = \begin{bmatrix} -\partial_y \sigma_{11} + \partial_x \sigma_{12} \\ -\partial_y \sigma_{12} + \partial_x \sigma_{22} \\ -\partial_y \sigma_{13} + \partial_x \sigma_{23} \\ \sigma_{12} \\ -\sigma_{11} + \sigma_{22} \\ \sigma_{23} \\ \sigma_{13} \end{bmatrix}$$

and

$$U = \begin{bmatrix} u_x^1 & u_y^1 & u_z^1 & u_{xx}^1 - u_{yy}^1 & u_{xy}^1 & u_{xz}^1 & -u_{yz}^1 \\ \vdots & \vdots & \vdots & \vdots & \vdots & \vdots & \vdots \\ u_x^N & u_y^N & u_z^N & u_{xx}^N - u_{yy}^N & u_{xy}^N & u_{xz}^N & -u_{yz}^N \end{bmatrix}.$$

Here, u^j is the voltage corresponding to the jth injection current, $u_x^j = \frac{\partial u^j}{\partial x}$, and σ is assumed to be a symmetric positive definite matrix. As in the harmonic B_z algorithm, we may use an iterative procedure to compute s in (3.148). Assuming that we have computed all seven terms of s, we can immediately determine $\sigma_{12}(\mathbf{r}) = s_4(\mathbf{r})$, $\sigma_{13}(\mathbf{r}) = s_7(\mathbf{r})$ and $\sigma_{23}(\mathbf{r}) = s_6(\mathbf{r})$. To determine σ_{11} and σ_{22} from s, we use the relation between s and σ:

$$\frac{\partial \sigma_{11}}{\partial x} = s_2 - \frac{\partial s_5}{\partial x} + \frac{\partial s_4}{\partial y} \quad \text{and} \quad \frac{\partial \sigma_{11}}{\partial y} = -s_1 + \frac{\partial s_4}{\partial x}. \tag{3.149}$$

The last component σ_{33} can be obtained by using the physical law $\nabla \cdot \mathbf{J} = 0$.

Numerical simulation results using a relatively simple two-dimensional model demonstrated that the algorithm can successfully reconstruct images of an anisotropic conductivity tensor distribution provided the B_z data has a high SNR. Unfortunately, this algorithm is not successful in practical environments since it is very weak against noise and the matrix U is ill-conditioned in the interior region.

3.10 Imaging Experiments

[Oh *et al.* (2003a)] conducted the first experimental study using the B_z-based MREIT method, and reconstructed multi-slice conductivity images, demonstrating the ability of the harmonic B_z algorithm to produce images of a three-dimensional conductivity distribution. Since then, imaging techniques in MREIT have advanced rapidly and now can offer conductivity imaging for animal and human experiments [Woo and Seo (2008); Seo and Woo (2011)]. Given a noise level of the MRI scanner with an adopted imaging method including RF coils and pulse sequence, the quality of a reconstructed conductivity image is mainly proportional to the product of the amplitude and duration of injection currents. It also depends on many other MR imaging parameters including the main magnetic field inhomogeneity, gradient linearity, and chemical shift artifacts. In animal or human experiments, internal regions such as bones, lungs, and gas-filled organs cause some difficulties, since the SNR could be low there due to the MR signal void phenomenon. Regarding the current injection apparatus, we should secure its amplitude stability and reduce its electronic noise, interference, and timing jitters. The position and size of electrodes must also be optimized since they influence the induced magnetic flux density signal.

In order to demonstrate that the conductivity image provides meaningful diagnostic information that is not available from other imaging modalities, we need accumulated experience and knowledge on how to interpret a conductivity image in relation with anatomy and pathology of a specific organ.

3.10.1 *Phantom experiment*

3.10.1.1 *Non-biological phantom imaging*

The J-substitution algorithm was used in the first experimental MREIT study [Khang *et al.* (2002)]. It produced a very crude image of a saline phantom. [Lee *et al.* (2003)] and [Oh *et al.* (2003)] tried conductivity image reconstructions of a cubic saline phantom including a cylindrical piece of sausage shown in Figure 3.29(a). Rotating the phantom twice in the bore of a 0.3 T MRI scanner, they

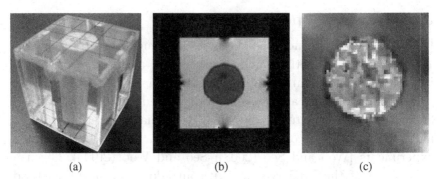

Fig. 3.29.   (a) Cubic saline phantom containing a cylindrical sausage, (b) MR magnitude image and (c) reconstructed resistivity (inverse of conductivity) image using the J-substitution algorithm [Lee *et al.* (2003)]. The experiment was performed using a 0.3 T MRI scanner.

measured $\mathbf{B}_1 = (B_{x,1}, B_{y,1}, B_{z,1})$ and $\mathbf{B}_2$ subject to two orthogonal current injections, I_1 and I_2, respectively. Computing corresponding current densities of $\mathbf{J}_1$ and $\mathbf{J}_2$, they used the J-substitution algorithm to reconstruct a cross-sectional image of the conductivity distribution inside the phantom. Compared with the MR magnitude image in Figure 3.29(b), the reconstructed conductivity image in Figure 3.29(c) well distinguished the sausage object but suffered from measurement noise and also numerous sources of errors involved in the rotation process. In Figure 3.29(b), we can observe the RF shielding artifacts near the electrodes. This observation led to the invention of the recessed electrode in later experimental MREIT studies.

[Oh *et al.* (2003)] conducted the first experimental study using the B_z-based MREIT method. They used a 0.3 T MRI scanner and an acrylic phantom equipped with four recessed electrodes. The phantom was filled with saline and included two polyacrylamide objects as shown in Figure 3.30(a)−(d). Reconstructed multi-slice conductivity images as shown in Figure 3.30(e)−(i) demonstrated the ability of the harmonic B_z algorithm to produce images of a three-dimensional conductivity distribution. Due to the large amount of noise from the 0.3 T MRI scanner and weak B_z signal around four corners of the phantom, they had to use a high degree of regularization. This resulted in smoothed pixel values around the peripheral regions.

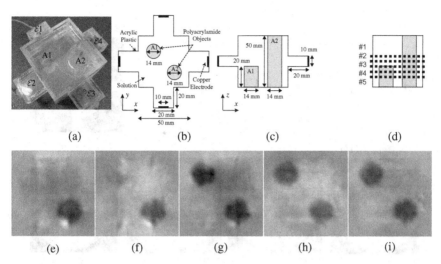

Fig. 3.30. Multi-slice conductivity images from a polyacrylamide phantom using the harmonic B_z algorithm. The experiment was performed using a 0.3 T MRI scanner. (a) Photo, (b) top view, (c) side view, and (d) slice positions of the phantom. (e)−(i) are reconstructed conductivity images at slices #1−5, respectively.

In order to improve the image quality, [Oh *et al.* (2004)] used a 3 T MRI scanner. They constructed a resolution phantom (shown in Figure 3.31) using two wedge-shaped sponges and cotton threads that produced an inhomogeneous three-dimensional conductivity distribution. By using the harmonic B_z algorithm, they reconstructed multi-slice conductivity images in Figure 3.31.

[Lee *et al.* (2006)] proposed the B_z-based MREIT method to image the breast. They constructed a three-dimensional breast phantom in Figure 3.32 (left) including three spherical anomalies with different conductivity values. Compared with the MR magnitude image of the breast phantom in Figure 3.32 (middle), the reconstructed conductivity image (right) clearly distinguished two anomalies that had higher and lower conductivity values compared with that of the background. The anomaly in the middle had a similar conductivity value as the background. Two different images in Figure 3.32 (middle and right) of the same imaging object demonstrate that MREIT provides new contrast information not available from conventional MRI technique.

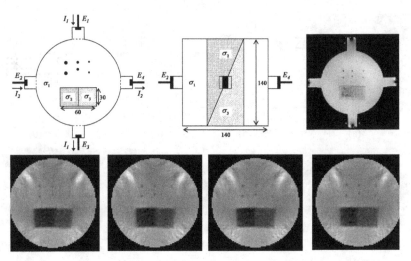

Fig. 3.31. Resolution phantom experiment using a 3 T MRI scanner [Oh *et al.* (2004)]. (Top) A top and side view of the phantom and MR magnitude image. (Bottom) Reconstructed multi-slice conductivity images using the harmonic B_z algorithm. The background region of σ_1 was filled with saline. Two regions of σ_2 and σ_3 were formed by using two wedge-shaped sponges with different densities. The six dots were cotton threads with diameters of 4 (left), 3 (middle), and 2 mm (right). Four recessed electrodes were attached to the middle of the phantom to inject currents.

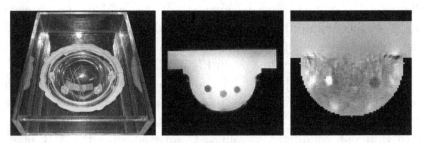

Fig. 3.32. Breast phantom experiment using a 3 T MRI scanner [Lee *et al.* (2006c)]. (left) Photo of the breast phantom, (middle) MR magnitude image and (right) reconstructed conductivity image using the harmonic B_z algorithm.

3.10.1.2 *Biological phantom imaging*

After numerous non-biological phantom imaging experiments, [Oh *et al.* (2005)] performed B_z-based MREIT experiments of biological tissue phantoms. They built phantoms containing chunks of meat

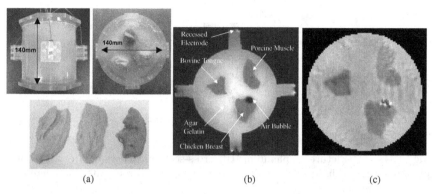

Fig. 3.33.   Biological tissue phantom imaging using a 3 T MRI scanner [Oh *et al.* (2005)]. (a) Photo of the phantom, (b) its MR magnitude image, and (c) reconstructed conductivity image using the harmonic B_z algorithm.

as shown in Figure 3.33(a). Compared with the MR magnitude image in Figure 3.33(b), the reconstructed conductivity image in Figure 3.33(c) showed excellent structural information as well as the conductivity information. They measured conductivity values of the meat beforehand and found that pixel values in the reconstructed conductivity image were close to the measured values. As shown in Figure 3.33(b), an air bubble was formed inside the phantom. The MR signal void in the air bubble caused the measured B_z data to be very noisy. From Figure 3.33(c), we can observe that the reconstructed conductivity image shows spurious spikes inside the region of the air bubble. Since this kind of technical problem can occur in a living body, the inpainting method was proposed by [Lee *et al.* (2006)].

3.10.1.3   *Contrast mechanism of apparent conductivity*

[Oh *et al.* (2011)] explained the contrast mechanism in MREIT by performing and analyzing a series of numerical simulations and imaging experiments. They built a stable conductivity phantom including a hollow insulating cylinder with holes. Filling both inside and outside the hollow cylinder with the same saline as shown in Figure 3.34, they controlled ion mobilities to create a conductivity contrast without being affected by an ion diffusion process. From numerical simulations and imaging experiments, they found that

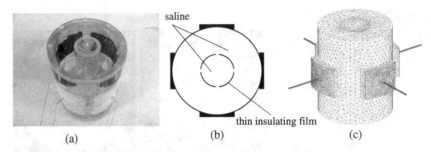

Fig. 3.34.   (a) Picture of phantom, (b) cross-sectional views of a conductivity phantom with a thin hollow cylindrical film having holes around its circumference, and (c) its mesh.

slopes of induced magnetic flux densities change with hole diameters and therefore conductivity contrasts. Associating the hole diameter with an apparent conductivity of the region inside the hollow cylinder with holes, [Oh *et al.*] experimentally validated the contrast mechanism in MREIT.

The conductivity phantom was placed inside the bore of a 3 T MRI scanner and the basic MREIT pulse sequence in Figure 3.4 was adopted. Through two pairs of opposing electrodes, they sequentially injected currents along two different directions to obtain induced magnetic flux density data B_{z1} and B_{z2}. Imaging parameters were as follows: TR/TE = 1200/30 ms, FOV = 180 × 180 mm^2, slice thickness = 6 mm, NEX = 8, matrix size = 128 × 128 and number of slices = 8. Using the harmonic B_z algorithm, conductivity images were reconstructed.

The pointwise conductivity in a microscopic scale was the same everywhere inside the phantom except the insulating film; that is, the conductivity inside the film was the same as that outside the film. Figure 3.35 shows reconstructed conductivity images of the phantom including the hollow cylinder with four holes of different diameters. The measured B_z data sets were used to reconstruct the images, which can be interpreted as apparent conductivity images, as well as ion mobility images. Note that the apparent conductivity inside the film is different from its pointwise conductivity.

As expected, ion mobilities are higher through the four holes. Ion mobilities inside the holes and also the internal region of the hollow

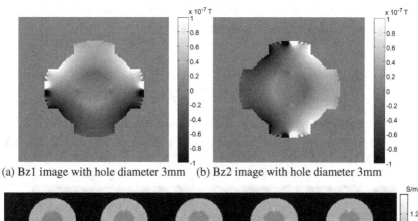

(a) Bz1 image with hole diameter 3mm   (b) Bz2 image with hole diameter 3mm

(c) conductivity images of various hole diameters

Fig. 3.35.   Reconstructed conductivity images of the phantom including the hollow cylinder with four holes of different diameters using measured B_z data sets.

cylinder increase as the hole diameter is enlarged. They estimated apparent conductivity values of the region inside the hollow cylinder as average pixel values within the region. These apparent conductivity values increased as the hole diameter was enlarged.

When the phantom includes a hollow insulating cylinder without holes, ions inside the cylinder are immobile under the low-frequency electric field and do not contribute to any current flow. Indeed, the hollow cylindrical anomaly without holes behaved as a solid insulator and produced abrupt deflections of B_z around the edge of the insulating anomaly. When the hollow cylinder has holes, ions are mobile through the holes. The holes make ions inside the cylinder mobile and these mobile ions contribute to the current flow throughout the cylindrical anomaly. From the conductivity images in Figure 3.35, we can see that current entered the cylindrical anomaly through the holes and this made the region inside the cylinder appear as a region with a non-zero conductivity value.

3.10.2 *Animal experiment*

3.10.2.1 *Postmortem animal imaging*

Figure 3.36 shows reconstructed multi-slice conductivity images of a postmortem canine brain by using a 3 T MRI scanner and 40 mA

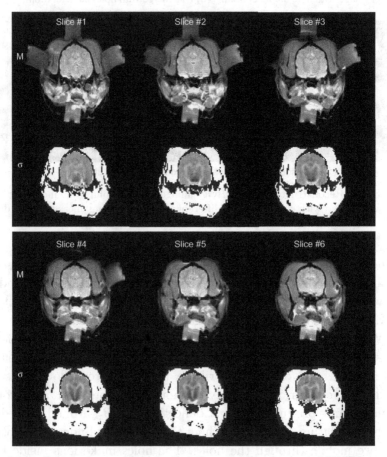

Fig. 3.36.   Postmortem animal imaging of a canine head using a 3 T MRI scanner [Kim *et al.* (2007)]. Multi-slice MR magnitude images of a canine head are shown in the top rows and reconstructed equivalent isotropic conductivity images of its brain are in the bottom rows.

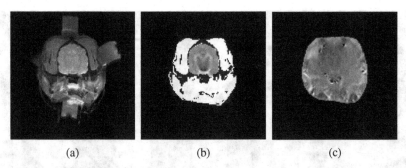

Fig. 3.37. Comparison of (a) MR magnitude image, (b) conductivity image of the brain only, and (c) conductivity image of the entire head from a postmortem canine head.

injection currents [Kim *et al.* (2007)]. Their primary goals were to produce high-resolution conductivity images of white and gray matter *in situ* and to enhance experimental techniques to undertake *in vivo* animal imaging studies. The images were reconstructed using the harmonic B_z algorithm, which does not handle the tissue anisotropy. Hence, the reconstructed conductivity images should be interpreted by the equivalent isotropic conductivity. They restricted conductivity image reconstructions to the brain region to avoid technical difficulties related with the skull. Reconstructed conductivity images with a pixel size of $1.4 \times 1.4\,\text{mm}^2$ showed a clear conductivity contrast between gray and white matter. The images in Figure 3.36 were the first MREIT images of an intact animal. Figure 3.37 compares an MR magnitude image in (a), conductivity image of the brain region only in (b), and conductivity image of the entire head in (c).

[Jeong *et al.* (2008)] proposed a thin and flexible carbon-hydrogel electrode to replace the bulky and rigid recessed electrode. They found that the new electrode produces a negligible amount of artifacts in MR and conductivity images and significantly simplifies the experimental procedure. The electrode can be fabricated in different shapes and sizes. Adding a layer of conductive adhesive, one can easily attach the electrode on an irregular surface with an excellent contact. Using a pair of carbon-hydrogel electrodes with a large contact area, the amplitude of an injection current can

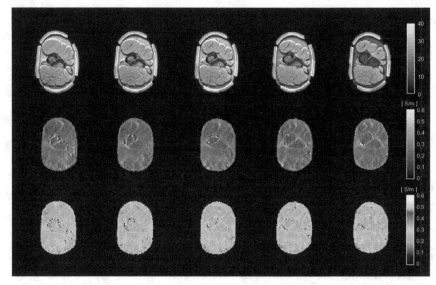

Fig. 3.38.   Postmortem animal imaging of a swine leg using a 3 T MRI scanner [Minhas *et al.* (2008)]. Multi-slice MR magnitude (top), conductivity (middle), and color-coded conductivity (bottom) images.

be increased primarily due to a reduced average current density underneath the electrodes. [Minhas *et al.* (2008)] evaluated the performance of the new electrode by conducting MREIT imaging experiments of five postmortem swine legs. Reconstructed equivalent isotropic conductivity images of a swine leg in Figure 3.38 show a good contrast among different muscles and bones. From the reconstructed images, we can observe spurious spikes in the outer layers of bones primarily due to the MR signal void there.

Figures 3.39(a) and (b) are MR magnitude and reconstructed conductivity images of a postmortem canine abdomen [Jeon *et al.* (2009b)]. Since the abdomen includes a complicated mixture of different organs, interpretation of a reconstructed conductivity image needs further investigation. They found that conductivity image contrast in the canine kidney is quite different from that of the MR magnitude image clearly distinguishing the cortex, internal medulla, renal pelvis, and urethra. The internal medulla of the kidney and the urethra appear to be significantly more conductive than the cortex of the kidney.

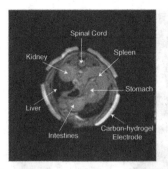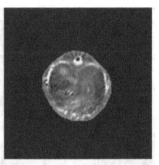

Fig. 3.39. (left) MR magnitude image and (right) reconstructed conductivity image from a postmortem canine abdomen [Jeon *et al.* (2009b)]. The conductivity image shows a significantly different image contrast compared with the MR magnitude image.

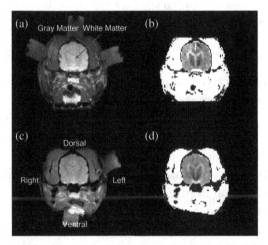

Fig. 3.40. (a) *In vivo* and (c) postmortem MR magnitude images of a canine head. (b) *In vivo* and (d) postmortem equivalent isotropic conductivity images of the brain. The same animal was used for both *in vivo* and postmortem experiments [Kim *et al.* (2008b)]. The image in (b) was obtained by using 5 mA injection currents whereas 40 mA was used in (d).

3.10.2.2 *In vivo animal imaging*

[Kim *et al.* (2008b)] described the first *in vivo* animal imaging experiment using a 3 T MRI scanner. They injected 5 mA currents into the head of an anesthetized dog. They imaged the canine brain before and after sacrificing it. Figure 3.40 compares *in vivo* and

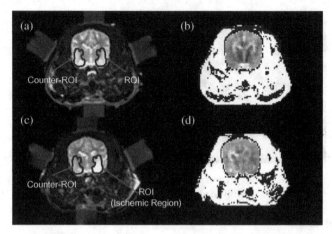

Fig. 3.41.   T$_2$-weighted MR images of a canine head (a) before and (c) after the embolization. Shown in (b) and (d) are corresponding equivalent isotropic conductivity images. The region-of-interest (ROI) defines the ischemic region and counter-ROI defines the symmetrical region in the other side of the brain [Kim *et al.* (2008b)].

postmortem conductivity images of a canine brain. Though the *in vivo* conductivity image is noisier than the postmortem image primarily due to the reduced amplitude of injection currents, the *in vivo* image clearly shows a contrast among white matter, gray matter, and other brain tissues. They also conducted *in vivo* imaging experiments of canine brains without and with a regional brain ischemia. As shown in Figure 3.41, the ischemia produced noticeable conductivity changes in reconstructed images.

Following the first *in vivo* imaging experiment of the canine brain by [Kim *et al.* (2008)], numerous *in vivo* animal imaging experiments have been conducted for imaging regions of extremities, upper and lower abdomen, pelvis, neck, thorax, and head. Animal models of various diseases were also tried. Accumulated results of these *in vivo* animal imaging experiments resulted in a proper design of *in vivo* human imaging experiments.

Figure 3.42 shows images of a canine chest. The reconstructed conductivity image reveals conductivity contrasts among the heart, longissimus thoracis muscle, and thoracic wall. Since MR signals from the lungs are weak, conductivity images of the lungs show peculiar noise patterns. The enlarged conductivity image of the heart

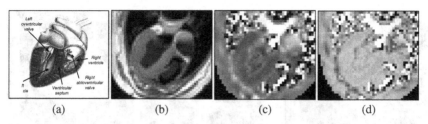

(a)   (b)   (c)   (d)

Fig. 3.42. Magnified images of the heart: (a) anatomy of the heart, (b) MR magnitude image, (c) reconstructed conductivity image, and (d) color-coded conductivity image. Conductivity images distinguish the ventricle, ventricular septum, and myocardium.

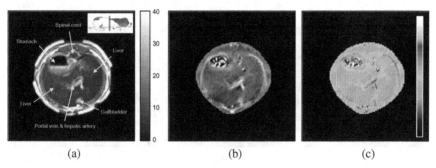

(a)   (b)   (c)

Fig. 3.43. Upper abdomen imaging: (a) MR magnitude image, (b) reconstructed conductivity image, and (c) color-coded conductivity image.

in Figure 3.42 well distinguishes the heart structure including the ventricle, ventricular septum, and myocardium.

Figure 3.43 shows images of a canine upper abdomen. Conductivity images reveal different organs including the liver, stomach, gallbladder, and blood vessels. Conductivity images distinguish organs in the lower abdomen including the spinal cord, peritoneal cavity, kidney, liver, large and small intestines, spleen, and stomach. The peritoneal cavity, which mainly consists of conductive fluids, shows a high conductivity value.

Figure 3.44 shows images of a canine pelvis. Conductivity images exhibit different contrasts for the prostate, sacrum, rectum, and surrounding muscles. Figure 3.45 shows enlarged images of the prostate. Compared with the MR magnitude image of the prostate, the corresponding conductivity image shows a clear contrast between

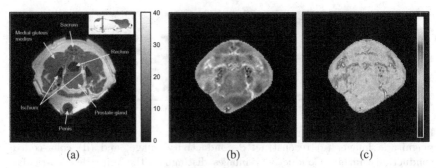

Fig. 3.44. Pelvis imaging: (a) MR magnitude image, (b) reconstructed conductivity image, and (c) color-coded conductivity image.

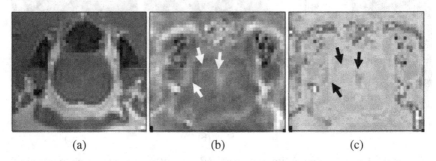

Fig. 3.45. (a) MR magnitude image of the prostate, (b) reconstructed conductivity image, and (b) color-coded conductivity image. Conductivity images distinguish the central and peripheral zones which are closely related to prostate cancer and benign prostatic hyperplasia. Arrows indicate the canine prostate structure.

the central and peripheral zones which are closely related with prostate cancer and benign prostatic hyperplasia.

[Kim *et al.* (2010)] performed *in vivo* disease model animal experiments to validate the MREIT technique in terms of its capability to produce a conductivity contrast corresponding to brain ischemia and abscess. Injecting 5 mA imaging currents into the head of an anesthetized dog, they collected induced magnetic flux density data using a 3T MRI scanner. Applying the harmonic Bz algorithm to the data, they reconstructed scaled conductivity images providing conductivity contrast information. To investigate any change of electrical conductivity due to brain diseases of ischemia and abscess, they scanned an animal with such a regional brain disease along with

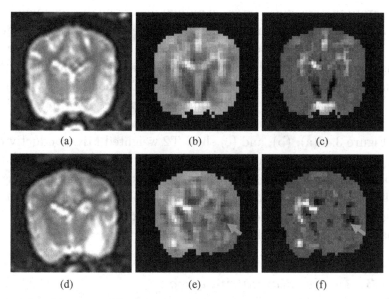

Fig. 3.46.   Shown in (a), (b), and (c) are T2 weighted MR, reconstructed conductivity, and color-coded images of the first normal canine brain, respectively. Shown in (d), (e), and (f) are corresponding images of the same canine brain after inducing a regional ischemia. The arrow in the right temporal lobe indicates a significantly decreased conductivity contrast.

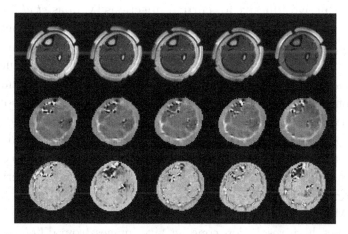

Fig. 3.47.   *In vivo* MREIT imaging experiment of a human leg using a 3 T MRI scanner [Kim *et al.* (2008c, 2009)]. Multi-slice MR magnitude images, reconstructed equivalent isotropic conductivity images, and color-coded conductivity images of a human leg are shown in the top, middle, and bottom rows, respectively.

a separate prior scan of the same animal having no disease model. In the brain ischemic region, conductivity images showed a significantly decreased contrast. The conductivity images of brain abscess showed a significantly increased contrast, which was not apparent in the normal brain. The results indicate that MREIT conductivity images have a potential to provide meaningful diagnostic information that is not available from other imaging modalities.

Figure 3.46(a), (b), and (c) show T2 weighted MR, conductivity, and color-coded conductivity images of a normal canine brain, respectively. Figure 3.46(d), (e), and (f) show corresponding images of the same canine brain with an abscess. Conductivity images show a significantly increased contrast in the left frontal lobe, which is not apparent in the normal brain.

3.10.3 *In vivo human imaging*

For the first *in vivo* human imaging experiment, [Kim *et al.* (2008c)] chose the lower extremity as the imaging region [Kim *et al.* (2008c, 2009)]. After a review of the institutional review board, they performed MREIT experiments of human subjects using a 3 T MRI scanner. They adopted thin and flexible carbon-hydrogel electrodes with conductive adhesive for current injections [Minhas *et al.* (2008)]. Due to their large surface area of $80 \times 60 \, mm^2$ and good contact with the skin, they could inject pulse-type currents with their amplitude of as much as 9 mA into the lower extremity without producing a painful sensation. Sequential injections of two currents in orthogonal directions were used to produce cross-sectional equivalent isotropic conductivity images in Figure 3.47 with 1.7 mm pixel size and 4 mm slice gap. The conductivity images effectively distinguished different parts of muscles and bones. The outermost fatty layer was also clearly shown in each conductivity image. Excessive noise was observed in the outer layers of two bones due to the MR signal void phenomenon there. Minhas *et al.* suggested further human imaging experiments to produce high-resolution conductivity images from different parts of the human body.

The *in vivo* human MREIT experiment of the calf has revealed two technical issues regarding the chemical shift artifact and noise in

B_z images [Kim *et al.* (2009)]. The chemical shift occurs in fat regions and results in misalignments of pixels along the frequency encoding direction. Reconstructed conductivity images using such data suffer from artifacts originated from signal void at one side and overlap at the other. Fat suppression methods should be avoided in MREIT since they weaken MR signals which carry information on the induced magnetic flux B_z. Acquiring k-space data at a wider bandwidth is also undesirable due to an increased noise level in MR signals. To improve the quality of conductivity images, we should use a chemical shift artifact correction method which can remove the artifact in both MR magnitude and phase images. The first step is to separate the MR image into water and fat images. Pixel misalignments are then corrected in the fat image. By adding the corrected fat image to the water image, we can produce an artifact-free MR image. The classical three-point Dixon's water-fat separation technique has been recently modified for MREIT to produce artifact-free B_z images [Minhas *et al.* (2009); Hamamura *et al.* (2009)]. Figure 3.48 shows the results with the chemical shift artifact correction method applied before conductivity image reconstructions [Minhas *et al.* (2009)].

3.10.4 *Challenging problems and future directions*

Conductivity images of an electrically conducting object with a pixel size of about 1 mm are provided by MREIT. It achieves such a high spatial resolution by adopting an MRI scanner to measure internal magnetic flux density distributions induced by externally injected imaging currents. Theoretical and experimental studies in MREIT demonstrate that it is expected to be a new clinically useful bio-imaging modality. Its capability to distinguish conductivity values of different biological tissues in their living wetted states is unique.

Following the *in vivo* imaging experiment of the canine brain [Kim *et al.* (2008b)], numerous *in vivo* animal imaging experiments are being conducted for imaging regions of extremities, abdomen, pelvis, neck, thorax, and head. Animal models of various diseases are also being tried. To reach the stage of clinical applications, *in vivo* human imaging experiments are also in progress [Kim *et al.* (2009)].

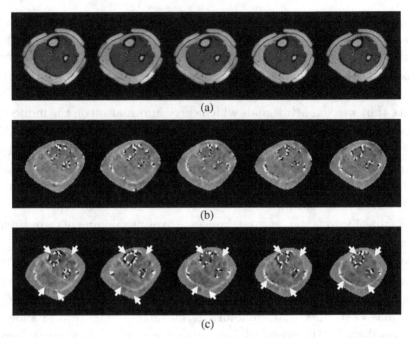

Fig. 3.48. (a) Multi-slice MR magnitude images of the calf. In (b) and (c) we see reconstructed conductivity images without and with the chemical shift artifact correction, respectively. Arrows in (c) regions of a significant conductivity contrast improvement as a result of noise removal using the chemical shift artifact correction.

These trials are expected to accumulate new diagnostic information based on *in vivo* conductivity values of numerous biological tissues.

The use of MREIT to overcome the ill-posed nature of the inverse problem in EIT and provide high-resolution conductivity images has been attempted. Even though current EIT images have a relatively poor spatial resolution, high temporal resolution and portability in EIT could be advantageous in several biomedical application areas [Holder (2005)]. Instead of competing in a certain application area, MREIT and EIT will be supplementary to each other. Taking advantage of the high spatial resolution in MREIT, [Woo and Seo (2008)] discuss numerous application areas of MREIT in biomedicine, biology, chemistry, and material science. We should note that it is possible to produce a current density image for any electrode configuration once the conductivity distribution is obtained.

Future studies should overcome a few technical barriers to advance the method to the stage of routine clinical uses. The biggest hurdle at present is the amount of injection current that may stimulate muscle and nerve. Reducing it down to a level that does not produce undesirable side effects is the key to the success of this new bio-imaging modality. This demands innovative data processing methods based on rigorous mathematical analysis as well as improved measurement techniques to maximize the SNR for a given data collection time.

Acknowledgments

Seo and Woo would like to thank all members of IIRC for participating in the MREIT project for the last 12 years. Those include Ohin Kwon, Rosalind Sadleir, Tonng In Oh, Hyung Joong Kim, Sungwhan Kim, Jeong-Rock Yoon, Chunjae Park, Yong Jung Kim, Suk-ho Lee, Chang-Ock Lee, Kiwan Jeon, Mourad Sini, Jijun Liu, Byung Il Lee, Atul Minhas and graduate students. Seo gratefully acknowledges an NRF grant from MEST.

References

Adler A, Arnold JH, Bayford R, Borsic R, Brown B, Dixon P, Faes TJC, Frerichs I, Gagnon H, Gräber Y, Grychtol B, Hahn G, Lionheart WRB, Malik A, Patterson RP, Stocks J, Tizzard A, Weiler N and Wolf GK (2009). *GREIT: a unified approach to 2D linear EIT reconstruction of lung images, Physiol. Meas.*, Vol. 30, pp. S35–S55.

Alessandrini G and Magnanini R (1992). *The index of isolated critical points and solutions of elliptic equations in the plane, Ann. Scoula. Norm. Sup. Pisa Cl Sci.*, Vol. 19, pp. 567–589.

Alessandrini G, Rosset E and Seo JK (2000). *Optimal size estimates for the inverse conductivity problem with one measurement, Proc. Amer. Math. Soc.*, Vol. 128, pp. 53–64.

Alessandrini G and Nesi V (2001). *Univalent σ-harmonic mappings, Arch. Rational Mech. Anal.*, Vol. 50, pp. 747–757.

Astala K and Päivärinta L (2006). *Calderon's inverse conductivity problem in the plane, Ann. Math.*, Vol. 163, pp. 265–299.

Barber DC and Brown BH (1984). *Applied potential tomography, J. Phys. E. Sci. Instrum.*, Vol. 17, pp. 723–733.

Bauman P, Marini A and Nesi V (2000). *Univalent solutions of an elliptic system of partial differential equations arising in homogenization, Indiana Univ. Math. J.*, Vol. 128, pp. 53–64.

Bensoussan A, Lions JL and Papanicolaou G (1978). *Asymptotic Analysis for Periodic Structures*, Elsevier, New York.

Berenstein C and Tarabusi EC (1991). *Inversion formulas for the k-dimensional Radon transform in real hyperbolic spaces, Duke Math. J.*, Vol 62, pp. 1–19.

Birgul O and Ider YZ (1995). *Use of the magnetic field generated by the internal distribution of injected currents for electrical impedance tomography, Proc. IXth Int. Conf. Elec. Bio-Impedance*, Heidelberg, Germany, pp. 418–419.

Birgul O and Ider YZ (1996). *Electrical impedance tomography using the magnetic field generated by injected currents, Proc. 18th Ann. Int. Conf. IEEE EMBS*, Amsterdam, pp. 784–785.

Birgul O, Eyuboglu BE and Ider YZ (2003). *Experimental results for 2D magnetic resonance electrical impedance tomography (MREIT) using magnetic flux density in one direction, Phys. Med. Biol.*, Vol. 48, pp. 3485–3504.

Birgul O, Hamamura MJ, Muftuler T and Nalcioglu O (2006). *Contrast and spatial resolution in MREIT using low amplitude current, Phys. Med. Biol.*, Vol. 51, pp. 5035–5049.

Borcea L (2002). *Electrical impedance tomography, Inverse Probl.*, Vol. 18, pp. R99–R136.

Briane M, Milton GW and Nesi V (2004). *Change of sign of the correctors determinant for homogenization in three-dimensional conductivity, Arch. Rational Mech. Anal.*, Vol. 173, no. 1, pp. 133–150.

Brown BH, Barber DC and Seagar AD (1985). *Applied potential tomography: possible clinical applications, Clin. Phys. Physiol. Meas.*, Vol. 6, pp. 109–121.

Brown R and Uhlmann G (1997). *Uniqueness in the inverse conductivity problem with less regular conductivities in two dimensions, Comm. Part. Diff. Eqns.*, Vol. 22, pp. 1009–1027.

Calderón AP (1980). *On an inverse boundary value problem*, In *Seminar on Numerical Analysis and its Applications to Continuum Physics*, Soc. Brasileira de Matemàtica, Rio de Janeiro, Brazil, pp. 65–73.

Cheney M, Isaacson D, Newell J, Goble J and Simske S (1990). *NOSER: An algorithm for solving the inverse conductivity problem, Int. J. Imag. Syst. Tech.*, Vol. 2, pp. 66–75.

Cheney M, Isaacson D and Newell JC (1999). *Electrical impedance tomography, SIAM Review*, Vol. 41, pp. 85–101.

Cheng KS, Isaacson D, Newell JC and Gisser DG (1989). *Electrode models for electric current computed tomography, IEEE Trans. Biomed. Eng.*, Vol. 36, pp. 918–924.

Colton D and Kress R (1998). *Inverse Acoustic and Electromagnetic Scattering Theory*, Second edition, Springer Verlag, Berlin.

Difazio G (1996). L^p *estimates for divergence from elliptic equations with discontinuous coefficients, Boll. Un. Mat. Ital. A*, Vol. 10, pp. 409–420.

Engl HW, Hanke M and Neubauer A (1996). *Regularization of Inverse Problems, Mathematics and its Applications*, Kluwer Academic Publishers, Dordrecht.

Eyuboglu M, Reddy R and Leigh JS (1998). *Imaging electrical current density using nuclear magnetic resonance, Elektrik*, Vol. 6, pp. 201–214.

Eyuboglu M, Birgul O and Ider YZ (2001). *A dual modality system for high resolution-true conductivity imaging, Proc. XI Int. Conf. Elec. Bioimpedance (ICEBI)*, pp. 409–413.

Folland GB (1976). *Introduction to Partial Differential Equations*, Princeton University Press, Princeton, NJ.

Fuks LF, Cheney M, Isaacson D, Gisser DG and Newell JC (1991). *Detection and imaging of electric conductivity and permittivity at low frequency, IEEE Trans. Biomed. Engr.*, Vol. 3, pp. 1106–1110.

Gabriel C, Gabriel S and Corthout E (1996). *The dielectric properties of biological tissues: I. literature survey, Phys. Med. Biol.*, Vol. 41, pp. 2231–2249.

Gabriel S, Lau RW and Gabriel C (1996). *The dielectric properties of biological tissues: II. measurements in the frequency range 10Hz to 20GHz, Phys. Med. Biol.*, Vol. 41, pp. 2251–2269.

Gamba HR and Delpy DT (1998). *Measurement of electrical current density distribution within the tissues of the head by magnetic resonance imaging, Med. Biol. Eng. Comput.*, Vol. 36, pp. 165–170.

Gao G, Zhu SA and He B (2005). *Estimation of electrical conductivity distribution within the human head from magnetic flux density measurement, Phys. Med. Biol.*, Vol. 50, pp. 2675–2687.

Gao N, Zhu SA and He B (2006). *New magnetic resonance electrical impedance tomography (MREIT) algorithm: the RSM-MREIT algorithm with applications to estimation of human head conductivity, Phys. Med. Biol.*, Vol. 51, pp. 3067–3083.

Geddes LA and Baker LE (1967). *The specific resistance of biological material: a compendium of data for the biomedical engineer and physiologist, Med. Biol. Eng.*, Vol. 5, pp. 271–293.

Geuze RH (1983). *Two methods for homogeneous field defibrillation and stimulation, Med. Biol. Eng. Comput.*, Vol. 21, pp. 518–520.

Ghiglia DC and Pritt MD (1998). *Two-dimensional phase unwrapping: Theory, algorithms, and software*, Wiley, New York.

Gisser DG, Isaacson D and Newell JC (1988). *Theory and performance of an adaptive current tomography system, Clin. Phys. Physiol. Meas.*, Vol. 9, Suppl. A, pp. 35–41.

Gisser DG, Isaacson D and Newell JC (1990). *Electric current computed tomography and eigenvalues, SIAM J. Appl. Math.*, Vol. 50, pp. 1623–1634.

Griffiths H (2001). *Magnetic induction tomography, Meas. Sci. Technol.*, Vol. 12, pp. 1126–1131.

Grimnes S and Martinsen OG (2000). *Bioimpedance and Bioelectricity Basics*, Academic Press, San Diego, CA.

Grisvard P (1985). *Elliptic Problems in Nonsmooth Domains.* Pitman, Boston.

Haacke EM, Petropoulos LS, Nilges EW and Wu DH (1991). *Extraction of conductivity and permittivity using magnetic resonance imaging, Phys. Med. Biol.*, Vol. 36, pp. 723–733.

Haacke EM, Brown RW, M. R. Thompson MR and Venkatesan R (1999). *Magnetic Resonance Imaging: Physical Principles and Sequence Design*, John Wiley, Hoboken, NJ.

Hamamura MJ, Muftuler LT, Birgul O and Nalcioglu O (2006). *Measurement of ion diffusion using magnetic resonance electrical impedance tomography*, Phys. Med. Biol., Vol. 51, pp. 2753–2762.

Hamamura MJ, Nalcioglu O and Muftuler LT (2009). *Correction of chemical shift artifact in magnetic resonance electrical impedance tomography*, Proc. Intl. Soc. Magn. Reson. Med., pp. 4658.

Hanke M and Brühl M (2003). *Recent progress in electrical impedance tomography*, Inverse Probl., Vol. 19, pp. S65–S90.

Hanke M, Harrach B and Hyvonen N (2011). *Justification of point electrode models in electrical impedance tomography*, Math. Models Methods Appl. Sci., Vol. 21, pp. 1395–1413.

Harrach B, Seo JK and Woo EJ (2010). *Physical justification of the factorization method in frequency-Difference electrical impedance tomography*, IEEE Trans. Med. Imag., Vol. 29, pp. 1918–1926.

Hasanov KF, Ma AW, Nachman AI and Joy MLG (2008). *Current density impedance imaging*, IEEE Trans. Med. Imag., Vol. 27, pp. 1301–1309.

Henderson RP and Webster JG (1978). *An impedance camera for spatially specific measurements of the thorax*, IEEE Trans. Biomed. Eng., Vol. 25, pp. 250–254.

Holder D (eds.) (2005). *Electrical Impedance Tomography: Methods, History and Applications*, IOP Publishing, Bristol.

Hoult DI (2000). *The principle of reciprocity in signal strength calculations — a mathematical guide*, Concepts Magn. Reson., Vol. 12, pp. 173–187.

Hoult DI and Richards RE (1976). *The signal-to-noise ratio of the nuclear magnetic resonance experiment*, J. Magn. Reson., Vol. 24, pp. 71–85.

Ider YZ and Birgul O (1998). *Use of the magnetic field generated by the internal distribution of injected currents for Electrical Impedance Tomography (MR-EIT)*, Elektrik, Vol. 6, no. 3, pp. 215–258.

Ider YZ and Onart S (2004). *Algebraic reconstruction for 3D magnetic resonance electrical impedance tomography (MREIT) using one component of magnetic flux density*, Physiol. Meas., Vol. 25, pp. 281–294.

Isaacson D and Isaacson E (1989). *Comment on Calderon's paper: 'On an inverse boundary value problem'*, Math. Comp., Vol. 52, pp. 553–559.

Isaacson D and Cheney M (1991). *Effects of measurement precision and finite numbers of electrodes on linear impedance imaging algorithms*, SIAM J. Appl. Math., Vol. 51, pp. 1705–1731.

Isaacson D and Cheney M (1996). *Process for Producing Optimal Current Patterns for Electrical Impedance Tomography*, U.S. Patent 5, 588, 429; Dec. 31.

Jeon K, Lee CO, Kim HJ, Woo EJ and Seo JK (2009a). *CoReHA: conductivity reconstructor using harmonic algorithms for magnetic resonance electrical impedance tomography (MREIT)*, J. Biomed. Eng. Res., Vol. 30, pp. 279–287.

Jeon K, Minhas AS, Kim TT, Jeong WC, Kim HJ, Kang BT, Park HM, Lee CO, Seo JK and Woo EJ (2009b). *MREIT conductivity imaging of the postmortem canine abdomen using CoReHA, Physiol. Meas.*, Vol. 30, pp. 957–966.

Jeong WC, Kim YT, Lee CO, Minhas AS, Kim HJ, Woo EJ and Seo JK (2008). *Design of carbon-hydrogel electrode for MREIT. Proc. 9th Conf. EIT*, Dartmouth, NH.

Joy M, Nachman A, Hasanov H, Yoon RS and Ma AW (2004). *A new approach to Current Density Impedance Imaging (CDII), Proceedings ISMRM*, no. 356, Kyoto, Japan.

Joy ML, Scott GC and Henkelman RM (1989). *In-vivo detection of applied electric currents by magnetic resonance imaging, Magn. Reson. Imaging*, Vol. 7, pp. 89–94.

Kenig C, Sjostrand J and Uhlmann G (2007). *The Calderon problem with partial data; Ann. Math.*, Vol. 165, pp. 567–591.

Khang HS, Lee BI, Oh SH, Woo EJ, Lee SY, Cho MH, Kwon O, Yoon JR and Seo JK (2002). *J-substitution algorithm in magnetic resonance electrical impedance tomography (MREIT): Phantom experiments for static resistivity images, IEEE Trans. Med. Imag.*, Vol. 21, no. 6, pp. 695–702.

Kim YJ, Kwon O, Seo JK and Woo EJ (2003). *Uniqueness and convergence of conductivity image reconstruction in magnetic resonance electrical impedance tomography, Inverse Probl.*, Vol. 19, pp. 1213–1225.

Kim HJ, Lee BI, Cho Y, Kim YT, Kang BT, Park HM, Lee SL, Seo JK and Woo EJ (2007). *Conductivity imaging of canine brain using a 3 T MREIT system: postmortem experiments, Physiol. Meas.*, Vol. 28, pp. 1341–1353.

Kim S, Lee J, Seo JK, Woo EJ and Zribi H (2008a). *Multi-frequency trans-admittance scanner: mathematical framework and feasibility, SIAM J. Appl. Math.*, Vol. 69, no. 1, pp. 22–36.

Kim HJ, Oh TI, Kim YT, Lee BI, Woo EJ, Seo JK, Lee SY, Kwon O, Park C, Kang BT and Park HM (2008b). *In vivo electrical conductivity imaging of a canine brain using a 3 T MREIT system, Physiol. Meas.*, Vol. 29, pp. 1145–1155.

Kim HJ, Kim YT, Jeong WC, Minhas AS, Woo EJ, Kwon OJ and Seo JK (2008c). *In vivo conductivity imaging of a human leg using a 3 T MREIT system, Proc. 9th Conf. EIT*, Dartmouth, NH.

Kim HJ, Kim YT, Minhas AS, Jeong WC, Woo EJ, Seo JK and Kwon OJ (2009). *In vivo high-resolution conductivity imaging of the human leg using MREIT: the first human experiment, IEEE Trans. Med. Imag.*, Vol. 28, pp. 1681–1687.

Kim HJ, Jeong WC, Kim YT, Minhas AS, Lee TH, Lim CY, Park HM, Seo JK and Woo EJ (2010). *In vivo conductivity imaging of canine male pelvis using a 3T MREIT system, J. Phys.: Conf. Ser.*, Vol. 224, no. 012020.

Kohn R and Vogelius M (1984). *Determining conductivity by boundary measurements, Comm. Pure Appl. Math.*, Vol. 37, pp. 113–123.

Ksienski DA (1992). *A minimum profile uniform current density electrode, IEEE Trans. Biomed. Eng.*, Vol. 39, no. 7, pp. 682–692.

Kwon O, Woo EJ, Yoon JR and Seo JK (2002a). *Magnetic resonance electrical impedance tomography (MREIT): simulation study of J-substitution algorithm, IEEE Trans. Biomed. Eng.*, Vol. 49, no. 2, pp. 160–167.

Kwon O, Lee JY and Yoon JR (2002b). *Equipotential line method for magnetic resonance electrical impedance tomography (MREIT), Inverse Probl.*, Vol. 18, pp. 1089–1100.

Kwon O, Park CJ, Park EJ, Seo JK and Woo EJ (2005). *Electrical conductivity imaging using a variational method in B_z-based MREIT, Inverse Probl.*, Vol. 21, pp. 969–980.

Kwon O, Pyo HC, Seo JK and Woo EJ (2006). *Mathematical framework for Bz-based MREIT model in electrical impedance imaging, computer and mathematics with applications*, Vol. 51, pp. 817–828.

Langberg E (1993). *Electrical Heating Catheter*, U.S. Patent 5, pp. 257–635.

Laugesen RS(1996). *Injectivity can fail for higher-dimensional harmonic extensions, Complex Variables*, Vol. 28, pp. 357–369.

Lee BI, Oh SH, Woo EJ, Lee SY, Cho MH, Kwon O, Seo JK, Lee JY and Baek WS (2003). *Three-dimensional forward solver and its performance analysis in magnetic resonance electrical impedance tomography (MREIT) using recessed electrodes, Phys. Med. Biol.*, Vol. 48, pp. 1971–1986.

Lee BI, Lee SH, Kim TS, Kwon O, Woo EJ and Seo JK (2005). *Harmonic decomposition in PDE-based denoising technique for magnetic resonance electrical impedance tomography, IEEE Trans. Biomed. Eng.*, Vol. 52, pp. 1912–1920.

Lee E, Seo JK, Woo EJ and Zhang T (2011). *Mathematical framework for a new microscopic electrical impedance tomography (micro-EIT) system, Inverse Probl.*, Vol. 27, 055008.

Lee JY (2004). *A reconstruction formula and uniqueness of conductivity in MREIT using two internal current distributions, Inverse Probl.*, Vol. 20, pp. 847–858.

Lee S, Seo JK, Park C, Lee BI, Woo EJ, Lee SY, Kwon O and Hahn J (2006). *Conductivity image reconstruction from defective data in MREIT: numerical simulation and animal experiment, IEEE Trans. Med. Imag.*, Vol. 25, pp. 168–176.

Lionheart W, Polydorides W and Borsic A (2005). *The reconstruction problem, Electrical Impedance Tomography: Methods, History and Applications*, IOP Publishing, Bristol.

Liu J, Pyo HC, Seo JK and Woo EJ (2006). *Convergence properties and stability issues in MREIT algorithm, Contemp. Math.*, Vol. 25, pp. 168–176.

Liu J, Seo JK, Sini M and Woo EJ (2007). *On the convergence of the harmonic B_z algorithm in magnetic resonance electrical impedance tomography, SIAM J. Appl. Maths*, Vol. 67, pp. 1259–1282.

Liu J, Seo JK and Woo EJ (2010). *A posteriori error estimate and convergence analysis for conductivity image reconstruction in MREIT, SIAM J. App. Math.*, Vol. 70, no. 8, pp. 2883–2903.

Meier T, Luepschen H, Karsten J, Leibecke T, Großherr M, Gehring and Leonhardt S (2008). *Assessment of regional lung recruitment and derecruitment during a PEEP trial based on electrical impedance tomography, Intens. Care Med.*, Vol. 34 , pp. 543–550.

Metherall P, Barber DC, Smallwood RH and Brown BH (1996). *Three-dimensional electrical impedance tomography, Nature*, Vol. 380, pp. 509–512.

Minhas AS, Jeong WC, Kim YT, Kim HJ, Lee TH and Woo EJ (2008). *MREIT of postmortem swine legs using carbon-hydrogel electrodes, J. Biomed. Eng. Res.*, Vol. 29, pp. 436–442.

Minhas AS, Kim YT, Jeong WC, Kim HJ, Lee SY and Woo EJ (2009). *Chemical shift artifact correction in MREIT, J. Biomed. Eng. Res.*, Vol. 30, pp. 461–468.

Mueller J, Siltanen S and Isaacson D (2009). *A direct reconstruction algorithm for electrical impedance tomography, IEEE Trans. Med. Imag.*, Vol. 21, no. 6, pp. 555–559.

Muftuler LT, Hamamura MJ, Birgul O and Nalcioglu O (2004). *Resolution and contrast in magnetic resonance electrical impedance tomography (MREIT) and its application to cancer imaging, Technol. Cancer Res. Treat.*, Vol. 3, pp. 599–609.

Muftuler LT, Hamamura MJ, Birgul O and Nalcioglu O (2006). *In vivo MRI electrical impedance tomography (MREIT) of tumors, Technol. Cancer Res. Treat.*, Vol. 5, pp. 381–387.

Nachman A (1988). *Reconstructions from boundary measurements, Ann. Math.*, Vol. 128, pp. 531–576.

Nachman A (1996). *Global uniqueness for a two-dimensional inverse boundary problem, Ann. Math.*, Vol. 143, pp. 71–96.

Nachman A, Wang D, Ma W and Joy M (2007a). *A local formula for inhomogeneous complex conductivity as a function of the RF magnetic field, ISMRM 15th Scientific Meeting & Exhibition*, Berlin: ISMRM. Available at: http://www.ismrm.org/07/Unsolved.htm, accessed 13 June 2013.

Nachman A, Tamasan A and Timonov A (2007b). *Conductivity imaging with a single measurement of boundary and interior data, Inverse Probl.*, Vol. 23, pp. 2551–2563.

Nachman A, Tamasan A and Timonov A (2009). *Recovering the conductivity from a single measurement of interior data, Inverse Probl.*, Vol. 25, 035014.

Nachman A, Tamasan A and Timonov A (2010). *Reconstruction of planar conductivities in subdomains from incomplete data, SIAM J. Appl. Math.*, Vol. 70 , no. 8, pp. 3342–3362.

Nam H and Kwon O (2010). *Optimization of multiply acquired magnetic flux density B_z using ICNE-Multiecho train in MREIT, Phys. Med. Biol.*, Vol. 55, pp. 2743–2759.

Newell JC, Gisser DG and Isaacson D (1988). *An electric current tomograph, IEEE Trans. Biomed. Engr.*, Vol. 35, pp. 828–833.

Oh SH, Lee BI, Woo EJ, Lee SY, Cho MH, Kwon O and Seo JK (2003). *Conductivity and current density image reconstruction using harmonic B_z algorithm in magnetic resonance electrical impedance tomography, Phys. Med. Biol.*, Vol. 48, pp. 3101–3016.

Oh SH, Lee BI, Park TS, Lee SY, Woo EJ, Cho MH, Kwon O and Seo JK (2004). *Magnetic resonance electrical impedance tomography at 3 Tesla field strength, Magn. Reson. Med.*, Vol. 51, pp. 1292–1296.

Oh SH, Lee BI, Woo EJ, Lee SY, Kim TS, Kwon O and Seo JK (2005). *Electrical conductivity images of biological tissue phantoms in MREIT, Physiol. Meas.*, Vol. 26, pp. S279–S288.

Oh TI, Kim YT, Minha A, Seo JK, Kwon O and Woo EJ (2011). *Ion mobility imaging and contrast mechanism of apparent conductivity in MREIT, Phy. Med. Bio.*, Vol. 56, pp. 2265–2277.

Onart O, Ider YZ and Lionheart W (2003). *Uniqueness and reconstruction in magnetic resonance-electrical impedance tomography (MR-EIT), Physiol. Meas.*, Vol. 24, pp. 591–604.

Park C, Kwon O, Woo EJ and Seo JK (2004a). *Electrical conductivity imaging using gradient B_z decomposition algorithm in magnetic resonance electrical impedance tomography (MREIT), IEEE Trans. Med. Imag.*, Vol. 23, pp. 388–394.

Park C, Park EJ, Woo EJ, Kwon O and Seo JK (2004b). *Static conductivity imaging using variational gradient B_z algorithm in magnetic resonance electrical impedance tomography, Physiol. Meas.*, Vol. 25, pp. 257–269.

Park C, Lee BI, Kwon O and Woo EJ (2006). *Measurement of induced magnetic flux density using injection current nonlinear encoding (ICNE) in MREIT, Physiol. Meas.*, Vol. 28, pp. 117–127.

Putensen C, Wrigge H and Zinserling J (2007). *Electrical impedance tomography guided ventilation therapy, Curr. Opin. Crit. Care*, Vol. 13, pp. 344.

Rahman ARA, Register J, Vuppala G and Bhansali S (2008). *Cell culture monitoring by impedance mapping using a multielectrode scanning impedance spectroscopy system (CellMap), Physiol. Meas.*, Vol. 29, pp. 227–239.

Rubinstein JT, Spelman FA, Soma M and Suesserman MF (1987). *Current density profiles of surface mounted and recessed electrodes for neural prostheses, IEEE Trans. Biomed. Eng.*, Vol. BME-34, pp. 864–874.

Sadleir R, Grant S, Zhang SU, Lee BI, Pyo HC, Oh SH, Park C, Woo EJ, Lee SY, Kwon O and Seo JK (2005). *Noise analysis in MREIT at 3 and 11 Tesla field strength, Physiol. Meas.*, Vol. 26, pp. 875–884.

Santosa F and Vogelius M (1990). *A back-projection algorithm for electrical impedance imaging, SIAM J. Appl. Math.*, Vol. 50, pp. 216–243.

Scott GC, Joy MLG, Armstrong RL and Henkelman RM (1991). *Measurement of nonuniform current density by magnetic resonance, IEEE Trans. Med. Imag.*, Vol. 10, no. 3, pp. 362–374.

Scott GC, Joy MLG, Armstrong RL and Henkelman RM (1992). *Sensitivity of magnetic-resonance current density imaging, J. Magn. Reson.*, Vol. 97, pp. 235–254.

Scott GC (1993). *NMR Imaging of Current Density and Magnetic Fields*, PhD thesis, University of Toronto, Canada.

Seo JK (1996). *On the uniqueness in the inverse conductivity problem, J. Fourier Anal. Appl.*, Vol. 2, pp. 227–235.

Seo JK, Yoon JR, Woo EJ and Kwon O (2003a). *Reconstruction of conductivity and current density images using only one component of magnetic field measurements, IEEE Trans. Biomed. Eng.*, Vol. 50, pp. 1121–1124.

Seo JK, Kwon O, Lee BI and Woo EJ (2003b). *Reconstruction of current density distributions in axially symmetric cylindrical sections using one component of magnetic flux density: computer simulation study, Physiol. Meas.*, Vol. 24, pp. 565–577.

Seo JK, Pyo HC, Park C, Kwon O and Woo EJ (2004). *Image reconstruction of anisotropic conductivity tensor distribution in MREIT: computer simulation study, Phys. Med. Biol.*, Vol. 49, pp. 4371–4382.

Seo JK, Lee J, Kim SW, Zribi H and Woo EJ (2008a). *Frequency-difference electrical impedance tomography (fdEIT): algorithm development and feasibility study, Physiol. Meas.*, Vol. 29, pp. 929–944.

Seo JK, Kim SW, Kim S, Liu J, Woo EJ, Jeon K and Lee CO (2008b). *Local harmonic B_z algorithm with domain decomposition in MREIT: computer simulation study, IEEE Trans. Med. Imag.*, Vol. 27, pp. 1754–1761.

Seo JK, Jeon K, Lee CO and Woo EJ (2011). *Non-iterative harmonic Bz algorithm in MREIT, Inverse Probl.*, Vol. 27, 085003.

Seo JK and Woo EJ (2011). *Magnetic Resonance Electrical Impedance Tomography (MREIT), SIAM Review*, Vol. 53, no. 1, pp. 40–68.

Seo JK and Woo EJ (2012). *Nonlinear Inverse Problems in Imaging*, Wiley, Chichester, UK.

Seo JK, Bera TK, Kwon H and Sadleir R (2013) *Effective admittivity of biological tissues as a coefficient of elliptic PDE, CMMM*, Vol. 2013, article id: 353849.

Somersalo E, Cheney M, Isaacson and Isaacson E (1991). *Layer stripping: A direct numerical method for impedance imaging, Inverse Probl.*, Vol. 7, pp. 899–926.

Somersalo E, Cheney M and Isaacson D (1992). *Existence and uniqueness for electrode models for electric current computed tomography, SIAM J. Appl. Math.*, Vol. 52, pp. 1023–1040.

Song Y, Lee E, Seo JK and Woo EJ (2011). *Optimal geometry toward uniform current density electrodes, Inverse Probl.*, Vol. 27, no. 7, p. 17.

Suesserman MF, Spelman FA and Rubinstein JT (1991). *In vitro measurement and characterization of current density profiles produced by nonrecessed, simple recessed and radially varying recessed stimulating electrodes. IEEE Trans. Biomed. Eng.*, Vol. 38, no. 5, pp. 401–408.

Sylvester J and Uhlmann G (1986). *A uniqueness theorem for an inverse boundary value problem in electrical prospection, Comm. Pure Appl. Math.*, Vol. 39, pp. 92–112.

Sylvester J and Uhlmann G (1987). *A global uniqueness theorem for an inverse boundary value problem, Ann. Math.*, Vol. 125, pp. 153–169.

Sylvester J and Uhlmann G (1988). *Inverse boundary value problems at the boundary-continuous dependence, Comm. Pure Appl. Math.*, Vol. 21, pp 197–221.

Thomas SR and Dixon RL (1986). *NMR in Medicine, American Institute of Physics*, pp. 549–563.

Tungjitkusolmun S, Woo EJ, Hong C, Tsai JZ, Vorperian VR and Webster G (2000). *Finite element analysis of uniform current density electrodes for radio-frequency cardiac ablation. IEEE Tans. Biomed. Eng.*, Vol. 47, no. 1, pp. 32–40.

Uhlmann G (2009). *Electrical impedance tomography and Calderon's problem, Inverse Probl.*, Vol. 25, 123011.

Vauhkonen PJ, Vauhkonen M, Savolainen T and Kaipio JP (1999). *Three-dimensional electrical impedance tomography based on the complete electrode model, IEEE Trans. Biomed. Eng.*, Vol. 46, pp. 1150–1160.

Verchota G (1984). *Layer potentials and boundary value problems for Laplace's equation in Lipschitz domains*, J. Func. Anal., Vol. 59, pp. 572–611.

Webster JG (1990). *Electrical Impedance Tomography*, Taylor & Francis, Oxford.

Wexler A, Fry B and Neiman MR (1985). *Impedance-computed tomography algorithm and system*, Appl. Opt., Vol. 24, pp. 3985–3992.

Wiley JD and Webster JG (1982). *Analysis and control of the current distribution under circular dispersive electrodes*, IEEE Trans. Biomed. Eng., Vol. BME-29, pp. 381–385.

Wiley JD and Webster JG (1982). *Distributed equivalent-circuit models for circular dispersive electrodes*, IEEE Trans. Biomed. Eng., Vol. BME-29, pp. 385–389.

Woo EJ, Hua P, Webster JG and Tompkins W (1993). *A robust image reconstruction algorithm and its parallel implementation in electrical impedance tomography*, IEEE Trans. Med. Imag., Vol. 12, pp. 137–146.

Woo EJ, Lee SY and Mun CW (1994). *Impedance tomography using internal current density distribution measured by nuclear magnetic resonance*, SPIE, Vol. 2299, pp. 377–385.

Woo EJ and Seo JK (2008). *Magnetic resonance electrical impedance tomography (MREIT) for high-resolution conductivity imaging*, Physiol. Meas., Vol. 29, pp. R1–R26.

Yorkey T, Webster JG and Tompkins W (1987). *Comparing reconstruction algorithms for electrical impedance tomography*, IEEE Trans. Biomed. Eng., Vol. 34, pp. 843–852.

Zhang N (1992). *Electrical Impedance Tomography based on Current Density Imaging*, MS Thesis, University of Toronto, Canada.

Chapter 4

MR-EPT

The idea of quantitatively extracting electric conductivity and permittivity from magnetic resonance (MR) images was first proposed in 1991 [Haacke *et al.* (1991)]. However, only recently, the electric properties of the human body have been introduced as a quantitative image contrast in standard magnetic resonance imaging (MRI) via electric properties tomography (EPT) [Katscher *et al.* (2006, 2009a); Wen (2003)]. EPT allows the determination of the conductivity and permittivity using the radio frequency (RF) transmit field map of a standard MR scan.

As discussed in the previous chapter, magnetic resonance electrical impedance tomography (MREIT) also takes advantage of the spatial encoding inherent to MRI, however, by applying external currents to the patient via mounted electrodes. In contrast, RF current density imaging (RF-CDI) makes electrode mounting obsolete by the application of a separate RF pulse for current induction, again taking advantage of MRI spatial encoding [Beravs *et al.* (1999); Scott *et al.* (1995); Wang *et al.* (2009)]. All these methods differ from the presented approach, which uses a standard MR system and requires neither electrode mounting nor the application of additional RF energy. Instead, the EPT approach employs post-processing the RF transmit field map of the imaging RF pulse. As illustrated in Figure 4.1, the electric properties of tissue distort the transmit field in a very dedicated way. This presents the chance that measuring the distorted transmit field allows reconstruction of the tissue's electric properties, which are responsible for the observed distortions.

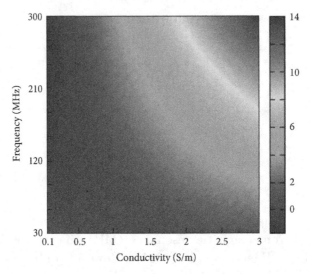

Fig. 4.1.   Impact of electric conductivity on phase of RF transmit field [Katscher *et al.* (2013)]. A tumor of radius 1.5 cm is located in a head model with mean conductivity of 0.4 S/m, corresponding to the mean conductivity of a healthy brain [Gabriel *et al.* (1996)]. Depending on the tumor conductivity and the applied Larmor frequency, the phase of the RF transmit field differs up to 14° compared with a tumor-free head. This presents the chance that measuring the distorted RF transmit field allows the reconstruction of the tissue's electric properties, which is the basic idea of EPT.

Since electrical properties are in general frequency dependent, EPT yields quantitative values for conductivity and permittivity at MR Larmor frequency. This frequency is significantly higher than the frequency used in classical bioimpedance studies. However, electric properties are not only of potential diagnostic value, but also central parameters in the field of RF safety. Here, the local heating of tissue is a major problem at high field MR, particularly in the framework of parallel transmission (see, e.g., [Graesslin *et al.* (2006); Zelinski *et al.* (2008)]). The acceptable local specific absorption rate (SAR), which is directly related to tissue heating, may limit the parameter space available for the application of specific MR sequences. Thus, an exact, patient-individual determination of local SAR is highly desirable. The EPT approach provides a step towards such patient-specific local SAR determination with sufficient accuracy and short computation time (see, e.g., [Katscher *et al.* (2008)]). For local SAR determination, it is mandatory to determine the electric properties at Larmor frequency of the MR system used, as is the case for MR-EPT.

This chapter starts with a discussion of the mathematical background of the different versions of EPT. Model assumptions underlying EPT are presented and potential means to overcome these assumptions are shown. Then, EPT results of numerous research groups around the world are summarized; i.e., simulations and studies of phantoms [Bulumulla *et al.* (2009); Cloos and Bonmassar (2009); Katscher *et al.* (2006); Zhang *et al.* (2010)], *ex vivo* animals [Wen (2003)], volunteers [Katscher *et al.* (2007); Voigt *et al.* (2011b)], and patients [Lier *et al.* (2011b, 2012c); Voigt *et al.* (2011a)].

4.1   Mathematical Model

4.1.1   *Central EPT equation*

The patient's electric properties are related to quantities that are accessible via MRI by EPT. The transmitted RF pulse is affected by the conductivity and permittivity of the tissue being imaged. This relation is achieved by a suitable arrangement of Maxwell's equations. Numerous possibilities exist for such arrangements. In the following, the method described in [Voigt *et al.* (2011b)] is depicted exemplarily.

The magnetic field strength vector $\mathbf{H}$ and the electric field vector $\mathbf{E}$, corresponding to the RF fields of the MR system, are assumed to be time-harmonic $\mathbf{H}, \mathbf{E} \sim e^{i\omega t}$. Using this assumption, Ampère's law is integrated along a closed path ∂A that delineates the border of A

$$\frac{1}{i\omega} \oint_{\partial A} \nabla \times \mathbf{H}(\mathbf{r}) \cdot d\mathbf{l} = \oint_{\partial A} \tau(\mathbf{r})\mathbf{E}(\mathbf{r}) \cdot d\mathbf{l}. \tag{4.1}$$

Here, ω is the Larmor frequency, $\tau = \epsilon - i\frac{\sigma}{\omega}$ denotes the complex permittivity with ϵ being the scalar permittivity and σ the electric conductivity, and $d\mathbf{l}$ is a line element. For the following derivations, τ is assumed to be isotropic. Then, Faraday's law reads

$$-i\omega\mu \int_A \mathbf{H}(\mathbf{r}) \cdot d\mathbf{S} = \oint_{\partial A} \mathbf{E}(\mathbf{r}) \cdot d\mathbf{l} \tag{4.2}$$

with μ being the (assumed to be constant) permeability and surface element $d\mathbf{S}$.

Now, we present a way to extract the quantity $\tau(\mathbf{r})$ from a partial knowledge of $\mathbf{H}(\mathbf{r})$. For ease of explanation, assume that the volume V is a small sphere centered at $\mathbf{r}_V$ and A is a cross-sectional area of V with its normal vector $\mathbf{n}_A$. We also assume that $\nabla\tau \approx 0$ in the volume V. Dividing (4.1) by (4.2) relates the electric properties to the magnetic fields

$$\frac{\oint_{\partial A} \nabla \times \mathbf{H}(\mathbf{r}) \cdot d\mathbf{l}}{\omega^2 \mu \int_A \mathbf{H}(\mathbf{r}) \cdot d\mathbf{S}} = \frac{\oint_{\partial A} \tau(\mathbf{r})\mathbf{E}(\mathbf{r}) \cdot d\mathbf{l}}{\oint_{\partial A} \mathbf{E}(\mathbf{r}) \cdot d\mathbf{l}} \approx \tau(\mathbf{r}_V). \qquad (4.3)$$

Equation (4.3) represents the EPT approach used in [Katscher *et al.* (2009a)]. Using Stokes theorem and the vector identity $\nabla \times \nabla \times \mathbf{H} = -\nabla^2 \mathbf{H}$ yields

$$\tau(\mathbf{r}_V) \approx \frac{\int_A \nabla \times \nabla \times \mathbf{H}(\mathbf{r}) \cdot d\mathbf{S}}{\omega^2 \mu \int_A \mathbf{H}(\mathbf{r}) \cdot d\mathbf{S}} = -\frac{\int_A \nabla^2 \mathbf{H}(\mathbf{r}) \cdot d\mathbf{S}}{\omega^2 \mu \int_A \mathbf{H}(\mathbf{r}) \cdot d\mathbf{S}}. \qquad (4.4)$$

Since A is an arbitrarily orientated disk inside the object that is imaged, this additional degree of freedom can be used to further reduce the required input quantities. With a disk A having its normal vector $\hat{\mathbf{x}}$, (4.4) leads to

$$\tau(\mathbf{r}_V) \approx -\frac{\int_A \nabla^2 H_x(\mathbf{r})dS}{\omega^2 \mu \int_A H_x(\mathbf{r})dS} \approx -\frac{\int_V \nabla^2 H_x(\mathbf{r})d\mathbf{r}}{\omega^2 \mu \int_V H_x(\mathbf{r})d\mathbf{r}}. \qquad (4.5)$$

Here, the second approximation is obtained by stacking the slice A along $\hat{\mathbf{x}}$-direction. By changing the direction of the slice A, we obtain the same approximation (4.5) for H_y and H_z

$$\tau(\mathbf{r}_V) \approx -\frac{\int_V \nabla^2 H_x(\mathbf{r})d\mathbf{r}}{\omega^2 \mu \int_V H_x(\mathbf{r})d\mathbf{r}} \approx -\frac{\int_V \nabla^2 H_y(\mathbf{r})d\mathbf{r}}{\omega^2 \mu \int_V H_y(\mathbf{r})d\mathbf{r}}$$

$$\approx -\frac{\int_V \nabla^2 H_z(\mathbf{r})d\mathbf{r}}{\omega^2 \mu \int_V H_z(\mathbf{r})d\mathbf{r}}. \qquad (4.6)$$

Now, we employ the new basis vectors $\mathbf{a}_+, \mathbf{a}_-, \mathbf{e}_z$ related to the standard Cartesian $\hat{\mathbf{x}}, \hat{\mathbf{y}}, \hat{\mathbf{z}}$ via

$$\mathbf{a}_+ = \frac{\hat{\mathbf{x}} + i\hat{\mathbf{y}}}{\sqrt{2}}, \quad \mathbf{a}_- = \frac{\hat{\mathbf{x}} - i\hat{\mathbf{y}}}{\sqrt{2}}, \quad \hat{\mathbf{z}} = \mathbf{e}_z,$$

which are mutually orthogonal.[1] On this basis, the magnetic field vector reads $\mathbf{H} = (H_+, H_-, H_z)^T$ with

$$H_+ = \mathbf{H} \cdot \mathbf{a}_+ = \frac{H_x + iH_y}{\sqrt{2}}, \quad H_- = \mathbf{H} \cdot \mathbf{a}_- = \frac{H_x - iH_y}{\sqrt{2}}. \quad (4.7)$$

All three components of this magnetic field vector enter (4.4) and are significant in MRI; however, only H_+ couples to the proton spins (here, assuming that the direction of $\mathbf{B}_0$ is pointing to $-\hat{\mathbf{z}}$), and thus, is accessible via MR. Hence, (4.4) should be reformatted to eliminate the inaccessible H_- and H_z. Combining (4.5) and (4.6), we have

$$\tau(\mathbf{r}_V) \approx -\frac{\int_V \nabla^2 H_+(\mathbf{r}) d\mathbf{r}}{\omega^2 \mu \int_V H_+(\mathbf{r}) d\mathbf{r}} = -\frac{\int_{\partial V} \nabla H_+ \cdot d\mathbf{S}}{\omega^2 \mu \int_V H_+(\mathbf{r}) d\mathbf{r}}. \quad (4.8)$$

In contrast to the approach of [Katscher *et al.* (2009a)], (4.8) depends only on the measurable H_+, i.e., the positively rotating component of the transmit field, as it is the case in [Bulumulla *et al.* (2009); Cloos and Bonmassar (2009); Haacke *et al.* (1991); Wen (2003)]. However, in contrast to the representation shown in these publications, (4.8) does not require the explicit calculation of the second spatial derivative, which is of crucial importance for numerical stability.

Please note that (4.3–4.8) provide absolute values of τ. Any scaling factors of the magnetic field's magnitude cancel out by dividing.

The same derivations shown here can also be applied to the RF signal emitted not by the RF coil but by the relaxing spins; i.e., to the spatial sensitivity profile H_- of the applied receive coil. However, since no exact methods are published yet to determine receive sensitivities, EPT is typically based on the use of RF transmit sensitivities.

---

[1] $\mathbf{a}_+ \cdot \bar{\mathbf{a}}_- = 0$, $\hat{\mathbf{z}} \cdot \bar{\mathbf{a}}_\pm = 0$ with $\bar{\mathbf{a}}$ being the complex conjugate of $\mathbf{a}$.

4.1.2 *Approximate EPT equation*

Based on the EPT equation derived in the previous section, we describe an approximate version of the EPT equation, which facilitates data acquisition and reconstruction considerably, for the price of an acceptable error. Again, the chapter follows exemplarily the method described in [Voigt *et al.* (2011b)].

In order to obtain separate equations for σ and ϵ, the differentiation in (4.8) is executed explicitly taking into account that $H_+(\mathbf{r}) = \mathcal{H}_+(\mathbf{r})e^{i\phi_+(\mathbf{r})}$. Here, $\mathcal{H}_+ = |H_+|$ represents the magnitude of the positively rotating component of the RF transmit field (i.e., its "active" component responsible for spin excitation) and ϕ_+ its phase. From direct computation of $\nabla^2(\mathcal{H}_+(\mathbf{r})e^{i\phi_+(\mathbf{r})})$, we get

$$\frac{\nabla^2 H_+}{\omega^2 \mu H_+} = \frac{1}{\omega^2 \mu}\left(\frac{\nabla^2 \mathcal{H}_+}{\mathcal{H}_+} - |\nabla\phi_+|^2\right)$$

$$+ i\frac{1}{\omega^2 \mu}(\nabla\phi_+ \cdot \nabla\ln\mathcal{H}_+ + \nabla^2\phi_+) \qquad (4.9)$$

and thus

$$\epsilon(\mathbf{r}) = \frac{1}{\omega^2\mu}\left[|\nabla\phi_+(\mathbf{r})|^2 - \frac{\nabla^2\mathcal{H}_+(\mathbf{r})}{\mathcal{H}_+(\mathbf{r})}\right], \qquad (4.10)$$

$$\sigma(\mathbf{r}) = \frac{1}{\omega\mu}[\nabla\phi_+(\mathbf{r}) \cdot \nabla\ln\mathcal{H}_+(\mathbf{r}) + \nabla^2\phi_+(\mathbf{r})]. \qquad (4.11)$$

As shown in detail below, (4.10) and (4.11) can be approximated for standard MRI by

$$\epsilon(\mathbf{r}) = \frac{-\nabla^2\mathcal{H}_+(\mathbf{r})}{\omega^2\mu\mathcal{H}_+(\mathbf{r})}, \qquad (4.12)$$

$$\sigma(\mathbf{r}) = \frac{\nabla^2\phi_+(\mathbf{r})}{\omega\mu}, \qquad (4.13)$$

yielding magnitude-based permittivity imaging and phase-based conductivity imaging. Corresponding expressions can also be derived in the framework of the integral formulation starting from (4.8)

$$\tau(\mathbf{r}_V) \approx \frac{-\int_{\partial V} \nabla H_+(\mathbf{r}) \cdot d\mathbf{S}}{\omega^2 \mu \int_V H_+(\mathbf{r}) d\mathbf{r}}$$

$$= -\frac{\int_{\partial V} e^{i\phi_+(\mathbf{r})} \nabla \mathcal{H}_+(\mathbf{r}) \cdot d\mathbf{S}}{\omega^2 \mu \int_V \mathcal{H}_+(\mathbf{r}) e^{i\phi_+(\mathbf{r})} d\mathbf{r}} - i \frac{\int_{\partial V} \mathcal{H}_+(\mathbf{r}) e^{i\phi_+(\mathbf{r})} \nabla \phi_+(\mathbf{r}) \cdot d\mathbf{S}}{\omega^2 \mu \int_V \mathcal{H}_+(\mathbf{r}) e^{i\phi_+(\mathbf{r})} d\mathbf{r}}$$

$$= -\frac{\int_V e^{i\phi_+(\mathbf{r})} [\nabla^2 \mathcal{H}_+(\mathbf{r}) - i\nabla \phi_+(\mathbf{r}) \cdot \nabla \mathcal{H}_+(\mathbf{r})] d\mathbf{r}}{\omega^2 \mu \int_V \mathcal{H}_+(\mathbf{r}) e^{i\phi_+(\mathbf{r})} d\mathbf{r}}$$

$$-i \frac{\int_V e^{i\phi_+(\mathbf{r})} \mathcal{H}_+(\mathbf{r}) [\nabla^2 \phi_+(\mathbf{r}) + i|\nabla \phi_+(\mathbf{r})|^2 + \nabla \phi_+(\mathbf{r}) \cdot \nabla \ln \mathcal{H}_+(\mathbf{r})] d\mathbf{r}}{\omega^2 \mu \int_V \mathcal{H}_+(\mathbf{r}) e^{i\phi_+(\mathbf{r})} d\mathbf{r}}.$$

Corresponding to the approximation leading to (4.12) and (4.13), this equation can be approximated by

$$\tau(\mathbf{r}_V) \approx -\frac{\int_V [\nabla^2 \mathcal{H}_+(\mathbf{r}) - i\nabla \phi(\mathbf{r}) \cdot \nabla \mathcal{H}_+(\mathbf{r})] \, d\mathbf{r}}{\omega^2 \mu \int_V \mathcal{H}_+(\mathbf{r}) d\mathbf{r}}$$

$$-i \frac{1}{\omega^2 \mu |V|} \int_V [\nabla^2 \phi_+(\mathbf{r}) + i|\nabla \phi_+(\mathbf{r})|^2$$

$$+ \nabla \phi(\mathbf{r}) \cdot \nabla \ln \mathcal{H}_+(\mathbf{r})] d\mathbf{r}.$$

Separating real and imaginary parts and applying divergence theorem yields,

$$\epsilon(\mathbf{r}_V) \approx \frac{1}{\omega^2 \mu} \left[|\nabla \phi_+(\mathbf{r})|^2 d\mathbf{r} - \frac{\int_{\partial V} \nabla \mathcal{H}_+(\mathbf{r}) \cdot d\mathbf{S}}{\int_V \mathcal{H}_+(\mathbf{r}) dV} \right] \qquad (4.14)$$

$$\sigma(\mathbf{r}_V) \approx \frac{1}{\omega \mu |V|} \left[\int_{\partial V} \nabla \phi(\mathbf{r}) \cdot d\mathbf{S} + 2 \int_V \nabla \phi_+(\mathbf{r}) \cdot \nabla \ln \mathcal{H}_+(\mathbf{r}) d\mathbf{r} \right]. \qquad (4.15)$$

Finally, as above, the conductivity can be expressed as a function of the phase only

$$\sigma(\mathbf{r}_V) \approx \frac{1}{\omega \mu |V|} \int_{\partial V} \nabla \phi(\mathbf{r}) \cdot d\mathbf{S} \qquad (4.16)$$

and the permittivity can be related to the magnitude only

$$\epsilon(\mathbf{r}_V) \approx \frac{-\int_{\partial V} \nabla \mathcal{H}_+(\mathbf{r}) \cdot d\mathbf{S}}{\omega^2 \mu \int_V \mathcal{H}_+(\mathbf{r}) d\mathbf{r}}. \tag{4.17}$$

A motivation of (4.16) and (4.17) can be based on plane waves in infinite, homogeneous media as a simple model for the RF penetration of patients. In this framework, the plane wave $H_+(z) = \mathcal{H}_+(z)e^{i\phi_+(z)}$ propagating in z-direction is a solution to $\frac{\partial^2}{\partial z^2}H^+ + \mu\omega^2\tau H^+ = 0$ that is related to (4.8). With $k = \sqrt{\mu\omega^2\tau}$ denoting the wave number, $k = \sqrt{\omega^2\mu\epsilon - i\omega\mu\sigma}$ is obtained. The root can be written as a sum of real and imaginary part (without loss of generality only one branch is used)

$$k = \sqrt{\frac{\omega\mu}{2}}\left[-\sqrt{\omega|\tau| + \omega\epsilon} + i\sqrt{\omega|\tau| - \omega\epsilon}\right]. \tag{4.18}$$

The imaginary part of (4.18) describes the transmit phase ϕ_+ and the real part describes the influence on the magnitude $\mathcal{H}_+$. Two regimes of applicability of the approximations (4.16) and (4.17) can be investigated as follows.

First, the observed applicability of the approximations (4.16) and (4.17) is motivated for the regime $\omega\epsilon \approx \sigma$, valid for most human tissue types. To this goal, the impact of σ and ϵ on the amplitude $\mathcal{H}_+$ is estimated by the corresponding derivatives of the real part of (4.18)

$$\frac{\partial\Re\{k\}}{\partial(\omega\epsilon)} = -\sqrt{\frac{\omega\mu}{8}}\frac{1}{\sqrt{\omega|\tau| + \omega\epsilon}}\left(\frac{\epsilon}{|\tau|} + 1\right), \tag{4.19}$$

$$\frac{\partial\Re\{k\}}{\partial\sigma} = -\sqrt{\frac{\omega\mu}{8}}\frac{\sigma}{\omega|\tau|\sqrt{\omega|\tau| + \omega\epsilon}}. \tag{4.20}$$

Using $\sigma = \omega\epsilon$ and forming the ratio of the norms of (4.19) and (4.20) yields

$$\left[\left\|\frac{\partial\Re\{k\}}{\partial(\omega\epsilon)}\right\| \Big/ \left\|\frac{\partial\Re\{k\}}{\partial\sigma}\right\|\right]_{\sigma=\omega\epsilon} = 1 + \sqrt{2} > 1. \tag{4.21}$$

Thus, changes in the real part and hence in the magnitude $\mathcal{H}_+$ are predominately induced by ϵ. A similar derivation can be applied to the imaginary part of (4.18). The derivatives are

$$\frac{\partial(\Im(k))}{\partial\sigma} = \sqrt{\frac{\omega\mu}{8}}\frac{\sigma}{\omega|k|\sqrt{\omega|k|-\omega\epsilon}}, \tag{4.22}$$

$$\frac{\partial(\Im(k))}{\omega\partial\epsilon} = \sqrt{\frac{\omega\mu}{8}}\frac{1}{\sqrt{\omega|k|-\omega\epsilon}}\left[\frac{\epsilon}{|k|}-1\right]. \tag{4.23}$$

The ratio of (4.22) and (4.23) at $\sigma = \omega\epsilon$ can be computed, yielding

$$\left.\left|\frac{\partial(\Im(k))}{\partial\sigma}\right|\right|_{\sigma=\omega\epsilon}\bigg/\left.\left|\frac{\partial(\Im(k))}{\omega\partial\epsilon}\right|\right|_{\sigma=\omega\epsilon} = \frac{1}{\sqrt{1-\sqrt{2}}} > 1. \tag{4.24}$$

Thus, changes in the imaginary part and hence in the transmit phase ϕ_+ are predominately induced by σ.

Second, the increased accuracy of the approximations (4.16) and (4.17) for the regime $\sigma \gg \omega\epsilon$ (body fluids) and for the regime $\omega\epsilon \gg \sigma$ will be motivated, again using the model of plane waves. For $\omega\epsilon \gg \sigma$, the approximation $\omega|\tau| = \sqrt{\omega^2\epsilon^2+\sigma^2} \approx \omega\epsilon$ can be used in (4.18), which yields

$$\Re(k) \approx -\omega\sqrt{\mu\epsilon}. \tag{4.25}$$

This equation motivates amplitude-based permittivity imaging for $\omega\epsilon \gg \sigma$, since its real part (and thus, the amplitude of H_+) is influenced by the permittivity only. For $\sigma \gg \omega\epsilon$, the approximation $\omega|k| - \omega\epsilon \approx \sigma$ is used to yield

$$\Im(k) \approx \sqrt{\frac{\omega\mu\sigma}{2}}. \tag{4.26}$$

This equation motivates phase-based conductivity imaging for $\sigma \gg \omega\epsilon$, since its imaginary part (and thus, the phase of H_+) is influenced by the conductivity only.

Phase-based conductivity imaging typically yields a bias towards higher values. This bias can be motivated by the observed interplay of convex magnitude and concave phase distribution of the RF transmission field. The resulting antiparallel gradients of $\mathcal{H}_+$ and ϕ_+ yield a negative dot product in (4.11), and thus, a negative contribution of the neglected component in (4.13). Magnitude-based reconstruction yields lower values than the exact approach, since the transition from (4.10) to (4.12) omits a component, which is quadratic, and thus, is always positive.

Figures 4.2 and 4.3 demonstrate the validity of the approximation given in (4.16) and (4.17) using a spherical phantom

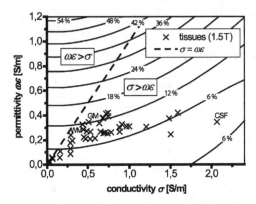

Fig. 4.2.   Conductivity normalized root-mean-square error (NRMSE) introduced by phase-based approximation for a spherical, homogeneous phantom [Voigt *et al.* (2011b)]. The dashed line separates the two regions $\omega\epsilon > \sigma$ and $\sigma > \omega\epsilon$. Highest errors in reconstructed conductivity are found for $\omega\epsilon \gg \sigma$. Dielectric properties of human tissue are indicated by crosses [Gabriel *et al.* (1996)]. For most tissues, NRMSE is of the order of 10%.

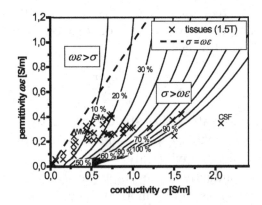

Fig. 4.3.   Permittivity NRMSE introduced by magnitude-based approximation for a spherical, homogeneous phantom [Voigt *et al.* (2011b)]. The dashed line separates the two regions $\omega\epsilon > \sigma$ and $\sigma > \omega\epsilon$. Highest errors in reconstructed permittivity are found for $\sigma \gg \omega\epsilon$. Dielectric properties of human tissue are indicated by crosses [Gabriel *et al.* (1996)]. For most tissues, except for highly conductive body fluids like blood and CSF, NRMSE is of the order of 20%.

(diameter = 20 cm) with uniform conductivity and permittivity 0 S/m $< \sigma <$ 2.5 S/m and 0 S/m $< \omega\epsilon <$ 1.2 S/m, covering the whole range of electric properties of human tissue at $B_0 = 1.5$ T. As discussed above, the approximation for conductivity is more valid for $\sigma \gg \omega\epsilon$ and the approximation for permittivity for $\omega\epsilon \gg \sigma$. For physiological tissue values at 1.5 T, roughly $2\omega\epsilon < \sigma < 10\omega\epsilon$ can be found. Consequently, the error in estimating the electric conductivity from phase information only is of the order of 5–15%. The error in estimating the permittivity from magnitude information only is of the order of 10–20% for most tissues, however, increases significantly for highly conductive tissues, e.g., the body fluids, cerebrospinal fluid (CSF), or blood.

Equations (4.12) and (4.13) or (4.16) and (4.17), respectively, are particularly favorable, since conductivity and permittivity imaging can be split into separate measurements. On one hand, in the case of permittivity imaging, only the magnitude has to be determined, skipping an additional phase measurement. On the other hand, for conductivity imaging, only the transmit phase has to be determined, skipping the magnitude measurement. This phase measurement can be significantly faster than the magnitude measurement. For instance, a conductivity study was presented where solving salt in water was measured in real time with EPT using a steady-state free-precession sequence [Stehning *et al.* (2011)].

4.1.3 *Boundary effects*

The full Helmholtz equation reads (see Chapter 2)

$$-\nabla^2 \mathbf{H}(\mathbf{r}) = \mu_0 \omega^2 \tau(\mathbf{r}) \mathbf{H}(\mathbf{r}) + i\omega (\nabla \tau(\mathbf{r})) \times \mathbf{E}. \tag{4.27}$$

The first term, which is the leading term for high frequencies, is equivalent to (4.8), the full EPT reconstruction. However, in opposition to (4.27), (4.8) does not contain an explicit second derivative, which increases the numerical reconstruction stability. Nevertheless, several EPT studies are performed using this "truncated" Helmholtz equation [Bulumulla *et al.* (2009); Cloos and Bonmassar (2009);

Haacke *et al.* (1991); Lier *et al.* (2010); Wen (2003)]

$$-\frac{\nabla^2 H_+(\mathbf{r})}{\mu_0 \omega^2 H_+(\mathbf{r})} = \tau(\mathbf{r}). \qquad (4.28)$$

However, as discussed above, neglecting the second term of (4.27) neglects variations of τ. Consequently, it typically leads to reconstruction artifacts along boundaries between compartments with different τ. These artifacts, frequently an over- or undershooting of the reconstructed τ along the compartment boundaries, are illustrated in Figure 4.4 in a numerical phantom. An increasing kernel size lowers the peaks of the artifacts, however, simultaneously increasing the affected area [Katscher *et al.* (2009a)].

These artifacts can be avoided by image segmentation prior to reconstruction, and performing separate reconstructions on the different compartments. Alternatively, the full Helmholtz equation, (4.27), can be taken into account. The occurring partial derivatives of τ act as additional unknowns. It was suggested that these additional unknowns can be solved using parallel transmission systems ("dual excitation algorithm" [Zhang *et al.* (2010)]):

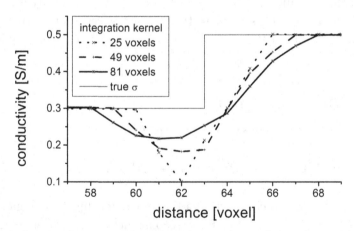

Fig. 4.4. Simulations using a phantom with two adjacent hemispheres of different conductivity [Katscher *et al.* (2009a)]. The variation of τ inside the integration area leads to an error along the hemisphere interface, which depends on the size of the integration area used. Profiles of the reconstructed conductivity along the central axis are plotted.

Assuming $H_z^1 = 0 = H_z^2$,

$$
\begin{bmatrix}
i\omega\mu H_x^1 & 0 & \dfrac{\partial H_y^1}{\partial x} - \dfrac{\partial H_x^1}{\partial y} & -\dfrac{\partial H_x^1}{\partial z} \\[2ex]
i\omega\mu H_x^1 & -\dfrac{\partial H_y^1}{\partial x} + \dfrac{\partial H_x^1}{\partial y} & 0 & -\dfrac{\partial H_x^1}{\partial z} \\[2ex]
i\omega\mu H_x^2 & 0 & \dfrac{\partial H_y^2}{\partial x} - \dfrac{\partial H_x^2}{\partial y} & -\dfrac{\partial H_x^2}{\partial z} \\[2ex]
i\omega\mu H_x^2 & -\dfrac{\partial H_y^2}{\partial x} + \dfrac{\partial H_x^2}{\partial y} & 0 & -\dfrac{\partial H_x^2}{\partial z}
\end{bmatrix}
\begin{bmatrix}
\tau \\[2ex]
\dfrac{\partial \ln \tau}{\partial x} \\[2ex]
\dfrac{\partial \ln \tau}{\partial y} \\[2ex]
\dfrac{\partial \ln \tau}{\partial z}
\end{bmatrix}
$$

$$
=
\begin{bmatrix}
-\nabla^2 H_x^1 \\[1.5ex]
-\nabla^2 H_y^1 \\[1.5ex]
-\nabla^2 H_x^2 \\[1.5ex]
-\nabla^2 H_y^2
\end{bmatrix}
$$

where $\mathbf{H}^1$ and $\mathbf{H}^2$ are the magnetic RF-field of the first and second transmit channel, respectively. Here, the comparison of different excitations of the same subject enables the determination of the unknown partial derivatives of τ. In this way, the artifacts along compartment boundaries can be significantly reduced. However, it was reported that large SNR is required to obtain reasonable results due to adverse noise figures in this algorithm [Zhang *et al.* (2010)]. This noise figure can be alleviated by adding more RF transmit channels.

An alternative solution to cope with varying τ was proposed by [Nachman *et al.* (2007)]:

$$
-\frac{\nabla^2 \mathbf{H}(\mathbf{r}) \cdot (\nabla \times \mathbf{H}(\mathbf{r}))}{\mu_0 \omega^2 \mathbf{H}(\mathbf{r}) \cdot (\nabla \times \mathbf{H}(\mathbf{r}))} = \tau(\mathbf{r}). \tag{4.29}
$$

However, this formulation requires the knowledge of all three spatial components of the magnetic field. Moreover, it shows singularities at

$$\mathbf{H}(\mathbf{r}) = \mathbf{0}, \tag{4.30}$$

$$\nabla \times \mathbf{H}(\mathbf{r}) = \mathbf{0}, \tag{4.31}$$

$$\mathbf{H}(\mathbf{r}) \cdot (\nabla \times \mathbf{H}(\mathbf{r})) = 0. \tag{4.32}$$

The first singularity (4.30) also appears in (4.28) and (mitigated by integration) in (4.8). However, it corresponds to a signal void in the underlying MR images (e.g., air, bone, or outside the field of view [FOV] of the applied RF coil), and thus, seems to be acceptable. The second singularity (4.31) corresponds to $\mathbf{E}(\mathbf{r}) = \mathbf{0}$, which is typically the case in the center of a birdcage coil (i.e., around the center of all corresponding MR images), which seems to be less benign than the first singularity (4.30). The third singularity (4.32) corresponds to the orthogonality between $\mathbf{H}(\mathbf{r})$ and $\mathbf{E}(\mathbf{r})$.

4.1.4 *Anisotropy*

In its general form, τ is given by a rank-2 tensor, including anisotropic cases of conductivity and permittivity

$$\tau(\mathbf{r}) = \begin{pmatrix} \tau_{xx}(\mathbf{r}) & \tau_{xy}(\mathbf{r}) & \tau_{xz}(\mathbf{r}) \\ \tau_{yx}(\mathbf{r}) & \tau_{yy}(\mathbf{r}) & \tau_{yz}(\mathbf{r}) \\ \tau_{zx}(\mathbf{r}) & \tau_{zy}(\mathbf{r}) & \tau_{zz}(\mathbf{r}) \end{pmatrix}.$$

In vivo, anisotropic cases can be found in tissue with preferred cell direction, e.g., in muscles and nerves [Epstein and Foster (1983); Gabriel *et al.* (1996)]. Measuring the anisotropy of the tissue's τ, and characterizing the underlying cell structure, might increase diagnostic information. In the mathematical model discussed above, an isotropic τ was assumed. A way to estimate anisotropy via EPT of τ was sketched by [Katscher *et al.* (2010a)]. This estimation is based on post-processing an acquired B1 map multiple with (4.3), using different orientations of the integration area A in this equation. For instance, assume that the tensor $\tau(\mathbf{r})$ is given by its eigenvectors $\mathbf{v}_1, \mathbf{v}_2, \mathbf{v}_3$ (unit vectors) and its corresponding eigenvalues τ_1, τ_2, τ_3, respectively. We further assume that $|\tau_1| \geq |\tau_2| \geq |\tau_3|$, V is a sphere centered at $\mathbf{r}_V$, and A is a cross-sectional disk centered at $\mathbf{r}_V$ with its normal vector $\mathbf{n}_A$ (see Section 4.1.1). It is crucial to note that the following quantity Φ in (4.3) for isotropic τ is independent of the direction $\mathbf{n}_A$, whereas, in the case of anisotropic τ, it depends on the direction of $\mathbf{n}_A$:

$$\Phi(\mathbf{H}; A) := \frac{\oint_{\partial A} \nabla \times \mathbf{H}(\mathbf{r}) \cdot d\mathbf{l}}{\mu_0 \omega^2 \int_A \mathbf{H}(\mathbf{r}) \cdot d\mathbf{S}} = \frac{\oint_{\partial A} \tau(\mathbf{r}) \mathbf{E}(\mathbf{r}) \cdot d\mathbf{l}}{\oint_{\partial A} \mathbf{E}(\mathbf{r}) \cdot d\mathbf{l}}.$$

Using the eigenvectors $\mathbf{v}_1, \mathbf{v}_2, \mathbf{v}_3$ of the matrix τ,

$$\tau(\mathbf{r}) \mathbf{E}(\mathbf{r}) = \tau(\mathbf{r}) \left[\sum_{j=1}^{3} E_j(\mathbf{r}) \mathbf{v}_j \right] = \sum_{j=1}^{3} \tau_j E_j(\mathbf{r}) \mathbf{v}_j$$

where $E_j = \mathbf{E} \cdot \mathbf{v}_j$. Then, the quantity $\Phi(\mathbf{H}; A)$ can be expressed as

$$\Phi(\mathbf{H}; A) = \frac{\oint_{\partial A} \sum_{j=1}^{3} (\tau_j E_j(\mathbf{r}) \mathbf{v}_j) \cdot d\mathbf{l}}{\oint_{\partial A} \mathbf{E}(\mathbf{r}) \cdot d\mathbf{l}} = \sum_{j=1}^{3} \tau_j f^j(\mathbf{E}; A) \qquad (4.33)$$

where

$$f^j(\mathbf{E}; A) = \frac{\oint_{\partial A} E_j(\mathbf{r}) \mathbf{v}_j \cdot d\mathbf{l}}{\oint_{\partial A} \mathbf{E}(\mathbf{r}) \cdot d\mathbf{l}} = \frac{\int_A \nabla E_j(\mathbf{r}) \times \mathbf{v}_j \cdot d\mathbf{S}}{\mu_0 \omega \int_{\partial A} \mathbf{H}(\mathbf{r}) \cdot d\mathbf{S}}.$$

For instance, if τ is isotropic, then $\tau_1 = \tau_2 = \tau_3$, and $\Phi(\mathbf{H}, A) = \tau$ regardless of the orientation of A; i.e., $\sum_{j=1}^{3} f^j = 1$.

Example 4.1. Consider the special case of $\tau_2 = \tau_3 = 0$. Then, the quantity $\Phi(\mathbf{H}; A)$ depends on the volume of a parallelepiped made by the three vectors $\mathbf{v}_1$, $\mathbf{n}_A$, and $\nabla E_1(\mathbf{r}_V)$:

$$\Phi(\mathbf{H}; A) = \tau_1 f^1(\mathbf{E}; A) \approx \tau_1 \frac{(\nabla E_1(\mathbf{r}_V) \times \mathbf{v}_1) \cdot \mathbf{n}_A}{\mathbf{H}(\mathbf{r}_V) \cdot \mathbf{n}_A}. \qquad (4.34)$$

For instance, if $\tau_1 = \tau_{xx}$, an orientation of $A = A_{yz}$ perpendicular to τ_{xx} yields zero conductivity

$$\frac{\oint_{\partial A_{yz}} \tau_{xx} E_x \, \hat{\mathbf{x}} \cdot d\mathbf{l}}{\oint_{\partial A_{yz}} \mathbf{E} \cdot d\mathbf{l}} = 0. \qquad (4.35)$$

On the other hand, non-zero results are expected for $A = A_{xy}$ or $A = A_{xz}$ parallel to τ_{xx}

$$\frac{\oint_{\partial A_{xz}} \tau_{xx} E_x \,\hat{\mathbf{x}} \cdot dl}{\oint_{\partial A_{xz}} \mathbf{E} \cdot dl} = \tau_{xx} f^1(\mathbf{E}). \tag{4.36}$$

Of course, this concept requires a modeling of the unknown magnetic field components H_-, H_z (like $H_- = H_z = 0$ for a quadrature volume coil), which introduces additional uncertainty to the reconstruction results. Nevertheless, the measurement of anisotropic effects in a straw phantom using the presented concept was reported [Katscher *et al.* (2010a)].

4.1.5 *Local SAR*

Tissue heating during MR measurements is a potential hazard at high-field MRI, and particularly in the framework of parallel RF transmission. The heating is directly related to the RF energy absorbed during an MR examination, i.e., the SAR, requiring reliable SAR estimation methods. Currently used SAR estimation methods are based on models which are neither patient specific nor take into account patient position and posture. This current practice of SAR simulations using a standardized subject shows several disadvantages. Particularly, standardized subject SAR simulations suffer from limited accuracy [Buchenau *et al.* (2009)], i.e., the actual local SAR pattern varies significantly with patient size and patient position. Another source of error can be a non-specific assignment of dielectric properties to the patient model. It has been shown that the exact value of electric properties is important for local SAR determination [Hurt *et al.* (2000)]. Thus, a sufficiently accurate determination of local SAR has to be based on patient-specific data. Furthermore, idealizing the RF transmit chain and coil can also be a source of error for SAR simulations. In real settings, imperfections or malfunctions along the transmit chain could lead to completely different RF and SAR patterns. Remaining model errors enforce large safety margins, and therefore, might lead to wasted imaging capabilities with respect to speed and/or SNR. An exact patient-specific determination of local SAR might help to fully leverage hardware capabilities.

Recently, direct local SAR measurements with EPT have been addressed in the framework of simulated data [Cloos and Bonmassar (2009)] and *in vivo* experiments [Voigt *et al.* (2009)] and validated using finite-difference time-domain (FDTD) simulations of a realistic coil model as well as a realistic patient model based on individual data. To this goal, the electric field is removed from the SAR definition by Ampère's law

$$\text{SAR}(\mathbf{r}) \sim \sigma(\mathbf{r})|\mathbf{E}(\mathbf{r})|^2 = \sigma(\mathbf{r}) \left| \frac{\nabla \times \mathbf{H}(\mathbf{r})}{\omega \tau(\mathbf{r})} \right|^2. \qquad (4.37)$$

Thus, first τ has to be determined as described above. Then, a model for the missing field components H_- and H_z has to be chosen. Again, for volume coils, the approximation $H_- = H_z = 0$ can be applied. In opposition to the EPT reconstruction of σ and ϵ, the absolute scaling of $\mathbf{H}$ is required to get the absolute scaling of the local SAR. This scaling (typically in the range of several μT) is usually provided by commercial MR scanners.

Figure 4.5 shows reconstructed local SAR for phantom [Katscher *et al.* (2009a)] and *in vivo* studies [Voigt *et al.* (2010a)]. The FDTD simulation shown for comparison is based on the segmented

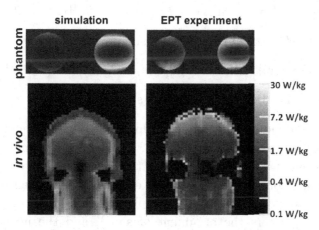

Fig. 4.5. Local SAR distribution for phantom (above; [Katscher *et al.* (2009a)]) and for *in vivo* study (below; [Voigt *et al.* (2010a)]). The results exhibit a high correlation between measured and simulated SAR, enabling the identification and localization of local SAR hot spots. However, the absolute scaling of the local SAR appears to be reduced as a consequence of neglecting unknown magnetic field components.

three-dimensional MR image of the individual volunteer. The shown SAR corresponds to $B_1 = 9\mu T$ and an RF duty cycle of 100% for demonstration purposes. The results exhibit a high correlation between measured and simulated SAR, enabling the identification and localization of local SAR hot spots. The absolute scaling of the local SAR appears to be reduced as a consequence of the assumption $H_- = H_z = 0$. The reconstruction of local SAR can also be applied to the phase-based conductivity reconstruction, assuming a constant permittivity. This procedure still maintains the overall spatial shape of the local SAR, however, further reduces its scaling [Voigt *et al.* (2010a)].

4.2   Data Collection Method

The equations discussed above are applied by EPT to the RF transmit field generated by the RF coil used in a standard MR system. In this chapter, methods to measure the (complex) RF transmit field are presented.

The MR signal is affected by the positive and negative rotating magnetic field components (H_+ and H_-, see Chapter 2 and (4.7)). Assuming a repetition time TR and echo time TE of TR $\gg T_1 \gg$ TE, the image signal S depends on H_+ and H_- via [Hoult (2000)]

$$S(\mathbf{r}) = V_1 M_0(\mathbf{r}) H_-(\mathbf{r}) \exp(i\phi_+(\mathbf{r})) \sin(V_2\alpha |H_+(\mathbf{r})|)$$

$$= V_1 M_0(\mathbf{r})| H_-(\mathbf{r})| \exp(i(\phi_+(\mathbf{r}) + \phi_-(\mathbf{r}))) \sin(V_2\alpha |H_+(\mathbf{r})|)$$

$$\equiv V_1 M_0(\mathbf{r})| H_-(\mathbf{r})| \exp(i\phi(\mathbf{r})) \sin(V_2\alpha |H_+(\mathbf{r})|). \qquad (4.38)$$

Here, α denotes the nominal flip angle of the sequence (i.e., chosen in the scanner user interface), and V_1, V_2 system-dependent constants. Furthermore, M_0 contains the (non-complex) dependence of the image contrast on relaxation effects and spin density. Only the modulus $\mathcal{H}_+ = |H_+|$ of the complex circular component $H_+ = \mathcal{H}_+ \exp(i\phi_+)$ enters the argument of $\sin(\cdot)$, and the image signal is proportional to the phase factor $\exp(i\phi_+)$. This study assumes the main magnetic field in negative z-direction, leading to the effective transmit sensitivity H_+ and H_- corresponding to the receive sensitivity.

4.2.1 *Amplitude*

The transmit magnitude $\mathcal{H}_+$, required for EPT, can be measured in a straightforward manner due to its non-linear impact on S. In this framework, numerous techniques for $\mathcal{H}_+$ mapping (also called B_1 mapping) are published (see, e.g., [Akoka *et al.* (1993); Nehrke and Börnert (2012); Sacolick *et al.* (2010); Stollberger and Wach (1996); Yarnykh (2007)]). In principle, EPT can be used in combination with any B_1 mapping method. The accuracy of EPT depends on the accuracy of this mapping, i.e., the most accurate B_1 mapping method leads to the most accurate EPT results. Studies independent of EPT have been performed to discuss the topic of optimum B_1 mapping (see, e.g., [Morrell and Schabel (2010)]).

4.2.2 *Phase*

For EPT, the knowledge of the transmit phase ϕ_+ is required. There is no standard method published yet to exactly determine ϕ_+. According to (4.38), the measured transceive phase $\phi = \phi_+ + \phi'_-$ contains both the transmit ϕ_+ and the receive phase ϕ'_-. The prime indicates that the coil used for reception is not necessarily identical (or identically driven) with the transmit coil.

To determine ϕ_+, the use of a birdcage-type RF coil is advantageous, i.e., a quadrature body coil (QBC) or corresponding head coil. A birdcage coil usually switches the polarization between transmission and reception, since the structure of the birdcage coil imposes that H_+ is substantially larger than H_-. This leads to a receive sensitivity close to H_+, as explained in the following [Hoult (2000); Katscher *et al.* (2009a)].

Using Cartesian basis vectors $\hat{\mathbf{x}}$ and $\hat{\mathbf{y}}$, the fields $\mathbf{H}_1$ and $\mathbf{H}_2$ of the two ports of the birdcage coil used are given by

$$\begin{aligned}
\mathbf{H}_1 &= H_{x1}\hat{\mathbf{x}} + H_{y1}\hat{\mathbf{y}}, \\
\mathbf{H}_2 &= H_{x2}\hat{\mathbf{x}} + H_{y2}\hat{\mathbf{y}}.
\end{aligned} \tag{4.39}$$

For transmission, these two ports are driven with a phase shift of $90°$, which is switched for reception. The resulting fields $\mathbf{H}_T$ and

$\mathbf{H}_R$ read

$$\mathbf{H}_T = \mathbf{H}_1 + i\mathbf{H}_2,$$
$$\mathbf{H}_R = i\mathbf{H}_1 + \mathbf{H}_2. \tag{4.40}$$

The active component during transmission is the positive circularly polarized component of $\mathbf{H}_T$, and the active component during reception is the negative circularly polarized component of $\mathbf{H}_R$

$$H_T^+ = (\mathbf{H}_1 + i\mathbf{H}_2)_x + i(\mathbf{H}_1 + i\mathbf{H}_2)_y = H_{x1} - H_{y2} + iH_{x2} + iH_{y1},$$
$$H_R^- = (i\mathbf{H}_1 + \mathbf{H}_2)_x - i(i\mathbf{H}_1 - \mathbf{H}_2)_y = i(H_{x1} - H_{y2} - iH_{x2} - iH_{y1}). \tag{4.41}$$

The two ports are designed to transmit two different Cartesian components in an empty coil, e.g., $H_{y1} = H_{x2} = 0$. Thus, in this case, the two fields differ only by a constant phase factor of 90°

$$H_T^+ = iH_R^-. \tag{4.42}$$

Loading the coil with material of finite τ leads to finite orthogonal components H_{y1} and H_{x2}, and thus, (4.42) is fulfilled approximately only (or in case of certain symmetries in the measured subject/object [Lee *et al.* (2010)]). The magnitude of these components generally increases with the material's τ and the main field applied. Figure 4.6 compares H_T^+ and H_R^- and for a bi-cylindrical phantom, showing only marginal differences at $B_0 = 1.5$T. The increase of this error with increasing B_0 is documented in [Lier *et al.* (2011a)].

Now assuming $H_+ \approx H_-$ for a switched birdcage coil, it can also be assumed that

$$\phi = \phi_+ + \phi_-' \approx 2\phi_+ \rightarrow \phi_+ \approx \phi/2. \tag{4.43}$$

This "transceive phase assumption" is the basis for the determination of ϕ_+ used in the full EPT reconstruction. However, in case of the approximate EPT (Section 4.1.2), any superposition of two physical phases leads to twice the reconstructed conductivity due to the linearity of (4.16). This justifies the assumption of (4.43) for arbitrary combinations of transmit and receive (surface) RF coils.

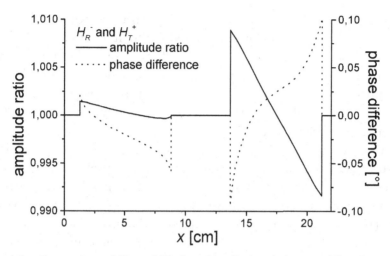

Fig. 4.6. Comparison of H_T and H_R for a bi-cylindrical phantom [Katscher *et al.* (2009a)]. The amplitude ratio and phase difference is plotted along the central axis. The marginal differences between the two fields justify the assumption underlying (4.43).

Before applying (4.43) to the measured transceive phase, the following three issues have to be taken into account.

(1) The transceive phase must not contain any contributions from B_0, i.e., any off-resonance effects. (In this respect, EPT can be seen as the opposite of quantitative susceptibility mapping, which uses only the off-resonance phase and removes all effects from B_1, essential for EPT.) The easiest way to exclude off-resonance effects is the use of refocusing pulses, i.e., sequences based on spin echoes (SE). In contrast, the transceive phase of field echo-based sequences includes off-resonance effects. In this case, these effects can be removed by any kind of B_0 mapping. In the easiest way, phase can be measured at two different echo time (TE) and extrapolated back to TE = 0. However, more sophisticated B_0 maps (for example, obtained in the framework of Dixon techniques; see, e.g., [Glover and Schneider (1991)]), can be applied.

(2) The transceive phase must not contain any contributions from eddy currents, particularly those induced in the tissue by gradient switching. This can be obtained by averaging two separate

measurements with inverted gradient polarization [King (2004)] or using sequences with balanced gradients [Stehning *et al.* (2011)].

(3) Lastly, before being cut in half, the transceive phase, now free of contributions from off-resonances and eddy currents, has to be unwrapped. This unwrapping in the three spatial dimensions can be facilitated by performing it separately for each spatial differentiation direction.

Using a parallel RF transmission system, it seems to be possible to distinguish ϕ_+ and ϕ_- by comparing reconstruction results from different transmit channels [Katscher *et al.* (2011); Sodickson (2010)]. These channels must yield identical electric properties, which gives a mean to separate ϕ_+ and ϕ_- of the different channels. The applicability of this method *in statu nascendi* has to be proven in future research.

4.3 Image Reconstruction

4.3.1 *SNR and calculus operation kernel*

Solving the EPT equations presented in Section 4.1 requires the numerical treatment of calculus operations. For the numerical computation of the integrals, adding voxels in a square region around the target voxel is usually performed. A standard method for numerical differentiation is Savitzky–Golay filtering, i.e., applying a set of convolution coefficients obtained by a local polynomial regression [Savitzky and Golay (1964)]. The number of convolution coefficients applied is typically higher in in-plane directions than in through-plane directions, according to typically non-isotropic voxel dimensions. The resulting three-dimensional kernel can be applied in k-space to reduce central processing unit (CPU) time. However, a fixed kernel size frequently leads to undefined voxels along region of interest (ROI) boundaries. Therefore, kernel size might be adjusted dynamically in the vicinity of ROI boundaries to minimize the number of undefined voxels. Remaining gaps in the conductivity and permittivity maps can be closed by a region-growing algorithm after the reconstruction.

A small kernel size causes a high spatial resolution and a low SNR of the reconstructed τ. Vice versa, a large kernel size causes a low

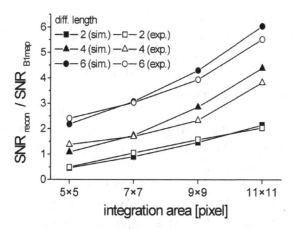

Fig. 4.7. Impact of numerical calculus operation on resulting SNR [Katscher *et al.* (2009a)]. The SNR of the reconstructed conductivity (normalized to the SNR of the underlying B_1 map) increases both with the differentiation length and integration area. This holds for simulated data (solid symbols) as well as for experimental data (open symbols).

spatial resolution and a high SNR of the reconstructed τ, and thus, is advantageous for a low SNR of the input B_1 map. Typically, 2–6 voxels in all spatial directions around the target voxel are involved for its reconstruction. Figure 4.7 shows the described trade-off for a phantom study [Katscher *et al.* (2009a)]. It reveals a noise figure, which causes the (effective) spatial resolution of an EPT map to be clearly lower than the spatial resolution of the original MR images.

4.3.2 *Main field strength and SNR*

Disregarding effects from kernel size, SNR of reconstructed permittivity is significantly lower than SNR of reconstructed conductivity due to the following two reasons: (1) The impact of the permittivity on the amplitude $\mathcal{H}_+$ is much lower than the impact of the conductivity on the phase ϕ_+; (2) The noise present in $\mathcal{H}_+$ maps is typically much higher than the noise present in the image phase. A too-low spatial resolution prohibits image segmentation prior to reconstruction, which might be used to circumvent the discussed neglection of the spatial variation of τ along ∂A. This problem can be addressed by improving SNR and/or spatial resolution of permittivity imaging via increasing the main field B_0. To assess the general feasibility of EPT at increased B_0, several effects have to be taken into account. On the one hand, according to the 4-Cole–Cole model [Gabriel *et al.* (1996)], conductivities increase and permittivities decrease with increasing B_0. On the other hand, increasing ω_0 leads to higher impact of dielectric properties on RF fields. The effect is linear in conductivity and quadratic in permittivity (cf (4.14), (4.15)), overcompensating the aforementioned permittivity decrease. This would improve the sensitivity of conductivity and permittivity measurements at high B_0.

For brain tissues, $\sigma \approx \omega\epsilon$ is observed at $B_0 = 2.3/3.7/14\,\mathrm{T}$ for gray matter (GM), white matter (WM), and CSF, respectively. Compared with $B_0 = 1.5\,\mathrm{T}$, this implies a better applicability of magnitude-based permittivity imaging (4.17) already at roughly $B_0 = 3\,\mathrm{T}$. For even higher field strength, the impact of ϵ on $\mathcal{H}_+$ further increases, eventually leading to $\omega\epsilon > \sigma$ for most tissue types. This is beneficial for the approximation underlying (4.17) for magnitude-based permittivity imaging, but simultaneously, hampers phase-based conductivity imaging. A systematic study on the impact of B_0 on EPT can be found in [Lier *et al.* (2011a)].

4.4 Numerical Simulations

4.4.1 *Head model*

Figures 4.8 and 4.9 show example results of an FDTD study using the visible human model [Voigt *et al.* (2011b)]. The head of the visible human was placed at the isocenter of a body coil at 1.5 T with electric properties according to [Gabriel *et al.* (1996)]. A resolution of $1 \times 1\,\mathrm{mm}^2$ in plane was used to simulate the magnetic fields. Magnitude $\mathcal{H}_+$ and phase ϕ_+ of the resulting transmit field were used for exact and approximate reconstruction according to (4.14) and (4.15), and (4.16) and (4.17), respectively. An additional reconstruction was performed with transceive phase assumption (4.43) mimicking the switched coil polarization performed for the experimental signal acquisition. The NRMSE was computed for 15 coronal slices to compare exact and approximate reconstruction results.

The comparison of full and approximated reconstruction shows little qualitative deviation (Figures 4.8 and 4.9). Residual errors in

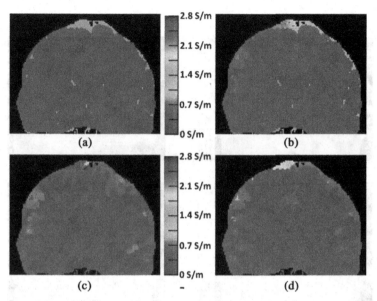

Fig. 4.8. Conductivity reconstruction of FDTD simulation of a realistic head model [Voigt *et al.* (2011b)]. (a) Conductivity distribution used in FDTD simulations. (b) Exact reconstruction using (4.14), i.e., based on complex H_+. (c) Approximated reconstruction using (4.16), i.e., based only on the transmit phase ϕ_+. (d) Approximated reconstruction based on the transceive phase assumption (4.43). A corresponding, quantitative analysis can be found in Table 4.1.

the exact reconstruction case are due to numerical effects. Fitting a second-order polynomial is particularly suitable for constant conductivity since in this case solving the inverse of (4.16) yields quadratic phase ϕ_+. This explains the higher accuracy achieved in simulations of homogeneous objects than in simulations of the heterogeneous head model. In the latter case, the use of higher-order polynomials improves the results. However, higher-order polynomials suffer from higher noise sensitivity, and thus, second-order polynomials are typically applied. The quantitative NRMSE introduced by the approximations is of the order of 10% for conductivity and 15% for permittivity reconstructions. In the case of permittivity imaging, the NRMSE is related to the CSF content present in the reconstructed slice; i.e., the more CSF present, the higher the error obtained. Quantitative values of conductivity and permittivity for full and approximate reconstruction are shown in Table 4.1.

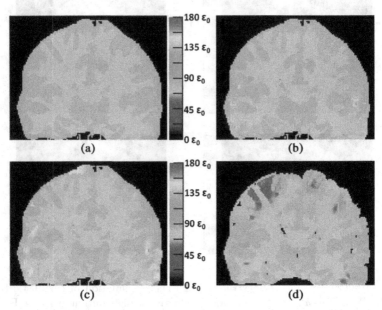

Fig. 4.9. Permittivity reconstruction of FDTD simulation data of a realistic head model [Voigt *et al.* (2011b)]. (a) Permittivity distribution used in FDTD simulations. (b) Exact reconstruction using (4.15), i.e., based on complex H_+. (c) Same as (b), however, based on the transceive phase assumption (4.43). (d) Approximated reconstruction using (4.17), i.e., based only on B_1 magnitude. The CSF is not shown in (d) since magnitude-based reconstruction of CSF permittivity violates $\omega\epsilon \gg \sigma$, and thus, does not yield a meaningful value (cf. Figure 4.3). A corresponding, quantitative analysis can be found in Table 4.1.

Table 4.1.   Analysis of FDTD results [Voigt *et al.* (2011b)]. Quantitative comparison of average values of conductivity and permittivity inside different regions of interest. Quantities were reconstructed from FDTD data. Corresponding images are shown in Figures 4.8 and 4.9.

	Conductivity [S/m]		Permittivity [ϵ_0]		Input value	
ROI	Exact	Approx.	Exact	Approx.	σ	ϵ
WM	0.30 ± 0.03	0.33 ± 0.04	68 ± 4	62 ± 6	0.29	67.8
GM	0.52 ± 0.06	0.57 ± 0.07	100 ± 9	89 ± 11	0.51	97.4
CSF	20.9 ± 0.12	2.19 ± 0.08	104 ± 12	n/a	2.07	97.3

These results confirm that approximate EPT seems to be feasible for the price of an acceptable error of roughly +10% (conductivity) or −10% (permittivity) as expected from theory (Section 4.1). These expectations are also confirmed by experimental results as will follow in the next section.

4.5   Experiments

4.5.1   *Phantom experiments*

Figure 4.10 shows an example phantom study to demonstrate the feasibility and accuracy of EPT [Katscher *et al.* (2009a, 2010b)]. To this goal, an iso-centric, bi-cylindrical phantom (diameters = 7.5 cm, height = 13 cm, cylinder axis distance = 12.5 cm) with different electric conductivities and permittivities was placed in a quadrature body coil at 64 MHz. The electric conductivity was adjusted $(0 < \sigma < 2\,\text{S/m})$ by the saline concentration and determined with an independent probe. Permittivity was adjusted $(18 < \epsilon_r < 80)$ via 2-propanol and determined via the mixing ratios applied. These electric properties roughly cover the physiological range [Gabriel *et al.* (1996)]. A suitable contrast agent was added to enhance the MR signal. Experiments were performed on a standard clinical MR system. B_1 maps were acquired using actual flip angle imaging (AFI) [Nehrke (2009); Yarnykh (2007)]. B_1 maps are derived from AFI by analyzing two fast field echo (FFE) images acquired in an interleaved fashion with the same flip angle, but

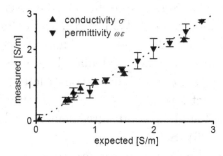

Fig. 4.10.   EPT phantom experiments [Katscher *et al.* (2009a, 2010b)]. A high correlation between *a priori* determined and EPT measured values is visible for (▲) conductivity and (▼) permittivity.

two different repetition times. This makes the approach independent from imperfect flip angle scaling arising from, e.g., non-linearities in the RF transmit chain. The phase ϕ_+ was obtained via (4.43) from the transceive phase of the long TR FFE image acquired for AFI. Additionally, to correct this phase for susceptibility artifacts and main field inhomogeneities, a B_0 map was acquired using a dual echo sequence ($\Delta\text{TE} = 10\,\text{ms}$), and the corresponding phase was subtracted. Conductivity reconstruction was performed according to (4.14) and (4.16) using a kernel of 5 pixels for in-plane derivatives and 4 pixels for through-plane derivatives. Permittivity reconstruction was performed according to (4.15) and (4.17) using 8 pixels in-plane and 6 pixels through-plane. Reconstructed conductivity and permittivity were averaged inside a circular region of interest and compared with the expected values. Quantitative results exhibit a correlation of roughly 99% between reconstructed and expected values for both conductivity and permittivity as well as for both full and approximate EPT reconstruction.

4.5.2   *Volunteer experiments*

In the following, example studies are described which apply EPT *in vivo* in the human head to investigate the electric properties of the brain. First, experiments are described with healthy volunteers at 1.5 T.

Detailed conductivity study with full reconstruction

In one of the volunteers, five different ROIs were defined based on the anatomic image: GM, WM, CSF, cerebellum, and corpus callosum [Voigt *et al.* (2009)]. Average values and standard deviation inside these compartments were calculated from the reconstructed electric conductivity. Conductivity reconstruction was performed according to the exact formula (4.14). The quantitative conductivity (see Table 4.2) is found in good agreement with literature values [Gabriel *et al.* (1996); Sekino *et al.* (2004)]. However, one has to keep in mind that literature values are frequently animal and/or *ex vivo* data, hampering a direct comparison with the human *in vivo* data.

Table 4.2. Volunteer's brain conductivity [Voigt *et al.* (2009)]. Mean values in five different compartments roughly match with literature values [Gabriel *et al.* (1996); Sekino *et al.* (2004)].

ROI	Conductivity σ	Literature
CSF	$1.85 \pm 0.87\,\text{S/m}$	$2.07\,\text{S/m}$
Cerebellum	$0.57 \pm 0.15\,\text{S/m}$	$0.72\,\text{S/m}$
Corpus callosum	$0.24 \pm 0.09\,\text{S/m}$	$0.21\,\text{S/m}$
WM	$0.32 \pm 0.12\,\text{S/m}$	$0.29\,\text{S/m}$
GM	$0.48 \pm 0.07\,\text{S/m}$	$0.51\,\text{S/m}$

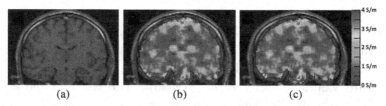

(a) (b) (c)

Fig. 4.11. Brain conductivity study [Voigt *et al.* (2011b)]. (a) SE image acquired to determine ϕ_+. (b) Exact reconstruction using (4.14), i.e., based on complex H_+. (c) Approximated reconstruction using (4.16), i.e., based only on the transmit phase ϕ_+.

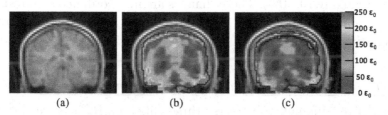

(a) (b) (c)

Fig. 4.12. Brain permittivity study [Voigt *et al.* (2011b)]. (a) FFE image acquired to determine $\mathcal{H}_+$. (b) Exact reconstruction using (4.15), i.e., based on complex H_+. (c) Approximated reconstruction using (4.17), i.e., based only on $\mathcal{H}_+$ magnitude.

Admittivity comparison, full/approximate reconstruction

In another volunteer, three different ROIs were defined based on the anatomic image: GM, WM, and CSF [Voigt *et al.* (2011b)]. Average values and standard deviation inside these compartments were calculated from the reconstructed conductivity and permittivity (Figures 4.11 and 4.12). Reconstructions were performed according

Table 4.3.   Analysis of *in vivo* study [Voigt *et al.* (2011b)]. Quantitative comparison of average values of conductivity and permittivity inside different ROIs. Values were reconstructed from measured data of a healthy volunteer. Corresponding images are shown in Figures 4.11 and 4.12.

ROI	Conductivity [S/m]		Permittivity [ϵ_0]	
	Exact formula	Phase-based approximation	Exact formula	Magnitude-based approximation
WM	0.39 ± 0.15	0.43 ± 0.15	72 ± 64	63 ± 66
GM	0.69 ± 0.14	0.72 ± 0.15	103 ± 69	91 ± 70
CSF	1.75 ± 0.34	1.82 ± 0.37	104 ± 21	98 ± 20

to the exact formulae (4.14) and (4.15) and the approximate formulae (4.16) and (4.17). Again, the quantitative conductivity and permittivity (see Table 4.3) is found in good agreement with literature values [Gabriel *et al.* (1996)]. The considerable errors found for permittivity imaging arise from the large-scale calculus operations smearing over different compartments. The phase-based reconstruction increases the conductivity results by roughly 5−10%. The magnitude-based reconstruction decreases the permittivity values by roughly 10−15%. These changes are in accordance with results from phantom simulations (Section 4.1.2) as well as FDTD brain simulation (Section 4.4.1).

Inter-subject conductivity variability, approximate reconstruction

In five different volunteers, three different ROIs were defined based on the anatomic image: GM, WM, and CSF [Voigt *et al.* (2011b)]. Average values and standard deviation inside these compartments were calculated from the reconstructed conductivity. Reconstructions were performed according to the approximate formula (4.16). The observed inter-subject variability is roughly 10% for gray and white matter and roughly 20% for CSF (see Table 4.4). The higher variability in CSF seems to be caused by the significantly lower number of voxels available for averaging conductivity values. Of course, the observed inter-subject variability contains two components, measurement errors and physiological

Table 4.4.   Inter-subject conductivity variability [Voigt *et al.* (2011b)]. The higher variability in CSF seems to be caused by the significantly lower number of voxels available for averaging conductivity values. These inter-subject variabilities contain two components, measurement errors and physiological differences between subjects.

	WM	GM	CSF
Volunteer 1	0.43 ± 0.15	0.72 ± 0.15	1.82 ± 0.37
Volunteer 2	0.33 ± 0.11	0.63 ± 0.25	1.00 ± 0.45
Volunteer 3	0.37 ± 0.15	0.74 ± 0.33	1.26 ± 0.28
Volunteer 4	0.37 ± 0.23	0.85 ± 0.3	1.85 ± 0.72
Volunteer 5	0.30 ± 0.18	0.70 ± 0.26	1.54 ± 0.59
Mean	$0.36 \pm 12.2\%$	$0.73 \pm 9.8\%$	$1.49 \pm 21.8\%$

Table 4.5.   Field strength dependence of permittivity [Katscher *et al.* (2010b)]. Values of a volunteer's brain reconstructed with EPT match literature expectations [Gabriel *et al.* (1996)] of a permittivity slightly higher at 1.5 T than at 3 T.

ROI	1.5 T		3 T	
	EPT	Literature	EPT	Literature
CSF	104 ± 21	97.3	102 ± 26	84.0
WM	72 ± 64	67.8	55 ± 27	52.5
GM	103 ± 69	97.4	79 ± 25	73.5

differences. Future studies shall work on separating these two components.

Field strength dependence

Last, a volunteer has been measured twice at 1.5 T and 3 T [Katscher *et al.* (2010b)]. Again, three different ROIs were defined based on the anatomic image: GM, WM, and CSF. Average values and standard deviation inside these compartments were calculated from the reconstructed permittivity. Reconstructions were performed according to the exact formula (4.15). The observed decrease of permittivity with increasing frequency is in accordance with literature (Table 4.5). Of course, in front of the large uncertainties reported, this result has to be confirmed by further studies.

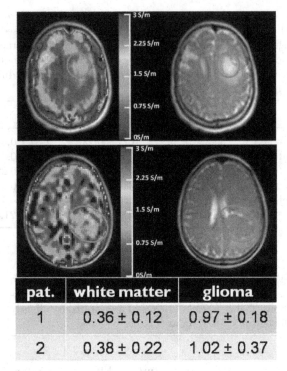

pat.	white matter	glioma
1	0.36 ± 0.12	0.97 ± 0.18
2	0.38 ± 0.22	1.02 ± 0.37

Fig. 4.13.   Tumor pilot study [Voigt *et al.* (2011a)]. Tumor conductivity appears to be pathologically increased by a factor of 2−3 compared with the surrounding white matter.

4.6   Medical Applications

Pilot studies have been performed applying EPT *in vivo* in the head of glioma patients at 1.5 T [Voigt *et al.* (2011a)] and higher field strengths [Lier *et al.* (2011b)]. Figure 4.13 shows results from the study at 1.5 T [Voigt *et al.* (2011a)]. In each patient, two different ROIs were defined based on the anatomic image: tumor and WM. Average values and standard deviation inside these compartments were calculated from the reconstructed electric conductivity. Conductivity reconstruction was performed according to the approximate formula (4.16). In both cases, the tumor conductivity seems to be pathologically increased by a factor of 2−3 compared with the surrounding white matter. Similar results have been reported from higher field strengths [Lier *et al.* (2011b)]. The factor of 2−3 is in the range of observations from surgically excised glioma samples [Lu *et al.* (1992)].

In 2010, initial results were also reported for a breast tumor [Borsic (2010)]. It is expected that more and more clinical studies will investigate the electric properties in tumors and other lesions in the near future.

4.7 Challenging Problems and Future Directions

The recently developed technique of MR-EPT has proven its principle feasibility. Numerous simulations and experiments confirm that MR-EPT is able to map electric conductivity and permittivity *in vivo* with high accuracy and high spatial resolution. The reconstruction technique of MR-EPT is comparatively simple, i.e, there is no need for any iteration, patient modeling, solving ill-posed inverse problems, or the like. However, MR-EPT is fighting with a couple of technical problems, which are currently under investigation in several research groups around the world.

(1) Determination of the transmit phase ϕ_+. The knowledge of ϕ_+ is required for accurately reconstructing τ. However, standard MR methods only allow mapping of the transceive phase. The extraction of ϕ_+ from this transceive phase is one of the central issues for MR-EPT. For a volume coil, ϕ_+ can be estimated by cutting the transceive phase in half. Approximate EPT depends linearly on the phase, and thus, it is sufficient to cut in half the reconstructed conductivity independently of the RF coils used. An analytical way to determine ϕ_+ might be given by using a parallel RF transmission system.

(2) Treatment of non-constant τ. Equations of EPT based on the truncated Helmholtz equation are failing in regions with strongly varying τ. Particularly along boundaries between compartments of different τ, erroneous oscillations of the reconstructed τ are observed. These oscillations can be avoided by separate reconstructions in the different compartments. Alternatively, the full Helmholtz equation can be used for reconstruction. Also in this framework, a parallel RF transmission system can help to obtain the missing partial derivatives of τ.

(3) Missing field components H_- and H_z. The knowledge of these components is not required to determine (constant) τ. However, it can be used to determine a non-constant τ as alternative to the determination of the missing partial derivatives of τ as discussed in (2). Furthermore, the knowledge of H_- and H_z is needed to accurately determine local SAR with MR-EPT. The assumption $H_- = H_z = 0$ seems to work well for quadrature volume coils; however, it gets problematic in the case of single transmit elements as found in a parallel RF transmission system.

From a technical point of view, future research will focus on the treatment of these three problematic points. Of course, researchers will also try to enlarge the functionality of MR-EPT, looking for additional information available with this technique. For instance, it seems to be worth elaborating the sketched method of measuring anisotropic τ in more detail. Also, methods to extend the single-frequency spectrum of MR-EPT would be very welcome.

On the other hand, studies have just started to clinically evaluate MR-EPT in its current status. To become a clinically accepted method, MR-EPT has to be able to answer diagnostic questions better than existing methods can (e.g., more accurately and/or with higher patient comfort). Up to now, no clinical standard modality exists to measure τ *in vivo*. This lack is responsible for the lack of knowledge about electric properties in human pathologies, at least *in vivo*. Thus, clinical MR-EPT studies have to cope not only with technical issues, but also with the bio-chemical relation between the investigated pathology and its observed electric properties. This makes MR-EPT a particularly interesting and exciting topic for future work.

Acknowledgments

Cordial thanks to Tobias Voigt for his substantial contributions to this chapter. Furthermore, we would like to thank, for many fruitful discussions: Christian Findeklee, Christian Stehning, and Philipp Karkowski, all of Philips Research Europe-Hamburg; as well as Nico van den Berg and Astrid van Lier, both of the University Medical Center, Utrecht.

References

Akoka S, Franconi F, Seguin F and Le Pape A (1993). *Radiofrequency map of an NMR coil by imaging, Magn. Reson. Imag.*, Vol. 11, pp. 437–441.

Balidemaj E, van Lier AL, Nederveen AJ, Crezee J and van den Berg CAT (2012). *Feasibility of EPT in the human pelvis at 3 T, Proc. 20th Annual Meeting of ISMRM*, Vol. 20, p. 3468.

Barker GJ, Simmons A, Arridge SR and Tofts PS (1998). *A simple method for investigating the effects of non-uniformity of radiofrequency transmission and radiofrequency reception in MRI, Br J. Radiol.*, Vol. 71, pp. 59–67.

Beravs K, Frangez R, Gerkis AN and Demsar F (1999). *Radiofrequency current density imaging of kainate-evoked depolarization, Magn. Reson. Med.*, Vol. 42, pp. 136–140.

Bernstein MA, King KF and Zhou XJ (2004). *Handbook of MRI Pulse Sequences*, Academic Press, San Diego, CA, pp. 316–331.

Borsic A (2010). *Imaging electrical properties of the breast–current experiences at Dartmouth, Proc. Int. Workshop on MR-based Impedance*, Seoul, Korea.

Buchenau S, Haas M, Hennig J and Zaitsev M (2009). *A comparison of local SAR using individual patient data and a patient template, Proc. 17th Annual Meeting of ISMRM*, Honolulu, Hawaii, USA, Vol. 17, p. 4798.

Bulumulla S and Hancu I (2012). *Breast permittivity imaging, Proc. 20th Annual Meeting of ISMRM*, Vol. 20, p. 2532.

Bulumulla SB, Yeo TB and Zhu Y (2009). *Direct calculation of tissue electrical parameters from B1 maps, Proc. 17th Annual Meeting of ISMRM*, Honolulu, Hawaii, USA, Vol. 17, p. 3043.

Bulumulla SB, Lee SK and Yeo TBD (2012). *Calculation of electrical properties from B1+ maps-a comparison of methods, Proc. 20th Annual Meeting of ISMRM*, Vol. 20, p. 3469.

Choi N, Ghim M, Yang S, Zho SY and Kim DH (2011). *In vivo conductivity mapping using double spin echo for flow effect removal, Proc. 19th Annual Meeting of ISMRM*, Vol. 19, p. 4466.

Cloos MA and Bonmassar G (2009). *Towards direct B1-Bsed local SAR estimation, Proc. 17th Annual Meeting of ISMRM*, Honolulu, Hawaii, USA, Vol. 17, p. 3037.

Epstein BR and Foster KR (1983). *Anisotropy in the dielectric properties of skeletal muscle, Med. Biol. Eng. Comput.*, Vol. 21, pp. 51–55.

Gabriel S, Lau RW and Gabriel C (1996). *The dielectric properties of biological tissues: III. Parametric models for the dielectric spectrum of tissues, Phys. Med. Biol.*, Vol. 41, pp. 2271–2293.

Gabriel S, Lau RW and Gabriel C (2011). *The dielectric properties of biological tissues: II. Measurements in the frequency range 10 Hz to 20 GHz, Phys. Med. Biol.*, Vol. 41, pp. 2251–2269.

Glover GH and Schneider E (1991). *Three-point Dixon technique for true water/fat decomposition with B0 inhomogeneity correction, Magn. Reson. Med.*, Vol. 18, pp. 371–383.

Graesslin I, Falaggis K, Vernickel P, Roeschmann P, Leussler C, Zhai Z, Morich M and Katscher U (2006). *Safety considerations concerning SAR during RF* amplifier malfunctions in parallel transmission, Proc. 14th Annual Meeting of ISMRM, Seattle, Washington, USA, p. 2041.

Grimnes S and Martinsen OG (2000). *Bioimpedance and Bioelectricity Basics*, Academic Press, San Diego, CA.

Haacke EM, Petropoulos LS, Nilges EW and Wu DH (1991). *Extraction of conductivity and permittivity using magnetic resonance imaging*, Phys. Med. Biol., Vol. 36, pp. 723–734.

Hoult DI (2000). *The principle of reciprocity in signal strength calculations-a mathematical guide*, Concept. Magn. Reson., Vol. 12, pp. 173–187.

Hurt W, Ziriax J and Mason P (2000). *Variability in EMF permittivity values: implications for SAR calculations*, IEEE Trans. Biomed. Eng., Vol. 47, pp. 396–401.

Joy ML, Scott GC and Henkelman RM (1989). *In vivo detection of applied electric currents by magnetic resonance imaging*, Magn. Res. Imaging, Vol. 7, pp. 89–94.

Katscher U, Hanft M, Vernickel P and Findeklee C (2006). *Electric Properties Tomography (EPT) via MRI*, Proc. 14th Annual Meeting of ISMRM, Seattle, Washington, USA, pp. 3035–3037.

Katscher U, Dorniok T, Findeklee C and Vernickel P (2007). *In vivo determination of electric conductivity and permittivity using Electric Properties Tomography (EPT)*, Proc. 15th Annual Meeting of ISMRM, Berlin, Germany, p. 1774.

Katscher U, Voigt T, Findeklee C, Nehrke K, Weiss S and Doessel O (2008). *Estimation of local SAR using B1 mapping*, Proc. 16th Annual Meeting of ISMRM, Toronto, Canada, p. 1191.

Katscher U, Voigt T, Findeklee C, Vernickel P, Nehrke K and Doessel O (2009a). *Determination of electric conductivity and local SAR via B1 mapping*, IEEE Trans. Med. Imag., Vol. 28, pp. 1365–1374.

Katscher U, Findeklee C and Voigt T (2009b). *Experimental estimation of local SAR in a multi-transmit system*, Proc. 17th Annual Meeting of ISMRM, Vol. 17, p. 4512.

Katscher U, Voigt T and Findeklee C (2010a). *Estimation of the anisotropy of Electric Conductivity via B1 Mapping*, Proc. 18th Annual Meeting of ISMRM, Vol. 18, p. 2866.

Katscher U, Karkowski P, Findeklee C and Voigt T (2010b). *Permittivity determination via phantom and in vivo B1 mapping*, Proc. 18th Annual Meeting of ISMRM, Vol. 18, p. 239.

Katscher U, Findeklee C and Voigt T (2011). *Single element SAR measurements in a multi-transmit system*, Proc. 19th Annual Meeting of ISMRM, Vol. 19, p. 494.

Katscher U, Findeklee C, Voigt T (2012). *B(1)-based specific energy absorption rate determination for nonquadrature radiofrequency excitation*, Magn. Reson. Med., Vol. 68, pp. 1911–1918.

Katscher U, Djamshidi K, Voigt T, Ivancevic M, Abe H, Newstead G and Keupp J (2012). *Estimation of breast tumor conductivity using parabolic phase fitting*, Proc. 20th Annual Meeting of ISMRM, Vol. 20, p. 3482.

Katscher U, van Lier A, van den Berg CAT and Keupp J (2012). *RF shimming improves phase-based conductivity imaging, Proc. 20th Annual Meeting of ISMRM*, Vol. 20, p. 3487.

Katscher U, Kim DH, and Seo JK (2013). *Recent progress and future challenges in MR electric properties tomography, Comput. Math. Methods Med.*, Article ID 546562.

Kim DH, Gho SM, Choi N and Liu C (2012). *Simultaneous electromagnetic property imaging using multiecho gradient echo, Proc. 20th Annual Meeting of ISMRM*, Vol. 20, p. 3464.

King KF (2004). *Eddy current compensation*, In: Bernstein MA, King KF and Zhou XJ, *Handbook of MRI Pulse Sequences*, Academic Press, San Diego, CA, pp. 316–331.

Lee J, Song Y, Choi N, Cho S, Seo JK and Kim DH (2013). *Noninvasive Measurement of Conductivity Anisotropy at Larmor frequency using MRI, Comput. Math. Methods Med.*, Vol. 2013, Article ID 421619.

Lee SK, Bulumulla SB, Dixon WT and Yeo DTB (2010). *B1 + phase mapping for MR-based electrical property measurement of a symmetric phantom, Proc. International Workshop on MR-based Impedance*, Seoul, Korea.

Leussler C, Karkowski P and Katscher U (2012). *Temperature dependant conductivity change using MR-based Electric Properties Tomography, Proc. 20th Annual Meeting of ISMRM*, Vol. 20, p. 3451.

Lu Y, Li B, Xu J and Yu J (1992). *Dielectric properties of human glioma and surrounding tissue, Int. J. Hypertherm.*, Vol. 8, pp. 750–760.

Morrell GR and Schabel MC (2010). *An analysis of the accuracy of magnetic resonance flip angle measurement methods, Phys. Med. Biol.*, Vol. 55, pp. 6157–6174.

Nachman AI, Wang D, Ma W and Joy MLG (2007). *A local formula for inhomogeneous complex conductivity as a function of the RF magnetic field, Proc. 15th Annual Meeting of ISMRM*. Available at http://www.ismrm. org/07/Unsolved.htm, accessed 13 June 2013.

Nehrke K (2009). *On the steady-state properties of actual flip angle imaging (AFI), Magn Reson Med.*, Vol. 61, pp. 84–92.

Nehrke K and Börnert P (2012). *DREAM-a novel approach for robust, ultrafast, multislice B(1) mapping, Magn. Reson. Med.*, Vol. 68, pp. 1517–1526.

Sacolick L, Wiesinger F, Hancu I and Vogel M (2010). *B1 mapping by Bloch-Siegert shift, Magn. Reson. Med.*, Vol. 63, pp. 1315–1322.

Savitzky A and Golay MJ (1964). *Smoothing and differentiation of data by simplified least square procedures, Analyt. Chem.*, Vol. 36, pp. 1627–1639.

Scott GC, Joy MLG, Armstrong RL and Henkelman RM (1991) *Measurement of nonuniform current density by magnetic resonance, IEEE Trans. Med. Imag.*, Vol. 10, pp. 362–374.

Scott GC, Joy LG, Armstrong RL and Henkelman RM (1995). *Rotating frame RF current density imaging, Magn. Reson. Med.*, Vol. 33, pp. 355–369.

Sekino H and Bartlett RJ (2004). *Relativistic coupled cluster calculations on neutral and highly ionized atoms, Neurol. Clin. Neurophysiol.*, Vol. 55, pp. 1–5.

Seo JK, Yoon JR, Woo EJ and Kwon O (2003). *Reconstruction of conductivity and current density images using only one component of magnetic field measurements, IEEE Trans. Biomed. Eng.*, Vol. 50, pp. 1121–1124.

Seo JK and Woo EJ (2011). *Magnetic resonance electrical impedance tomography (MREIT), SIAM Review*, Vol. 53, pp. 40–68.

Seo JK, Kim MO, Lee J, Choi N, Woo EJ, Kim HJ, Kwon OI and Kim DH (2012). *Error analysis of nonconstant admittivity for MR-based electric property imging, IEEE Trans. Med. Imag.*, Vol. 31, pp. 430–437.

Setsompop K, Wald LL, Alagappan V, Gagoski B, Hebrank F, Fontius U, Schmitt F and Adalsteinsson E (2006). *Parallel RF transmission with eight channels at 3 Tesla, Magn. Reson. Med.*, Vol. 56, pp. 1163–1171.

Shin J, Lee J, Seo JK and Kim DH (2012). *Quantification error in MREPT due to B1 map inaccuracy, Proc. 20th Annual Meeting of ISMRM*, Vol. 20, p. 2533.

Sodickson D (2010). *Addressing the challenges of electrical property mapping with magnetic resonance, Proc. International Workshop on MR-based Impedance*, Seoul, Korea.

Sodickson DK, Alon L, Deniz CM, Brown R, Zhang B, Wiggins GC, Cho GY, Eliezer Noam Ben, Novikov DS, Lattanzi R, Duan Qi, Sodickson LA and Zhu Y (2012). *Local Maxwell tomography using transmit-receive coil arrays for contact-free mapping of tissue electrical properties and determination of absolute RF phase, Proc. 20th Annual Meeting of ISMRM* Vol. 20, p. 387.

Stehning C, Voigt TR and Katscher U (2011). *Real-time conductivity mapping using balanced SSFP and phase-based reconstruction, Proc. 19th Annual Meeting of ISMRM*, Montreal, Canada, Vol. 19, p. 128.

Stehning C, Voigt T, Karkowski P and Katscher U (2012a). *Electric properties tomography (EPT) of the liver in a single breathhold using SSFP, Proc. 20th Annual Meeting of ISMRM*, Vol. 20, p. 386.

Stehning C, Voigt TR and Katscher U (2012b). *Reproducibility study of 3D SSFP phase-based brain conductivity imaging, MAGMA*, Vol. 25, pp. S197–S198.

Stollberger R and Wach P (1996). *Imaging of the active B1 field in vivo, Magn. Reson. Med.*, Vol. 35, pp. 246–251.

van Lier AL, Raaijmakers AJ, Brunner DO, Klomp DW, Pruessmann KP, Lagendijk JJ and van den Berg CAT (2010). *Propagating RF phase: a new contrast to detect local changes in conductivity, Proc. 18th Annual Meeting of ISMRM*, Stockholm, Sweden, p. 2864.

van Lier AL, Voigt T, Katscher U and van den Berg CAT (2011a). *Comparing Electric Properties Tomography at 1.5, 3 and 7 T, Proc. 19th Annual Meeting of ISMRM*, Vol. 19, p. 125.

van Lier AL, Hoogduin JM, Polders DL, Boer VO, Hendrikse J, Robe PA, Woerdeman PA, Lagendijk JJW, Luijten PR and van den Berg CAT (2011b). *Electrical conductivity imaging of brain tumours, Proc. 19th Annual Meeting of ISMRM*, Vol. 19, p. 4464.

van Lier AL, Katscher U, Raaijmakers A and van den Berg CAT (2012a). *Wavenumber imaging at 7T: increasing accuracy of EPT at high field strengths, Proc. 20th Annual Meeting of ISMRM*, Vol. 20, p. 3466.

van Lier AL, Brunner DO, Pruessmann KP, Klomp DW, Luijten PR, Lagendijk JJ and van den Berg CAT (2012b). *B1(+) phase mapping at 7T and its application for in vivo electrical conductivity mapping, Magn. Reson. Med.* Vol. 67, pp. 552–561.

van Lier AL, Kolk A, Brundel M, Hendriske J, Luijten P, Lagendijk J and van den Berg CAT (2012c). *Electrical conductivity in Ischemic stroke at 7.0 Tesla: A case study, Proc. 20th Annual Meeting of ISMRM,* Vol. 20, p. 3484.

Vernickel P, Roeschmann P, Findeklee C, Luedeke KM, Leussler C, Overweg J, Katscher U, Graesslin I and Schuenemann K (2007). *Eight-channel transmit/ receive body MRI coil at 3T, Magn. Reson. Med.,* Vol. 58, pp. 381–389.

Voigt T, Doessel O and Katscher U (2009). *Imaging conductivity and local SAR of the human brain, Proc. 17th Annual Meeting of ISMRM,* Honolulu, Hawaii, USA, p. 4513.

Voigt T, Homann H, Katscher U and Doessel O (2010a). *Patient-specific in vivo local SAR Estimation and Validation, Proc. 18th Annual Meeting of ISMRM,* Vol. 18, p. 3876.

Voigt T, Nehrke K, Doessel O and Katscher U (2010b). *T1 corrected B1 mapping using multi-TR gradient echo sequences, Magn. Reson. Med.,* Vol. 64, pp. 725–733.

Voigt T, Vaeterlein O, Stehning C, Katscher U and Fiehler J (2011a). *In vivo glioma characterization using MR conductivity imaging, Proc. 19th Annual Meeting of ISMRM,* Vol. 19, p. 127.

Voigt T, Katscher U and Doessel O (2011b). *Quantitative conductivity and permittivity imaging of the human brain using electric properties tomography, Magn. Reson. Med.,* Vol. 66, pp. 456–466.

Voigt T, Schuster A, Ishida M, Stehning C, Katscher U, Chiribiri A, Nagel E and Schaeffer T (2012). *Conductivity imaging of an ischemic pig heart model using electric properties tomography, Proc. 20th Annual Meeting of ISMRM,* Vol. 20, p. 3483.

Wang D, DeMonte TP, Ma W, Joy ML and Nachman AI (2009). *Multislice radio-frequency current density imaging, IEEE Trans. Med. Imag.,* Vol. 28, pp. 1083–1092.

Wen H (2003). *Noninvasive quantitative mapping of conductivity and dielectric distributions using RF wave propagation effects in high-field MRI, Proc. SPIE,* Vol. 5030, pp. 471–477.

Woo EJ, Lee SY and Mun CW (1994). *Impedance tomography using internal current density distribution measured by nuclear magnetic resonance, SPIE,* Vol. 2299, pp. 377–385.

Woo EJ and Seo JK (2008). *Magnetic resonance electrical impedance tomography (MREIT) for high-resolution conductivity imaging, Physiol. Meas.,* Vol. 29, pp. R1–R26.

Yarnykh VL (2007). *Actual flip-angle imaging in the pulsed steady state: a method for rapid three-dimensional mapping of the transmitted radiofrequency field, Magn. Reson. Med.,* Vol. 57, pp. 192–200.

Zelinski AC, Angelone LM, Goyal VK, Bonmassar G, Adalsteinsson E and Wald LL (2008). *Specific absorption rate studies of the parallel transmission of inner-volume excitations at 7T*, J Magn Reson Imaging, Vol. 28, pp. 1005–1018.

Zhang X, Zhu S and He B (2010). *Imaging electric properties of biological tissues by RF field mapping in MRI*, IEEE Trans. Med. Imag., Vol. 29, pp. 474–481.

Chapter 5

Quantitative Susceptibility Mapping

5.1 Introduction

Every material acquires a magnetic moment when it is put in a magnetic field $\mathbf{H}$. Magnetic susceptibility χ, defined by the relationship $\mathbf{M} = \chi\mathbf{H}$ with $\mathbf{M}$ the magnetic moment per unit volume (magnetization), is an intrinsic property of the material, reflecting its electronic perturbation by the applied magnetic field. The strong intrinsic magnetic moment of unpaired electrons makes most materials paramagnetic $(\chi > 0)$, while the magnetic moment associated with electron orbits makes some materials diamagnetic. This material's magnet moment is not on resonance and does not contribute direct signal in magnetic resonance imaging (MRI), in contrast to the much weaker nuclear magnetic moment of free water that is on resonance and contributes direct signal in MRI. To mark this distinction, the material magnetic moment is also referred to as the bulk magnetic moment. Statistical quantum mechanics may allow calculation of susceptibility for some materials of given configuration. Very important for biomedical practice is the relation between tissue magnetic susceptibility and disease, and an experimental method to measure tissue susceptibility.

Conceptual understanding can be obtained from the simple classical description. Tissue magnetic susceptibility can be decomposed of a paramagnetic component and a diamagnetic component. The paramagnetic part comes from contributions of unpaired electrons in biomaterial molecules that have intrinsic magnetic moments $\mu = \sqrt{\frac{1}{2}(1 + \frac{1}{2})}\mu_B$ a thousand times larger than nuclear magnetic

231

moments. These electronic magnetic moments tend to be aligned with the $\mathbf{B}_0$ field to be at the lowest energy state, and thermal motion at temperature $\mathcal{T}$ disrupts this alignment, reaching an equilibrium paramagnetic magnetization M described by Boltzmann's law for n_s spins per unit volume (Curie): $M = (n_s\mu^2 B_0)/(k_B\mathcal{T})$. The diagmagnetic component comes from the response of the orbiting electrons, even though their spins are paired evenly up and down producing no net spin. The simple electron ($\sharp n_e$, charge q_e, mass m_e) orbit (radius r) model provides a quantum mechanically correct result for explaining tissue diamagnetism (Langevin): $M = -\frac{n_e q_e^2}{6m_e}\langle r^2\rangle B_0$. As the diamagnetism/paramagnetism is about $\frac{k_B T}{\langle \frac{1}{2}m_e v^2\rangle} \sim 10^{-2} \ll 1$, biomaterials with unpaired electrons always have net paramagnetic magnetization.

Physiology and disease processes involve changes in tissue magnetic susceptibilities, so study of tissue susceptibility offers insight into life processes in health and disease. One important magnetic biomolecule is hemoglobin, where about 60% of body irons in Fe^{2+} are embedded for important oxygen transportation function. Hemoglobin without oxygen, deoxyhemoglobin, is strongly paramagnetic because its iron ions have four unpaired three-dimensional (3d) electrons. When oxygen combines with deoxyhemoglobin, the oxygen pulls the iron ion into the center of the pornpheryn circle, which splits iron's 3d orbits with six electrons pairing in three orbits at the lower energy level. Consequently, iron ions in oxyhemoglobin lose paramagnetism, and oxyhemoglobin is weakly diamagnetic [Pauling (1977)]. Another important magnetic biomolecule is ferritin which stores 30% of body iron in Fe^3+ that is readily for use when the body needs it and is highly paramagnetic with five unpaired 3D electrons. For example, the widely known functional MRI (fMRI) for studying brain function is based on the magnetic properties of oxyhemoglobin being paramagnetic and deoxyhemoglobin diamagnetic. Hemorrhage, neurodegenerative diseases, and various other diseases affecting iron transport, cause deposits of irons known to have large susceptibility. Depositions of calcium of negative susceptibility are associated with bone composition and breast cancer.

Magnetic susceptibility measurements of biomaterials have been investigated using a superconducting quantum interference device (SQUID) [Brittenham *et al.* (1982); Sepulveda *et al.* (1994); Allen *et al.* (2000); Nielsen *et al.* (2000); Carneiro *et al.* (2005)] and signal phase in magnetic resonance imaging [Chu *et al.* (1990); Weisskoff and Kiihne (1992); Holt *et al.* (1994); Wang *et al.* (1999); Li (2001); Langham *et al.* (2009); Fernandez-Seara *et al.* (2006); de Rochefort *et al.* (2008a)]. A 3D susceptibility distribution may be reconstructed by using a composite of multiple detectors [Sepulveda *et al.* (1994)] in a manner similar to the inversion used in magnetoencephalography (MEG) [Hämäläinen *et al.* (1993)]. Using superconducting detection coils, SQUID can detect small flux of the magnetic field of an object magnetized by a primary field. Each voxel in MRI is analogous to a self-contained SQUID coil, with its signal phase capable of detection of local magnetic fields associated with the magnetization of susceptible materials polarized by $\mathbf{B}_0$ of the magnetic (MR) scanner. Though superconducting coils have superior sensitivities to MRI voxels, the SQUID approach is severely limited for imaging by the number of detectors deployable to image a patient and by the detector positions that are outside of the object. The large number of voxels in 3D MRI overcomes these problems specific to SQUID, offering a very promising opportunity for *in vivo* quantitative susceptibility mapping (QSM).

The basic approach for estimating susceptibility of an object is to put the object in a known magnetic field and measure the field associated with the magnetization induced in the object. Susceptibility imaging of an arbitrary distribution is a long sought-after goal [Sepulveda *et al.* (1994)]. Deriving susceptibility from a measured field is easy only when the object has a uniform susceptibility distribution, which leads to a simple direct relation between field and susceptibility when the object geometry is known, such as measured from MRI [de Rochefort *et al.* (2008a)]. The magnetic fields of several uniform objects may be added linearly according to the superposition principle [Feynman *et al.* (1965); Jackson (1999)]. The volumetric magnetic susceptibilities for most objects are much smaller than one, and accordingly their mutual magnetizing effects may be ignored. Then the problem of determining susceptibilities of several uniform objects can be solved. However, the general inversion from field to susceptibility has been an unsolved problem or plagued with severe artifacts until recent work using susceptibility structural information in MRI [de Rochefort *et al.* (2010)].

5.2   Mathematical Model for Relating MRI Signal to Tissue Susceptibility

In this section, we first describe the forward problem from tissue magnetization to magnetic field, which follows the standard static magnetism physics applied to the specific MRI situation. Then we describe strategies to solve the inverse problem from magnetic field to susceptibility source.

5.2.1   *The forward problem description*

5.2.1.1 *Formulation of the forward problem from tissue magnetization to MRI measured field*

We formulate here the exact relation between tissue magnetization and magnetic field directly from the fundamental Maxwell equation [Salomir *et al.* (2003); Marques and Bowtell (2005); de Rochefort *et al.* (2008b)]. For a given magnetization distribution $\mathbf{M}(\mathbf{r})$ of tissue in an MR scanner, the corresponding macroscopic magnetic field $\mathbf{B}(\mathbf{r})$ can be derived from the Maxwell equation of static magnetism,

$$\nabla \cdot \mathbf{B} = 0 \tag{5.1}$$

$$\nabla \times \mathbf{B} = \mu_0 \nabla \times \mathbf{M}. \tag{5.2}$$

It should be noted that MRI phase measures the local field $\mathbf{B}_\ell$ experienced by water spins, which is different from the macroscopic field $\mathbf{B}$ because of the susceptible materials surrounding the water spin. The Lorentz sphere correction model may be used, which gives [Haacke *et al.* (1999); Jackson (1999)]

$$\mathbf{B}_\ell(\mathbf{r}) = \mathbf{B} - \frac{2}{3}\mu_0\mathbf{M}. \tag{5.3}$$

For all tissues, $\chi \ll 1$. The relation between magnetic susceptibility and magnetization can be simplified as

$$\chi(\mathbf{r}) = \frac{\mu_0}{B_0} M_z(\mathbf{r}) \tag{5.4}$$

where $\mathbf{B}_0 = B_0\hat{\mathbf{z}}$ is the main magnetic field of the MRI scanner. The equilibrium directions of magnetization and magnetic fields are along the z-axis, so we will focus on the z-component of the magnetic field that can be detected from the MR signal phase. For notational convenience, we introduce the relative difference field

$$\psi_b(\mathbf{r}) = (B_{\ell z} - B_0)/B_0. \tag{5.5}$$

Assume that

$$\mathbf{B}_\ell(\mathbf{r}) \approx \mathbf{B}_0 + \psi_b(\mathbf{r})\hat{\mathbf{z}}.$$

To derive an interrelation between χ and ψ_b, we will solve (5.1)–(5.2) first and then apply the Lorentz correction (5.3). The two first-order differential equations in (5.1)–(5.2) can be combined into a single second-order differential equation,

$$-\nabla^2\mathbf{B} = \mu_0[\nabla(\nabla \cdot \mathbf{M}) - \nabla^2\mathbf{M}]. \tag{5.6}$$

Taking the Fourier transform to (5.6), differentiation becomes multiplication by $\mathbf{k}$, the k-space position vector:

$$\mathbf{k}|^2 \mathcal{F}[\mathbf{B}](\mathbf{k}) = \mu_0[|\mathbf{k}|^2 \mathcal{F}[\mathbf{M}](\mathbf{k}) - \mathbf{k}(\mathbf{k} \cdot \mathcal{F}[\mathbf{M}](\mathbf{k}))] \tag{5.7}$$

where $\mathcal{F}[\mathbf{B}](\mathbf{k}) = \int e^{-2\pi i \mathbf{k}\cdot\mathbf{r}} d\mathbf{r}$. Therefore, after applying the Lorentz correction (5.3),

$$|\mathbf{k}|^2 \mathcal{F}[\mathbf{B}_\ell](\mathbf{k}) = \mu_0 \left[\frac{1}{3}|\mathbf{k}|^2 \mathcal{F}[\mathbf{M}](\mathbf{k}) - \mathbf{k}\left(\mathbf{k} \cdot \mathcal{F}[\mathbf{M}](\mathbf{k})\right) \right]. \tag{5.8}$$

Noting that $\mathcal{F}[\mathbf{B}_\ell](0) = \int \mathbf{B}_\ell(\mathbf{r})d\mathbf{r} \approx \int \mathbf{B}_0(\mathbf{r})d\mathbf{r} = (0,0,B_0) \int 1d\mathbf{r}$, (5.8) becomes

$$\mathcal{F}[\mathbf{B}_\ell](\mathbf{k}) = \underbrace{B_0\hat{\mathbf{k}}_z\delta(\mathbf{k})}_{\mathcal{F}[\mathbf{B}_0](\mathbf{k})} + \mu_0 \left[\frac{1}{3}\mathcal{F}[\mathbf{M}](\mathbf{k}) - \frac{\mathbf{k}}{|\mathbf{k}|^2}(\mathbf{k} \cdot \mathcal{F}[\mathbf{M}](\mathbf{k})) \right] \tag{5.9}$$

where $\hat{\mathbf{k}}_z$ is the unit vector in k_z-direction and $\delta(\mathbf{k})$ is the Dirac delta function of $\mathbf{k}$. According to (5.9) with (5.4) and (5.5), Fourier transform $\Psi(\mathbf{k}) = \mathcal{F}(\psi)$ can be simply expressed as

$$\Psi(\mathbf{k}) = \mathcal{F}\underbrace{\left(\frac{B_{\ell z} - B_0}{B_0}\right)}_{\psi} = \underbrace{\left(\frac{1}{3} - \frac{k_z^2}{|\mathbf{k}|^2}\right)}_{\mathcal{D}(\mathbf{k})} \underbrace{\frac{\mu_0}{B_0} M_z(\mathbf{k})}_{\mathcal{X}(\mathbf{k})} = \mathcal{D}(\mathbf{k})\mathcal{X}(\mathbf{k})$$

(5.10)

where $\mathcal{X}(\mathbf{k})$ is the Fourier domain susceptibility $\chi(\mathbf{r}) = \mathcal{F}^{-1}[\mathcal{X}]$. Using the identity $\mathcal{F}[f * g] = (\mathcal{F}[f])(\mathcal{F}[g])$ in Fourier transform [Lifshitz *et al.* (1982)], the corresponding formulation of (5.10) in image space is

$$\psi_b(\mathbf{r}) = \int d(\mathbf{r} - \mathbf{r}')\chi(\mathbf{r}')d\mathbf{r}'$$

(5.11)

where

$$d(\mathbf{r}) = \mathcal{F}^{-1}[\mathcal{D}(\mathbf{k})] = \mathcal{F}^{-1}\left[\frac{1}{3} - \frac{k_z^2}{|\mathbf{k}|^2}\right] = \frac{3\cos^2\theta_{\mathbf{r}} - 1}{4\pi|\mathbf{r}|^3}$$

(5.12)

and $\theta_{\mathbf{r}}$ is the angle between the vector $\mathbf{r}$ and z-axis. The kernel d, called the dipole kernel or the unit dipole response field, relates susceptibility to the measured relative field in (5.11) or its Fourier form (5.10):

$$d(\mathbf{r}) = \frac{1}{4\pi}\frac{3(\hat{\mathbf{z}} \cdot \hat{\mathbf{r}}) - 1}{|\mathbf{r}|^3} = \frac{1}{4\pi}\frac{2z^2 - x^2 - y^2}{|\mathbf{r}|^5}.$$

(5.13)

It should be noted that there is an alternative and equivalent way to derive the forward problem (5.11) using the magnetic field formula for a single dipole [Jackson (1999)]. The superposition principle gives the field of an arbitrary distribution $\mathbf{M}(\mathbf{r})$ as summation over all dipole contributions. The z-component along $\mathbf{B}_0$ direction for the macroscopic magnetic field is [Li and Leigh (2004)]:

$$B_z(\mathbf{r}) - B_0 = \int \frac{\mu_0 M_z(\mathbf{r}')}{4\pi} \left[\frac{3\cos^2\theta_{\mathbf{rr}'} - 1}{|\mathbf{r} - \mathbf{r}'|^3} + \frac{8\pi}{3}\delta(\mathbf{r} - \mathbf{r}') \right] d\mathbf{r}'$$

(5.14)

which leads to (5.11) as its second term is canceled by the Lorentz correction in (5.3).

5.2.1.2 *Inverse problem and mathematical analysis*

The inverse problem of QSM is to recover χ from the knowledge of ψ with

$$\psi(\mathbf{r}) = d * \chi(\mathbf{r}) = \int d(\mathbf{r} - \mathbf{r}')\chi(\mathbf{r}')d\mathbf{r}'. \qquad (5.15)$$

The corresponding Fourier transform to (5.15) is

$$\Psi(\mathbf{k}) = \mathcal{D}(\mathbf{k})\mathcal{X}(\mathbf{k}). \qquad (5.16)$$

Since $\mathcal{D}(\mathbf{k}) = \mathcal{F}[d](\mathbf{k}) = (k_x^2 + k_y^2 - 2k_z^2)|\mathbf{k}|^{-2}$, (5.16) is the Fourier transform of the following partial differential equation (PDE):

$$\left(\frac{1}{3}\nabla^2 - \frac{\partial^2}{\partial z^2} \right) \chi(\mathbf{r}) = \nabla^2\psi(\mathbf{r}). \qquad (5.17)$$

Since the kernel $d(\mathbf{r} - \mathbf{r}')$ has a point singularity at $\mathbf{r} = \mathbf{r}'$, proper care should be taken to interpret the convolution $d * \chi$. Indeed, the convolution $d * \chi$ does not make any sense classically. The following expression of ψ avoids the singularity of the kernel $d(\mathbf{r} - \mathbf{r}')$ at $\mathbf{r} = \mathbf{r}'$.

Theorem 5.1. *If χ is twice differentiable in the imaging domain Ω, then ψ satisfies*

$$\psi(\mathbf{r}) = \int_\Omega \frac{-1}{4\pi|\mathbf{r} - \mathbf{r}'|} \left(\frac{1}{3}\nabla^2 - \frac{\partial^2}{\partial z^2} \right) \chi(\mathbf{r}')d\mathbf{r}' + Harmonic \qquad (5.18)$$

where "Harmonic" is a harmonic function in Ω with a boundary data depending only on the quantities of χ and $\nabla\chi$ on the boundary $\partial\Omega$.

Proof. Direct computation yields

$$\left(\frac{1}{3}\nabla^2 - \frac{\partial^2}{\partial z^2}\right)\left(\frac{-1}{4\pi|\mathbf{r}|}\right) = d(\mathbf{r}) \quad \text{if } \mathbf{r} \neq 0. \tag{5.19}$$

Next, we need to check the singular behavior of $d(\mathbf{r})$ at $\mathbf{r} = 0$. From the divergence theorem, we have

$$\lim_{s\to 0^+}\underbrace{\int_{|\mathbf{r}|=s}\frac{1}{3}\mathbf{n}\cdot\nabla\left(\frac{-1}{4\pi|\mathbf{r}|}\right)dS_{\mathbf{r}}}_{\int_{|\mathbf{r}|<s}\frac{1}{3}\nabla^2\left(\frac{-1}{4\pi|\mathbf{r}|}\right)dr}$$

$$= \frac{1}{3} = \lim_{s\to 0^+}\underbrace{\int_{|\mathbf{r}|=s}n_z\frac{\partial}{\partial z}\left(\frac{-1}{4\pi|\mathbf{r}|}\right)dr}_{\int_{|\mathbf{r}|<s}\frac{\partial^2}{\partial z^2}\left(\frac{-1}{4\pi|\mathbf{r}|}\right)dr},$$

and therefore

$$\lim_{s\to 0^+}\int_{|\mathbf{r}|<s}\left(\frac{1}{3}\nabla^2 - \frac{\partial^2}{\partial z^2}\right)\left(\frac{-1}{4\pi|\mathbf{r}|}\right)dr = 0. \tag{5.20}$$

The expression (5.18) follows from (5.19), (5.20) and a simple integrating by parts. □

Next, we will derive an explicit representation for $\mathcal{X}$ under the assumption that Ψ is differentiable on the cone $\Gamma_0 := \{\mathbf{k} : k_x^2 + k_y^2 = 2k_z^2\}$ in **k**-space. Note that

$$-\frac{2}{3} \leq \mathcal{D}(\mathbf{k}) \leq \frac{1}{3} \quad \text{for all } \mathbf{k} \neq 0.$$

For given $-\frac{2}{3} \leq \alpha \leq \frac{1}{3}$, define

$$\Gamma_\alpha := \underbrace{\{\mathbf{k} : (1-3\alpha)(k_x^2 + k_y^2) = (2+3\alpha)k_z^2\}}_{\{\mathbf{k}:\mathcal{D}(\mathbf{k})=\alpha\}}. \tag{5.21}$$

We should note that $\cup\{\Gamma_\alpha : -\frac{2}{3} \leq \alpha \leq \frac{1}{3}\}$, the union of cones, covers the entire three-dimensional space.

Theorem 5.2. (Representation formula) *Assume that* $\frac{\partial}{\partial k_z}\Psi$
exists in $\mathbf{k}$*-space. Then,* $\mathcal{X}(\mathbf{k})$ *in (5.16) has the following representation formula:*

$$
\mathcal{X}(\mathbf{k}) =
\begin{cases}
\dfrac{1}{\alpha}\Psi(\mathbf{k}) & \text{if } \mathbf{k} \in \Gamma_\alpha \left(\alpha \neq 0, -\dfrac{2}{3} \leq \alpha \leq \dfrac{1}{3} \right) \\[2ex]
-\dfrac{9k_z}{4}\dfrac{\partial}{\partial k_z}\Psi(\mathbf{k}) & \text{if } \mathbf{k} \in \Gamma_0 \backslash \{0\}
\end{cases}
$$

$$(5.22)$$

Moreover, $\mathcal{X}$ *satisfies*

$$
\left(\frac{2(2+3\alpha)(3\alpha-1)}{9k_z} + \alpha\frac{\partial}{\partial k_z} \right) \mathcal{X}(\mathbf{k}) = \frac{\partial\Psi}{\partial k_z}(\mathbf{k}) \quad \text{for } \mathbf{k} \in \Gamma_\alpha
$$

$$(5.23)$$

where $-\frac{2}{3} \leq \alpha < \frac{1}{3}$.

Proof. If $\alpha \neq \frac{1}{3}$, the partial derivative of (5.16) with respect to k_z leads to

$$
\frac{\partial\Psi}{\partial k_z}(\mathbf{k}) = \frac{\partial\mathcal{D}}{\partial k_z}(\mathbf{k})\mathcal{X}(\mathbf{k}) + \mathcal{D}(\mathbf{k})\frac{\partial\mathcal{X}}{\partial k_z}(\mathbf{k}). \tag{5.24}
$$

Then, (5.23) follows from (5.24) and the fact that

$$
\frac{\partial}{\partial k_z}\mathcal{D}(\mathbf{k}) = \frac{2(2+3\alpha)(3\alpha-1)}{9k_z} \quad \text{for } \mathbf{k} \in \Gamma_\alpha \left(\alpha \neq \frac{1}{3} \right). \tag{5.25}
$$

Next, we will show the representation formula (5.22). For $\mathbf{k} \in \Gamma_\alpha$ with $\alpha \neq 0$, the identity (5.16) directly gives $\mathcal{X}(\mathbf{k}) = \frac{1}{\alpha}\Psi(\mathbf{k})$. For $\mathbf{k} \in \Gamma_0$, it follows from l'Hospital's rule and (5.25) that

$$
\mathcal{X}(\mathbf{k}) = \underbrace{\lim_{h\to 0} \frac{\Psi(\mathbf{k}+h\hat{\mathbf{k}}_z)}{\mathcal{D}(\mathbf{k}+h\hat{\mathbf{k}}_z)}}_{\lim_{h\to 0}\mathcal{X}(\mathbf{k}+h\hat{\mathbf{k}}_z)} = \frac{\frac{\partial\Psi}{\partial k_z}(\mathbf{k})}{\frac{\partial\mathcal{D}}{\partial k_z}(\mathbf{k})} = -\frac{9k_z}{4}\frac{\partial\Psi}{\partial k_z}(\mathbf{k}). \tag{5.26}
$$

$\square$

According to the Fourier inversion formula, (5.22) determines χ directly provided Φ is noise free and differentiable. Unfortunately, the reconstruction method using (5.22) is not robust against noise in Ψ near Γ_0 because small errors in data Ψ near Γ_0 produce large errors in the solution $\mathcal{X}$. Hence, the major issue of the inverse problem is to deal with this ill-conditioned structure near the zero cone Γ_0. This issue will be discussed in the next section.

5.2.1.3 *Ill-poised issue of the inverse problem from measured field to magnetization source*

In the case of ideal field data without noise and available in continuous space, the dipole kernel defined in (5.14) may be regarded as well conditioned for the field to source the inverse problem of (5.11) or (5.14) [Li and Leigh (2004)]. This point may be appreciated in the following manner of examining (5.11). When the dipole kernel in k-space is non-zero, susceptibility can be obtained by direct division of the dipole kernel as in (5.22). At locations where the dipole kernel become zero, the field also becomes zero [Haacke *et al.* (2005)], and l'Hospital's rule (5.26) may be used to estimate susceptibility by taking the derivative along a direction of kernel variation [Li *et al.* (2011)]. When there is noise in field data (and there is always noise in real data), the derivative of the noisy data tends to amplify noise, and it will generate severe noise artifacts [Kressler *et al.* (2010)]. The zeroes of the dipole kernel at $3k_z^2 = |\mathbf{k}|^2$ form two opposing cone surfaces at the magic angle (54.70° from the main magnetic field, Figure 5.1(a). Derivative (in k-space) of noise in the neighborhood of these cone surfaces Γ_0 disturbs robust determination of susceptibility. This may cause the ill-posedness of the inverse problem [Hanke and Hansen (1993); Bertero and Boccacci (1998); Aster *et al.* (2013)]. This theoretical analysis is exemplified in a case

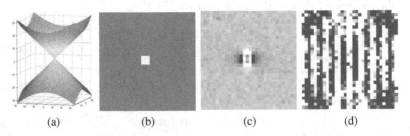

(a)   (b)   (c)   (d)

Fig. 5.1.   (a) The zero cone surfaces of the dipole kernel in k-space. (b) Susceptibility source. (c) Field map derived at SNR = 20. (d) Direct inversion image [Kressler *et al.* (2010)].

illustrated in Figure 5.1(c)−(d) when the straightforward k-space division (5.22) is used for inversion from field to source to reconstruct susceptibility map. A little noise added in the phase map (signal-to-noise [SNR] = 20) leads to a totally corrupted image of susceptibility that bears no physical resemblance to the true susceptibility source [Kressler *et al.* (2010)].

To get a sense of noise propagation, we can examine the condition number of the dipole kernel that characterizes the upper bound of noise propagation,

$$\text{cond}(\mathcal{D}) = \frac{\max_{\mathbf{k} \in \mathcal{A}} \mathcal{D}(\mathbf{k})}{\min_{\mathbf{k} \in \mathcal{A}} \mathcal{D}(\mathbf{k})} \propto \frac{1}{\text{dist}(\mathcal{A}, \Gamma_0)} \tag{5.27}$$

where $\mathcal{A}$ is the set of sampling points and dist $(\mathcal{A}, \Gamma_0)$ is the closest distance from sampling points to the zero cone surface Γ_0. Therefore, this condition number is large, resulting in large noise propagation.

5.2.2 *Solutions to the inverse problem*

5.2.2.1 *Morphology enabled dipole inversion (MEDI)*

The measured magnetic field is the convolution of the tissue magnetic source with the dipole kernel. For tissue characterization, we need to deconvolve the field information. The deconvolution to recover the susceptibility source is an ill-posed inverse problem since the dipole kernel is zero on the magic cone Γ_0 so that small errors in data near Γ_0 produce large errors in the solution. Additional information is required to deal with the inherently ill-posed characteristic. This amount of prior information required to solve the inverse problem may depend on data noise. Since the prior information may not be precise for describing the imaging situation, the use of prior information may also contribute to error in the final solution. Therefore, the inversion problem of incorporating prior information may have a solution with an error dependent on both data noise and information inaccuracy.

Prior information may naturally come from the magnitude images coexisting with the phase data, as well as from other morphologic images acquired in the same MRI exam. We refer to this information-guided inversion as morphology enabled dipole inversion

(MEDI) [Liu *et al.* (2011)]. It can be proved mathematically that the prior information of restricting the susceptibility edge locations to the locations of edges in the magnitude images allows a susceptibility solution with bounded error [Liu *et al.* (2012)]. That is to say, if most susceptibility edges are located within the set of locations of edges in the morphology images, there exists a sufficiently accurate solution for susceptibility distribution within the MEDI approach. This mathematical theorem allows us to search for an inverse solution but does not tell how to construct the solution. While we will describe in detail later on the susceptibility map reconstruction algorithm, here we would like to touch on the following immediate questions: How good is the prior information we can achieve in MEDI? How can we algorithmically express the prior information in MEDI?

According to Maxwell's equation (5.2), interfaces of bulk magnetization of susceptibility source polarized in an MR scanner cause inhomogeneous local fields. These local fields modify the phases of water proton spins in MRI and affect the detect signal. The local field effects on the MRI signal include the so-called dephasing, which increases with echo time and forms the widely known T2* hypointensity contrast in magnitude images of gradient echo MRI. Do all susceptibility edges show up at the locations of edges in the magnitude images? For a given echo time, most edges in susceptibility maps will show up in the magnitude image. There is the possibility that some susceptibility edges' effects are compensated by variation in proton spin density, causing them to go missing in the magnitude image at that given echo time. This possibility can be avoided using an additional magnitude image at a different echo time, where the susceptibility effects will be different enough to reveal that missing susceptibility edge. A multiple echo gradient echo sequence can be used to acquire images at many echo times. Mathematically, the degree of ill condition of the dipole inversion depends on the amount of noise, and an accurate solution may not require the prior information of all edge locations. Therefore, for a physically meaningful solution to the field source inverse problem, we can use the *a priori* information that most locations of susceptibility interfaces are accompanied by interfaces in the magnitude images of gradient echo (GRE) MRI.

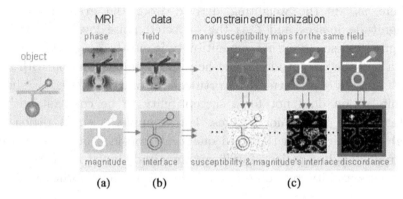

Fig. 5.2. Illustration of the MEDI approach to solve the field-to-source inverse problem in MRI. (a) Gradient echo (GRE) MRI is performed on the object to obtain both phase (top) and magnitude (bottom) images. (b) Local field (top) is estimated from phase by removing background field, and tissue interface mask (bottom) is generated from the magnitude image by inverting its gradient. (c) Susceptibility map is obtained by fitting susceptibility with local field data via Maxwell's equation and constraining susceptibility interfaces with tissue interfaces via their least discordance. Three possible solutions are illustrated in (c): zero padded k-division (left), L2 (middle), and L1 (right) minimization of the discordance, with L1 minimization providing the sparsest discordance and the most accurate susceptibility map.

A specific implementation of this MEDI approach is illustrated in Figure 5.2. We can mathematically express the prior information as follows. Edges in the susceptibility map that are not accompanied by edges in the magnitude images should be sparse. To promote the sparsity, a weighted L1 minimization can be employed to constrain edges in the susceptibility map to the locations of all known edges determined from all magnitude images and to fit susceptibility to the field information determined from all phase images in GRE MRI. Then the formulation for this particular form of prior information is

$$\arg\min_{\chi} \|w_m \nabla \chi\|_1, \tag{5.28}$$

and the formulation for the particular form of the inverse problem illustrated in Figure 5.2 is:

$$\begin{aligned} &\arg\min_{\chi} \|w_m \nabla \chi\|_1 \\ &\text{subject to the constraint } \|w(\psi - d * \chi)\|_2 < \zeta \end{aligned} \tag{5.29}$$

where w_m is the weighting derived from the gradients of all magnitude images and ζ is the expected noise level. Simulation (Figure 5.2) suggests that susceptibility is mostly localized by phase data and the magnitude images help to select the solution with the least amount of artifacts. It is worthwhile noting that the constrained minimization does not force susceptibility to be constant within interfaces of magnitude images. For example, a small region of high susceptibility in the third quadrant (top left) of the image in Figure 5.2 is in a region of uniform magnitude but it is recovered in the susceptibility map due to phase data in its neighborhood.

5.2.2.2 *Other forms of prior information for dipole inversion*

Various forms of prior information have been discussed in recent literature [de Rochefort *et al.* (2008a); Kressler *et al.* (2010); Wharton *et al.* (2010); Shmueli *et al.* (2009)]. Of interest are two that give simple inverse solutions. One is the k-space division with threshold, which is equivalent to using the truncated dipole kernel where the dipole kernel is set to a constant when it falls below a threshold [Shmueli *et al.* (2009); Wharton *et al.* (2010)]:

$$\text{Set } \mathcal{D}(\mathbf{k}) = \zeta \quad \text{when} \quad \mathbf{k} \in \Gamma_\alpha \quad \text{and} \quad \alpha < \zeta. \tag{5.30}$$

The corresponding inverse problem has a simple closed form solution:

$$\mathcal{X}(\mathbf{k}) = \begin{cases} \Psi(\mathbf{k})/\zeta & \text{if } \mathcal{D}(\mathbf{k}) < \zeta \\ \Psi(\mathbf{k})/\mathcal{D}(\mathbf{k}) & \text{otherwise} \end{cases}. \tag{5.31}$$

The drawback of this prior information is that it contains substantial inaccuracy. As the measured field information in the k-space neighborhood that $\mathcal{D}(\mathbf{k}) = 0$ is essentially noise, so this threshold solution (5.31) assigns in this zero dipole kernel neighborhood just noise to susceptibility with zero actual susceptibility value. This leads to underestimation in susceptibility values and streaking artifacts in the susceptibility map.

Another form of prior information is the piecewise constant model [de Rochefort *et al.* (2008a)], which approximates the object as a sum of regions of constant susceptibility:

$$\chi(\mathbf{r}) = \chi_p \quad \text{for } \mathbf{r} \in \text{region } p \tag{5.32}$$

where Ω_p is a local region. The corresponding inverse problem has a simple solution. Let d_p be the geometric factor representing the total dipole field at observation point $\mathbf{r}$ due to susceptibility source in region Ω_p, i.e., the convolution of the dipole kernel over region Ω_p,

$$d_p(\mathbf{r}) = \int_{\text{region } p} d(\mathbf{r} - \mathbf{r}')d\mathbf{r}'. \tag{5.33}$$

Then the forward problem (5.11) becomes

$$\sum_p \chi_p d_p(\mathbf{r}) = \psi(\mathbf{r}). \tag{5.34}$$

Because there are so many voxels with spins to detect the magnetic field, (5.34) is an over-determined problem, which can be rapidly solved using the weighted least squares method:

$$\chi = (D^T W D)^{-1} D^T W \psi \tag{5.35}$$

where the vector χ has elements χ_p, the matrix D has elements $d_p(\mathbf{r})$, the matrix W has only non-zero diagonal elements $w(\mathbf{r})$, and the vector ψ has elements $\psi(\mathbf{r})$, the measured relative field. The prior information in (5.32) may have applications in situations where there is a strong uniformly distributed contrast agent such as contrast enhanced blood in magnetic resonance arthrography (MRA) [de Rochefort *et al.* (2008b)].

5.2.2.3 *Condition the inverse problem well for precise solution − Calculation of Susceptibility using Multiple Orientation Sampling (COSMOS)*

The susceptibility indeterminacy at the zero cone surfaces of the k-space dipole kernel can be overcome by the multiple orientation sampling method [Marques and Bowtell (2005)]. Let $\psi_\theta(\mathbf{r})$ be the field map measured at object orientation angle θ, and $k_{z\theta}$ the k_z

value at angle θ, and N the total number of orientations, then the forward problem (5.10) becomes

$$\underbrace{(1/3 - k_{z\theta}^2/|\mathbf{k}|^2)}_{\mathcal{D}_\theta(\mathbf{k})}\mathcal{X}(\mathbf{k}) = \mathcal{F}[\psi_\theta](\mathbf{k}), \qquad \theta = \theta_1, \ldots, \theta_N. \qquad (5.36)$$

For example, the $k_{z\theta}$ with θ rotation around the x axis ($\perp \mathbf{B}_0$) is

$$k_{z\theta} = k_z \cos\theta + k_y \cos\theta.$$

This problem (5.36) can be solved for susceptibility at any $\mathbf{k}_\theta$ location, as long as one of the coefficients $\mathcal{D}_\theta(\mathbf{k}) := (1/3 - k_{z\theta}^2/|\mathbf{k}|^2)$ is sufficiently larger than zero. Here, data from different orientations can be registered spatially using a well-established rigid body registration algorithm [Ashburner and Friston (2007)]. For most susceptibility values, $\mathcal{X}(\mathbf{k})$ is over-determined and can be solved using a weighted least squares solver:

$$\mathcal{X} = \arg\min_{\mathcal{X}} \sum_{j=1}^{N} \|w_\theta(\psi_{\theta_j} - \mathcal{F}^{-1}[\mathcal{D}_{\theta_j}\mathcal{X}])\|_2^2 \qquad (5.37)$$

where the weighting factor w_θ is the signal magnitude at the θth orientation ($\propto$ phase SNR [Kressler *et al.* (2008); Conturo and Smith (1990)]) to account for measurement noise. An algorithm for sparse linear equations and sparse least squares (LSQR) can be used to solve (5.37) iteratively [Paige and Saunders (1982); Bjork (1996)]. This iteration converges rapidly (30 iterations in a few minutes in our preliminary 3D data on a Pentium 4 PC using Matlab), because the problem in (5.37) is well conditioned.

The condition number, indicating an upper bound on the relative error propagation in the inversion [Boyd and Vandenberghe (2004)], can be used to measure the stability of the inversion. The inverse problem for (5.37) can be reformulated using a block diagonal matrix. For N rotations around the x axis ($\perp \mathbf{B}_0$), the diagonal block is $[\mathcal{D}_{\theta_1}, \mathcal{D}_{\theta_2}, \ldots, \mathcal{D}_{\theta_N}]$ with $k_{z\theta} = k_z \cos\theta + k_y \cos\theta$. The condition number of a matrix is defined as the ratio between the maximum and the minimum singular value of that matrix:

$$\text{cond}(\mathcal{D}_{\theta_1,\ldots,\theta_N}) = \frac{\max_{\mathbf{k}} \sum_{j=1}^{N} [1/3 - (k_z \cos \theta_j + k_y \cos \theta_j)^2/|\mathbf{k}|^2]^2}{\min_{\mathbf{k}} \sum_{j=1}^{N} [1/3 - (k_z \cos \theta_j + k_y \cos \theta_j)^2/|\mathbf{k}|^2]^2}.$$

(5.38)

The optimal set of sampling orientations $(\theta_1, \ldots, \theta_N)$ is defined as the one achieving minimal condition number $\text{cond}(\mathcal{D}_{\theta_1,\ldots,\theta_N})$. Data acquisition at additional orientations vastly reduces the number (improving inversion) compared to single orientation [Wharton and Bowtell (2010)]. The optimal sampling orientations are $0°$, $60°$, $120°$ for $N = 3$ (corresponding minimal $\text{cond}(\mathcal{D}_{\theta_1,\ldots,\theta_N}) = 2.03$ for a $128 \times 128 \times 64$ image), consistent with the intuition that uniformly distributed orientations may perform the best.

This COSMOS method can serve as a gold standard for quantitative susceptibility mapping, because COSMOS does not use any prior information that may introduce regularization model error. However, the COSMOS method has major limitations: it is not practical or impossible to rotate a patient in a standard closed bore MRI scanner or to rotate a mouse/rat in a small bore animal scanner. And multiple orientation samples prolong the scanning time.

5.3 Data Acquisition Method

The local field information (the relative difference field) can be obtained from the phase image of gradient echo MRI. Non-invasive MRI provides very rich tissue contrasts and high spatial resolution, and is widely available. The MRI signal is sensitive to magnetic source of both linear and non-linear magnetic susceptibilities. So MRI offers a major advantage in data acquisition over other devices for measuring tissue susceptibilities, such as SQUID which is poor at spatial resolution [Farrell *et al.* (2007)], and magnetic particle imaging that only sensitizes non-linear susceptibilities [Gleich and Weizenecker (2005)].

Gradient echo sequence is a standard sequence on all MRI scanners. The phase image in gradient echo MRI, which typically is not saved in a clinical protocol, needs to be saved, in addition to the magnitude images. For sensitizing high susceptibility with good SNR, short echo time is preferred to preserve the signal against strong T2* signal loss at long echo time. For sensitizing low susceptibility with high SNR, long echo time is preferred to generate sufficient phase for detection. Both short and long echo times are naturally acquired simultaneously in the multiple echo gradient echo sequence. High field strength and multiple channel RF coils are preferred for generating high SNR in signal detection. Typical imaging parameters on a 3T MRI scanner for human brain imaging include 10 TEs of uniform TE spacing = 5 ms; TR = 60 ms; voxel size = $1 \times 1 \times 2$ mm3; matrix size = $240 \times 240 \times 50$; BW = ± 31.25 kHz, FA = $20°$, NEX = 1 and acceleration factor R = 2. The scan time is 6 min.

5.4   Image Reconstruction Method

Image reconstruction for quantitative susceptibility mapping requires two important elements: (1) remove the background field in the measured local field data and (2) find the solution of the inverse problem. For continuity of algorithm development, we describe first the algorithm for solving the inverse problem, and then discuss how to remove the background field when data is input into the inversion algorithm.

5.4.1   *The MEDI reconstruction algorithm*

Among various methods for generating susceptibility maps discussed in the above mathematical model discussed in Section 5.2.1, the image reconstruction for susceptibility distribution is straightforward except for the MEDI method, and arguably the MEDI method is the most practical and accurate method. So we focus on the MEDI reconstruction, with its inverse problem defined by the constrained minimization formulas (5.29), which belongs to the constrained convex optimization problem. A powerful method to solve the constrained problem is to turn it into the unconstrained Lagrangian problem with a properly chosen parameter λ:

$$\chi = \arg \min_{\chi} E(\chi, \lambda) := \lambda \|W(\psi - F_D\chi)\|_2 + \|M\nabla\chi\|_1. \qquad (5.39)$$

Here, quantities in (5.39) are expressed as vectors and matrices for numerical implementation: W is a $N \times N$ weighting matrix (N being the number of voxels in χ) compensating for the non-uniform phase noise, which can be derived from the magnitude of the complex MRI data [Kressler *et al.* (2008)]; F_D is the discrete version of $\mathcal{F}^{-1}\mathcal{D}\mathcal{F}$, M is a $3N \times 3N$ binary diagonal matrix generated from the gradient of a morphological image such as the magnitude image by assigning 0 to gradients representing substantial edges and 1 to all other gradients; and ∇ can be viewed as a non-diagonal gradient matrix with operating on susceptibility map χ expressed as a vector form. The first term is referred to as the data fidelity term, and the second term the constraint term.

In the classical method of the Lagrange multiplier, the first-order derivatives against the parameters in the cost function $E(\chi, \lambda)$ are set to zero to obtain the value of λ and to obtain the solution χ. This is only possible when the analytical expression is manageable under a small number of parameters in the cost function. With the million elements in χ (dimension of susceptibility map), (5.39) has to be solved numerically. A practical and robust method is the following iteration procedure.

The λ value is determined by solving (5.39) with various λ and then choosing a λ value such that the error in the data fidelity term is equal to the noise in data, $\|W(\psi - F_D\chi)\| \approx \zeta$ [Lustig *et al.* (2007)]. This choice is consistent with the rationale that the amount of prior information needed for dipole inversion is determined by data noise. Because the dipole inversion is fairly well conditioned as discussed in Section 5.1, we expect that the data fidelity term dominates the cost function with the λ value very high (on the order of several hundred as found in numerical simulation).

For a given λ, (5.39) is solved by setting the first-order derivative against χ to zero as in the standard Lagrange multiplier:

$$0 = \nabla_\chi E(\chi, \lambda) = 2\lambda (WF_D)^T(WF_D\chi - W\psi) + (M\nabla)^T \frac{\nabla\chi}{\|\nabla\chi\|}.$$
(5.40)

This non-linear system can be solved using a fixed point iteration method [Vogel and Oman (1996)]. Note that $-\nabla_\chi E(\chi, \lambda)$ is the direction of the steepest descent at the vector χ, and (5.40) is equivalent to $L\chi = L\chi - \nabla_\chi E(\chi, \lambda)$ where $L := 2\lambda(WF_D)^T WF_D$. With these observations, we have following iterative scheme

$$\chi_{n+1} = \chi_n - L^{-1}\nabla_\chi E(\chi_n, \lambda). \tag{5.41}$$

Here at each iteration, the matrix inversion in (5.27) is computed using the conjugate gradient method that is known to be robust in handling the inversion of a large matrix [Hestenes and Stiefel (1952)]. The conjugate gradient method is widely used in solving large systems of linear equations in many applications and the method details can be found in many texts, including [Seo and Woo (2012)].

5.4.2 *Background field removal without affecting local fields*

Accurate field mapping is necessary to minimize errors in the inverse solution. The phase of MRI raw data may require unwrapping, and effective unwrapping algorithms are available to accomplish this task [Ghiglia and Pritt (1998)]. Background field has to be removed, and existing methods include: (1) geometrical modeling that uses the Maxwell equations to remove background field according to the brain anatomy and a simple model for brain susceptibility [Neelavalli *et al.* (2009)]. However, this method suffers from the error in brain anatomy model and unknown field source outside imaging volume; (2) commonly used high pass filtering by removing a low spectral component such as a low spatial frequency or a lower-order polynomial component from the measured field map [Haacke *et al.* (2009); Langham *et al.* (2009)], which also filters out local field components at the low spectrum, leading to underestimation of local susceptibility source. Ineffective background field removal is a major source of error for quantitative susceptibility mapping.

We have observed that the dipole field from a source in a region of interest (ROI) is approximately orthogonal to the dipole field from a source outside the ROI, except near the ROI boundaries. Accordingly, we developed a new approach for the optimal estimation of the background field (ψ_b) by projecting the measured total field

(ψ) onto the subspace spanned by the external dipole source (χ_e) as in the Hilbert space projection theorem:

$$\psi_b(\mathbf{r}) = \min_{\chi_e} \sum_{\mathbf{r} \in ROI} ||w(\mathbf{r})(\psi(\mathbf{r}) - d * \chi_e(\mathbf{r}))||^2. \qquad (5.42)$$

Our preliminary data on phantom of known background field and *in vivo* imaging indicates that effective dipole fitting provides accurate background removal without affecting local field, far superior to the geometric modeling and high pass filtering method [Liu *et al.* (2010)].

For background field ψ_b with source outside the ROI, it obeys the Laplace equation with harmonic function as its solution. Averaging ψ_b over a sphere or shell is identical to ψ_b value at the spherical center. Let A be the averaging operator over a sphere or shell centered at the point, $(1 - A)\psi_b = 0$. This allows the following alternative spherical harmonic mean (SHM) method [Li (2001); Li and Leigh (2004); Schweser *et al.* (2010)]: the local field ψ_l can be estimated from the measured total field ψ by $\psi_l = (1 - A)^{-1} M(1 - A)\psi$, where first $1 - A$ filters out the background field, followed by its inversion to recover the local field. We will optimize the radius choice in A and compare SHM with probability density function (PDF) to form an optimal background removal method.

5.5 Numerical Simulation

As discussed in the image reconstruction in Section 5.4, the numerical simulation will focus on investigating the practical and accurate MEDI method.

A 3D numerical phantom was generated to evaluate the accuracy of the proposed method, to investigate the influence of SNR and the contrast-to-noise ratio (CNR) of the MR image, and to optimize regularization parameters. A phantom with nine spheres of the same size with increasing magnetic susceptibilities (ranging from 0.5 to 4.0 ppm) was placed in a background with zero susceptibility (Figure 5.3(a)). A magnitude image (Figure 5.3(b)) was constructed by assigning a uniform identical signal to each of the nine spheres that was twice that of the background, except for two spheres.

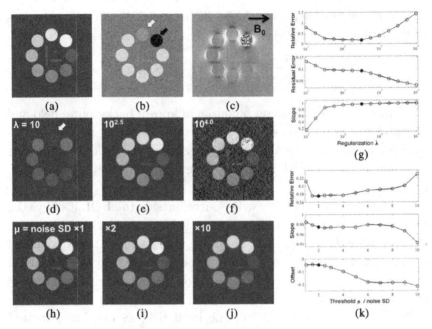

Fig. 5.3.   Selection of regularization and thresholding parameters. (a) Simulated susceptibilty map, (b) image magnitude, and (c) field map at a central section of a numerical phantom. Gaussian noise with SNR = 10 relative to the background was added. The parameter λ regulizes the susceptiblity map fidelity against the constraint term. QSM reconstructed with three representative λ are shown in (d–f). Relative error, residual error and linear regression slope obtained with a series of λ (10 $10^{4.0}$) are plotted in (g). The optimal choice of λ ($10^{2.5}$) generated the relative error that was minimal and the residual error that matched noise level. QSMs obtained with three representative thresholds $\hbar$ in generating the binary weighting are shown in (h–j). Relative error, linearity (linear regression slope and offset) obtained with various $\hbar$ ($1\sim 10$ times of the simulated noise SD) and $\lambda = 10^{2.5}$ are plotted in (k). The reconstructed QSM is quite robust against the choice of the threshold $\hbar$, and a choice for $\hbar$ at $2\sim 4$ times of the noise SD generates a minimal relative error and good linearity [Liu *et al.* (2012)].

One sphere (Figure 5.3(b), black arrow) had a zero magnitude signal (mimicking a hemorrhagic lesion of non-zero susceptibility but without MR signal), while the second (Figure 5.3(b), white arrow) had a signal that was only 30% higher than that of the background. Three small cylindrical tubes were placed perpendicular to each other in the central region of the phantom and were assigned a susceptibility of 0.5 ppm and a low magnitude signal of 10% of the background signal. The local magnetic field was computed from the described 3D susceptibility distribution according to (5.11). The phase map was generated from the local magnetic field using the relationship $\phi = \gamma B_0 TE \Delta B(\mathbf{r})$, where ϕ denotes the phase, γ the water gyromagnetic ratio, the field strength (1.5 T), and the echo time (4.5 ms). The combination of the simulated image magnitude m and phase ϕ generated a complex MR image, to which we added a complex Gaussian noise $n_c : me^{i\phi} + n_c = \tilde{m}e^{i\tilde{\phi}}$. Then, the phase $\tilde{\phi}$ of this noisy complex MR image was used to compute the local magnetic field (shown in Figure 5.3(c)), which was then used as the input for the QSM method. Results with SNR $= 10$ are illustrated as examples.

Various values for the parameter λ were used for calculating a susceptibility map to identify the optimal choice of λ. Similarly, various values of the threshold $\hbar$ for generating the binary mask M from the magnitude image were tested to determine an optimal choice. Optimality was defined in terms of the relative error of the reconstructed susceptibility map χ_r compared to the expected true susceptibility map χ_e and calculated as $\frac{\|\chi_e - \chi_r\|_2}{\|\chi_e\|_2}$. The residual error was calculated as $\frac{\|W(F_D\chi - \psi)\|_2}{\sqrt{N}}$, where N is the number of the voxels that contribute to the numerator. The nine spheres were chosen as ROIs. To assess accuracy, a linear regression was performed between the reconstructed susceptibilities and the true values. Results without using the weighting M, as well as those obtained with L_1-norm and L_2-norm minimization, were obtained for comparison.

The Lagrangian parameter λ controlled the fidelity of the reconstructed QSM as demonstrated in Figure 5.3(d–g). A small λ enforced the minimization of L_1-norm term (5.9), resulting in a smooth map with an underestimation of the susceptibility values of each of the nine spheres (Figure 5.3(d)). The structures with low CNR (the sphere indicated by the white arrow and the small tubes at the center) were barely seen, because the weighting M imposed the same value as the background. A large λ enforced the data fidelity at the cost of streaking artifacts (Figure 5.3(f)). The optimal QSM, shown in Figure 5.3(e) and highlighted with a solid black dot in Figure 5.3(g), corresponded to the minimum relative error (0.175), with a residual error (0.092) close to the simulated noise standard deviation (SD) (0.1). The linear regression indicated a high accuracy (slope = 0.98, offset −0.05 ppm) between the reconstructed and the known susceptibilities in the nine ROIs.

As shown in Figure 5.3(h−k), various $\hbar$ values ranging from two to eight times the noise SD provided roughly similar results in terms of susceptibility map quality, slope of the linear regression, and relative error. The smallest relative error with the fewest salt and pepper artifacts and the sharpest susceptibility edges were achieved for $\hbar = 2$ times of the noise SD. This scheme for choosing λ and $\hbar$ in the numerical simulation was then used for QSM reconstruction of the phantom and brain, as well as for the different minimization methods described in the following paragraph.

Four QSM reconstruction methods were compared: L_2-norm minimization method without the weighting M (denoted as L_2- in Figure 5.4(a)), L_2-norm minimization with the binary weighting M (WL_2- in Figure 5.4(b)), L_1-norm minimization without M (L_1 in Figure 5.4(c)), and L_1-norm minimization with M (WL_1 in Figure 5.2(d)). We observed significant improvements by applying the prior weighting M to the L_2-norm minimization. However, the susceptibility calculated using the weighted L_2 method in the region with low image CNR had a lower accuracy due to the insufficient definition of edges (white arrows in Figure 5.3(b) and Figure 5.4(b), and the outlier on Figure 5.4(j)). Both the L_1 and the weighted L_1 methods provided a more accurate susceptibility map with less streaking artifacts, and the weighting M in the L_1 method showed obvious improvement (Figure 5.4(d,h,m) versus Figure 5.4(c,g,k)) including clearer defined contours, a better accuracy (regression slope was 0.98 versus 0.97, and offset −0.05 versus 0.15), and a smaller relative error (0.175 versus 0.200). The WL_1 method (Figure 5.4(d)) showed good precision and accuracy even in regions with reduced magnitude signal and unreliable phase signal (black arrow in Figure 5.3(b)), as well as regions with a poor CNR (white arrow in Figure 5.3(b)). However, the mapping of susceptibility showed greater errors for the three small tubes at the center of the phantom in all methods (Figure 5.4); these tubes were small in size, had a low susceptibility, and a low SNR and CNR.

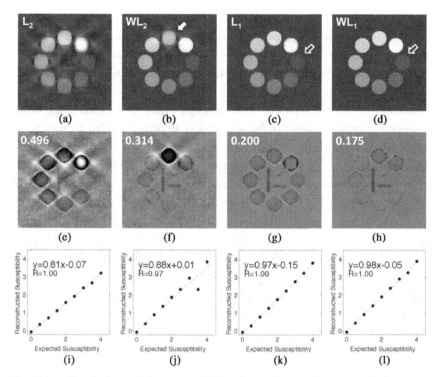

Fig. 5.4. Simulation validation of QSMs obtained with L2-norm minimization without (L_2, first column) and with weighting (WL_2, second column), and L1-norm minimization without (L_1, third column) and with weighting (WL_1, fourth column). The first row (a–d) shows the QSM, the second row (e–h) shows corresponding error maps with the number in the top left corner indicating the relative error, and the third row (i–l) shows the linear regression. Significant improvements are observed when applying the weighting M to L2 method (WL2 versus L2), but substantial errors in the region of low CNR remain (white arrow in b with black intensity in f indicating underestimation error in f). The errors were reduced in both L_1 and WL_1 (c and d). Applying weighting to L_1 further reduced the errors (g versus h) [Liu *et al.* (2012)].

5.6 Experimental Validation

5.6.1 *Validation of the reference standard COSMOS method*

Magnetic resonance imaging on a phantom with various gadolinium concentrations obtained a field map showing a conspicuous dipole pattern surrounding the vials with different gadolinium

concentrations. The COSMOS method provided good susceptibility images, clearly resolving different Gd concentrations with
no streaking artifacts. Linear regression analysis demonstrated
that COSMOS-estimated and prepared susceptibilities agree well
(R2 = 0.9997, slope is 0.96). An MRI on *in vitro* swine bone
embedded in gel generated bone susceptibility map. Compact bone
susceptibility was found to be -2.44 ± 0.89 ppm relative to water, in
fair agreement with previous *in vitro* work ($\chi_{bone-water} = -2.39$ ppm)
[Chieregato *et al.* (2003); Langham *et al.* (2009)]. The *in vitro* iron
quantification result in a chicken breast meat using COSMOS
is illustrated in Figure 5.5. The bright regions corresponding to
the $2\,\mu$L, $3\,\mu$L, and $4\,\mu$L iron-oxide injections are visible on this
image ($1\,\mu$L region not contained in this slice). Measured iron
masses are $1.23\,\mu$g, $2.09\,\mu$g, $3.32\,\mu$g, and $4.34\,\mu$g. The relation
between the estimated and prepared total iron oxide mass is plotted
in Figure 5.5(d). (For Ferridex, the conversion between susceptibility
and mass is $\chi_{Ferridex}/\rho = \mu_0 M_{Fe}(B_0)/B_0 = 64.7$pp μL/μg [Boyd and
Vandenberghe (2004)].) Again, linear regression indicated excellent
agreement between COSMOS estimated and the prepared (expected)
Fe mass.

Healthy subjects (n = 7) were imaged at three different orientations under the instruction to rotate their heads in the coronal plane
by bringing the head towards first the left and then the right shoulder.
Typically rotations from $-20°$ to $+20°$ were achieved, together
with images acquired in neutral position forming 3-rotation data
set for COSMOS processing. Some veins suppressed by geometry

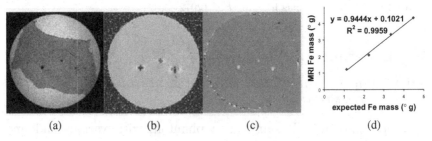

Fig. 5.5.   (a) Magnitude image. (b) Corresponding b(r). (c) Susceptibility map.
(d) MRI estimated iron-oxide mass versus implanted iron-oxide mass.

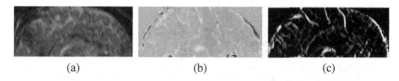

(a)   (b)   (c)

Fig. 5.6. Brain COSMOS: (a) magnitude, (b) phase, (c) susceptibility images.

factors in the convolution of (5.15) as depicted in the phase image (Figure 5.6(b)) are recovered in the susceptibility images. The susceptibility image (Figure 5.6(c)) demonstrates primary deoxy-homoglobin in veins. Susceptibility measured from superior sagittal sinus was $0.32 + 0.02$ ppm, suggesting 64% oxygen saturation level in venous blood assuming Hematocrit (Hct) is 0.4, which is in very good agreement with the literature: 65%+10% [Kressler *et al.* (2010)]. However, it was uncomfortable for subjects to maintain a tilted head position for a long time in the scanner.

5.6.2 *Validation of the MEDI method*

Phantom validation for MEDI quantification of SPIO (Figure 5.7). Neither the magnitude nor the local phase provided absolute super paramagnetic iron oxide nanoparticles (SPIO) quantification. There were substantial blooming effects in the phase and R2* map (Figure 5.7(a)). The QSM reconstructed by MEDI quantitatively mapped the amounts of SPIO without the blooming artifacts. Based on the magnitude images across all the echoes, R2* was measured and converted into a SPIO mass. The R2* quantification showed a non-linear relationship between estimated and prepared SPIO, especially a saturation at high doses (Figure 5.7(b)). By contrast, the linear regression between MEDI estimated SPIO and prepared SPIO showed a slope $= 1.08$ close to unity and an intercept $= 0.53$ close to zero. Noise propagation analysis demonstrated that the detection limit of MEDI was 5 pg/nL $Fe^{3}+$ at SNR $= 30$, similar to that of T2* contrast by the Rose model [Heyn *et al.* (2005)].

In vivo **validation by comparing with COSMOS for human brain QSM (Figure 5.8).** Because COSMOS reconstructs QSM from overdetermined data without any assumption,

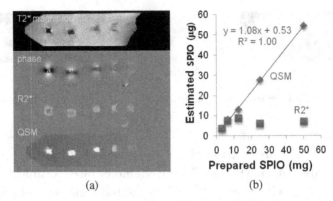

(a)   (b)

Fig. 5.7. (a) T2* magnitude/phase/R2*/QSM of a SPIO phantom. The blooming artifacts are eliminated in QSM. (b) QSM/R2* measurement of Fe is in excellent/poor agreement with prepared Fe in this phantom.

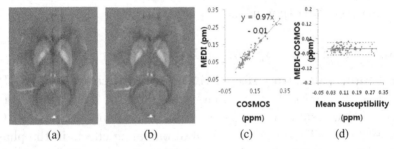

(a)   (b)   (c)   (d)

Fig. 5.8. (a) MEDI and (b) COSMOS generate similar QSM, as confirmed by (c) linear regression and Bland−Altman test (dashed lines indicate two standard deviations) [Liu *et al.* (2011)].

COSMOS can be used to validate MEDI. Both linear regression and Bland−Altman analysis (d) demonstrate excellent agreement between MEDI and COSMOS.

Animal model validation for MEDI quantification (Figure 5.9). The accuracy of the MEDI method was demonstrated in quantifying exogenous SPIO in mice imaging. We injected 35.5, 74.7, and 112 ng of SPIO into the right hemispheres of three mouse brains (Figure 5.9). Neither the magnitude nor the phase image provided direct quantification of the SPIO masses. By contrast, QSM illustrated SPIO masses in the three mouse brains of, respectively, 31.8, 69.4 and 103.6 ng, corresponding to 10%, 7.1%, and 7.5%

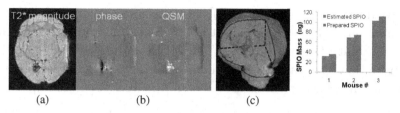

(a)   (b)   (c)

Fig. 5.9.   (a) T2* magnitude/phase/QSM of SPIO in a mouse brain. (b) Volume-rendered view of QSM. (c) Agreement between QSM estimated SPIO and microinjection prepared SPIO.

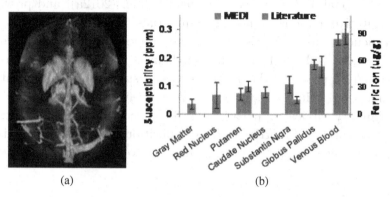

(a)   (b)

Fig. 5.10.   QSM reconstructed by MEDI in volume-rendered view (a) are in agreement with available literature values (b) from postmortem (putamen, substantia nigra and globus pallidus) or catheterization (venous blood).

underestimation possibly due to the loss of contrast agent during needle withdrawal. This experiment demonstrated QSM is potentially useful for quantitative dosimetry in targeted drug delivery.

Deoxyhemoglobin and iron mapping in human brain to validate MEDI by comparing with invasive literature values (Figure 5.10). The MEDI method was validated in quantifying endogenous iron and deoxyhemoglobin in human brain imaging ($n = 9$) by comparing with literature values [Riederer *et al.* (1989)] and a reference standard [Liu *et al.* (2009)] (Figure 5.10). The MEDI showed that the susceptibility of the venous blood was 0.2670.02 parts per million (ppm) higher than that of the arterial blood, corresponding to a net reduction in oxygenation saturation of 29.52%, which was in good agreement with 31.73.9% measured by invasive catheterization in an age-matched (22.92.4 years) group of volunteers [Gibbs *et al.* (1942)]. Furthermore, susceptibility allows estimation of [Fe^3+] assuming it is the dominant contributor to the susceptibility (Figure 5.10(b)). The MEDI estimated [Fe^3+] in the substantia nigra, putamen and globus pallidus were in the same range as those in postmortem measurements [Riederer *et al.* (1989)].

5.6.3 *Clinical applications*

Quantitative susceptibility mapping can remove blooming artifacts in traditional T2* weighted imaging [Li *et al.* (2012a)] and provide quantitative mapping of magnetic materials. Materials showing very conspicuous susceptibilities include iron deposition (ferritin) in deep brain nuclei and basal ganglia, deoxyhemoglobin in the veins, blood degradation products (hemosiderin in late stage), and concentrated calcification. Clinical applications are actively being developed, and preliminary clinical applications include accurate characterization of calcification, hemorrhage, iron deposition and iron metabolism pathology, as exemplified in the following five applications.

5.6.3.1 *Cerebral microhemorrhage*

Accurate universal depiction of cerebral microhemorrhage (or cerebral microbleed, CMB) and calcification. T2* weighted GRE MRI is the method of choice for studying CMB [Greenberg *et al.* (2009); Werring (2011)], but its appearance depends on imaging parameters including TE, field strength, orientation, etc. [Li *et al.* (2012a); Greenberg *et al.* (2009)], which can be overcome using QSM. The susceptibility value in QSM reconstructed from all echoes within a given TE was fairly independent of TE (fourth column in Figure 5.11(a)), in sharp contrast with the sensitive TE dependence of hypointensity in the magnitude and SMI images and moderate dependence in R2* map (first and second columns in Figure 5.11(a)). While both iron and calcium deposits appeared hypointense in magnitude/susceptibility weighted imaging (SWI) images and positive in R2* map, the foci of positive susceptibility on QSM (red arrows in Figure 5.11(a)) indicated iron (hemosiderin) deposits in CMB [Greenberg *et al.* (2009)], and the foci of negative

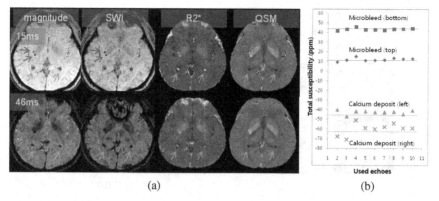

(a)   (b)

Fig. 5.11. (a) CMB appearances (red arrows) change with TE drastically in magnitude, SWI, and moderately R2* map but little in QSM. (b) QSMs reconstructed using various echoes confirm its invariance with TE.

susceptibility in the lateral ventricles (green arrows in Figure 5.11(a)) were interpreted as deposits of highly concentrated calcification, the only experimentally confirmed endogenous biomarkers with negative susceptibility [Liu *et al.* (2009)]. This patient study suggests that QSM, as an absolute quantification of biomarkers' susceptibility independent of imaging parameters, can serve as a standardized measure of CMB for definitive cross-study comparisons [Liu *et al.* (2012)].

5.6.3.2 *Hemorrhage*

Accurate measurement of hemorrhage volume. T2* weighted GRE MRI is very sensitive for imaging intracerebral hemorrhage (ICH) [Kidwell *et al.* (2004)], but it is very difficult to measure hematoma volume that is an essential clinical parameter for managing ICH patients [Burgess *et al.* (2008)]. Hematoma can be defined by QSM in GRE MRI of ICH patients by comparing magnitude and SWI images at various TEs and R2* map and QSM reconstructed from all echo data within given TEs (Figure 5.12). The hematoma border appears as a rim of hypointensity at short TE in magnitude image, and the whole hematoma becomes hypointense at long TE magnitude or in SWI. Hematoma appears as bright intensity in both R2* map and QSM. The hypointensity region increases drastically with TE in

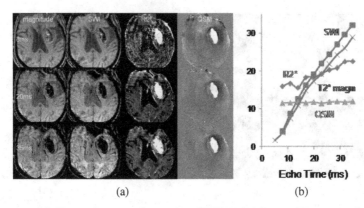

(a)   (b)

Fig. 5.12. (a) Hemorrhage appearance at $TE = 8/20/35$ ms in magnitude (first column)/SWI (second column)/R2* (third column)/QSM (fourth column). (b) Hematoma volume measurements vs. TE in the 4 image types.

magnitude image and is further enhanced by SWI. R2* removes some blooming artifacts but not all of them. With appearance and value invariant with echoes, QSM maps ICH, providing a standardized measure of hematoma volume in GRE MRI.

5.6.3.3 *Deep brain stimulation*

Conspicuous depiction of deep brain stimulation targets with iron deposition. Deep brain stimulation (DBS) for advanced Parkinson's disease (PD) requires placing an electrode in the subthalamic nucleus or the globus pallidus interna. While the precise mechanism of DBS effects on the brain remains to be found out, DBS is an effective surgical treatment of the medication-resistant disabling symptoms of advanced PD. Unfortunately, these structures are difficult to define in traditional MRI (T2 or T2* weighted imaging, T2W, T2*W), but fortunately they are prominently defined on QSM (Figure 5.13). This is because the water is fairly uniform around these deep brain structures, but iron is very selectively deposited in these structures. The CNR increases six-fold from traditional T2W to QSM, and QSM is becoming a method of choice for visualizing these DBS targets.

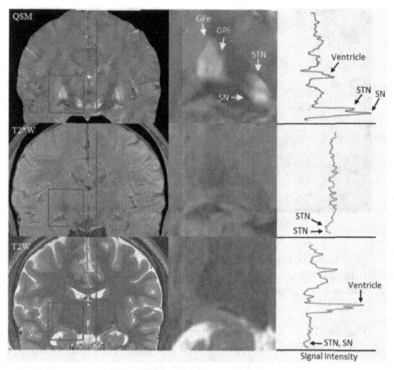

Fig. 5.13. Coronal imaging of the subthalamic nucleus (STN), obtained using three different imaging modalities: QSM, T2*W, and T2W. Zoomed view (blue square) is shown in the middle, conspicuously depicting globus pallidus interna (GPi) and subthalamic nucleus (STN). Sample vertical line is drawn through the left STN; the corresponding 1D signal intensity plot is shown on the right. The double dip in signal intensity — distinguishing the STN from the substantia nigra — is seen on the T2*W and QSM 1D plots, but not on the T2W plot, where only a single dip appears.

5.6.3.4 *Parkinson's disease*

Iron quantification in PD. A prominent pathophysiologic feature for PD is the increased nigral iron content. The pathogenesis of PD is not fully known yet; it involves pathologic variation of brain iron homeostasis. Iron overload associated with PD may be both a cause and consequence of PD. Traditional MRI methods for estimating iron in substantia nigra (SN) include phase and R2* ($1/T2^*$), which are theoretically inaccurate and experimentally erroneous (8). Precise measurements of SN iron concentration are enabled by

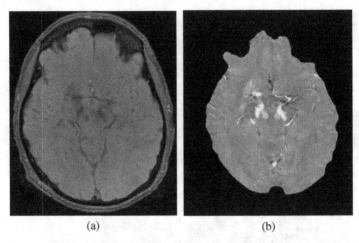

(a)   (b)

Fig. 5.14. (a) T2*W and (b) QSM of the substantia nigra (arrow). Not only
are the deep brain structures, including substantia nigra and red nuclei, better
visualized in QSM, but also QSM is quantitative, allowing a direct measure of
iron content in these structures.

QSM (Figure 5.14). Our preliminary data shows that QSM is more
sensitive than R2* for detecting the pathological changes in SN of
PD patients, suggesting QSM as a potential tool for diagnosing and
assessing PD.

5.6.3.5 *Multiple sclerosis*

Iron dynamics in multiple sclerosis (MS). Multiple sclerosis
is a devastating disease affecting predominantly Caucasian women
from 20 to 50; other populations are also susceptible to MS. As
with all neurodegenerative diseases, MS pathogenesis is not fully
understood and there is no cure for MS at this moment. Traditional
T2W imaging (with fluid attenuation, FLAIR) is the current gold
standard for imaging MS and defining MS lesion spatial distribution (Figure 5.15(a)). A hallmark of MS is demyelination, which
involves or is executed by activated microglia/macrophage. During
microglia/macrophage activation, there is iron accumulation in
microglia/macrophage (Figure 5.15(b)), though this pathologic alter-
ation of brain iron metabolism is not well understood. Measurement
by QSM (Figure 5.15(c)) demonstrates that there is no iron in

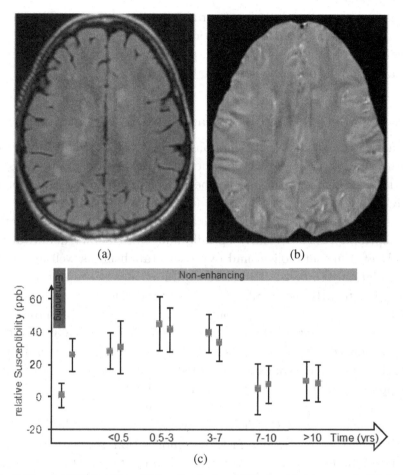

Fig. 5.15. (a) T2 FLAIR traditionally depicts MS lesions (white spots). (b) QSM depicts magnetic susceptibility (interpreted as iron) distribution in MS lesions. (c) Iron content in MS lesion at various ages measured by QSM in a cross-sectional study. The susceptibility value is relative to neighboring or contralateral normal appearing white matter. The blue measurement is the baseline QSM, and red from the follow-up QSM (separated by 0.5 yr). Lesion age is estimated from its first appearance in patient's serial MRI (error time interval between consecutive scans).

the MS lesion before, and at T-cell invasion (T1+Gd enhancing) iron increases rapidly, immediately following T1+Gd enhancing (during activated microglia/macrophage). As microglia/macrophage activation goes away, iron accumulation stops, iron content MS lesion remains constant and dissipates gradually over the years. Therefore, QSM provides additional information about MS lesion dynamics not available in traditional T2W MRI, and the rate of iron increase may be a biomarker of active demyelination in MS.

5.7   Challenging Problems and Future Directions

Quantitative susceptibility mapping, QSM, is a very young and highly active field. Tissue magnetic susceptibility property is a contrast mechanism that has not been exploited before in traditional MRI, which consists of relaxation (T1T2), motion (diffusion, perfusion and flow/motion), and chemical shift (spectroscopy). Magnetic susceptibility is molecularly specific and QSM allows quantitative study of iron metabolism and oxygen metabolism, as well as blood degradation products. Therefore, QSM is a very important contribution to MRI with valuable clinical and scientific applications. QSM techniques are being continuously developed and improved. The new information revealed by QSM is being actively digested and absorbed into approaches for medical and biological problems by clinicians and biomedical scientists. Quantitative susceptibility mapping is based on solving an ill-posed inverse problem, which is far more complex than traditional Fourier transform for image reconstruction in MRI. There are various technical challenges to make QSM accurate and fast. As information revealed by QSM is novel and has never been used before, it may take time to fully assess the clinical and scientific value and adopt QSM into practices. Future directions of the QSM field would include efforts to address these challenges. The future is full of surprises and new horizons beyond our power of prediction. We have attempted here to illustrate examples of what we can see right now as unmet challenges. While, arguably, QSM will become the method of choice for *in vivo* non-invasive measurement of iron contents in tissue, we need to develop a clear role for iron imaging for managing most neurodegenerative diseases, which will assess disease severity and monitor therapeutic outcome. Advancements in understanding disease pathophysiology and in disease therapeutics are needed to establish QSM's clinical role, and QSM can be a tool for pushing these advancements. Large clinical trials may be needed. Demyelination imaging is an urgent clinical need and motivation to fully develop QSM of myelin. The magnetic susceptibility anisotropy exhibited by myelin uniquely reflects the molecule lipid anisotropy and the macroscopic organization order of lipids in myelin and white matter tracks [Li *et al.* (2012b); Liu *et al.* (2012); Wisnieff *et al.* (2013); Sukstanskii and Yablonskiy (2013); Sati *et al.* (2012)]. Magnetic anisotropy needs to be described by a susceptibility tensor, whose determination from experimental data requires sampling from at least three orientations [Wisnieff *et al.* (2013); Liu (2010); Li *et al.* (2012c)]. These orientations are difficult to perform in clinical practice and may be insensitive to certain tensor components causing susceptibility tensor estimation error [Wisnieff *et al.* (2013)]. Innovation is needed to address these problems and make QSM of myelin susceptibility anisotropy feasible in practice. It has already been recognized that continuous improvement in QSM is needed to translate QSM into clinical practice in terms of improving accuracy and speed [Bilgic *et al.* (2012); Schweser *et al.* (2012a,b); Tang *et al.* (2012); Liu *et al.* (2013)]. Proper noise consideration [Liu *et al.* (2013)] may be critical for dealing with lesions with small SNRs, including hemorrhages. Better formulation of structure consistency with all available tissue structure data may improve accuracy. Flow compensation may be needed for studying deoxyhemoglobin in the veins. Fat signal needs to have proper account of chemical shift-induced phase when applying to tissue with fat. Non-linear phase evolution due to multiple tissue components in a voxel remains a challenge. As QSM is moving into clinical practice, new issues related to clinical practice such as shortening scan time must be addressed continuously.

Acknowledgments

One of the authors (YW) acknowledges grant support from NIH. He is very grateful to his (former) gifted postdoc/students including Drs. Ludovic de Rochefort, Bryan Kressler, Jing Liu, and Tian Liu for contributing to technical developments described in this chapter, and to his dedicated clinician collaborators including Drs. Shixin

Chang, Weiwei Chen, Susan Gauthier, Brain Kopell, Min Lou, and John Tsiouris for contributing to the clinical developments described in this chapter.

References

Allen PD, St Pierre TG, Chua-anusorn W, Strom V and Rao KV (2000). *Low-frequency low-field magnetic susceptibility of ferritin and hemosiderin*, Biochim. Biophys. Acta, Vol. 1500, no. 2, pp. 186–196.

Ashburner J and Friston K (2007). *Rigid body registration.*, In: *Ashburner J, Friston K and Penny W (ed), The Analysis of Functional Brain Images*, Academic Press, London, pp. 49–62.

Aster RC, Bochers B and Thurber CH (2013). *Parameter Estimation and Inverse Problems*, Academic Press, Oxford, UK.

Bertero M and Boccacci P (1998). *Introduction to Inverse Problems in Imaging*, IOP Publishing, Bristol, UK.

Bilgic B, Pfefferbaum A, Rohlfing T, Sullivan EV and Adalsteinsson E (2012). *MRI estimates of brain iron concentration in normal aging using quantitative susceptibility mapping*, Neuroimage, Vol. 59, no. 3, pp. 2625–2635.

Bjork A (1996). *Numerical methods for least squares problems*, SIAM, Philadelphia, PA, pp. 165–186.

Boyd S and Vandenberghe L (2004). *Convex Optimization*, Cambridge University Press, Cambridge.

Brittenham GM, Farrell DE, Harris JW, Feldman ES, Danish EH, Muir WA, Tripp JH and Bellon EM (1982). *Magnetic-susceptibility measurement of human iron stores*, N. Engl. J. Med., Vol. 307, no. 27, pp. 1671–1675.

Burgess RE, Warach S, Schaewe TJ, Copenhaver BR, Alger JR, Vespa P, Martin N, Saver JL and Kidwell CS (2008). *Development and validation of a simple conversion model for comparison of intracerebral hemorrhage volumes measured on CT and gradient recalled echo MRI*, Stroke, Vol. 39, pp. 2017–2020.

Carneiro AA, Fernandes JP, de Araujo DB, Elias J Jr., Martinelli AL, Covas DT, Zago MA, Angulo IL, St Pierre TG and Baffa O (2005). *Liver iron concentration evaluated by two magnetic methods: magnetic resonance imaging and magnetic susceptometry*, Magn. Reson. Med., Vol. 54, no. 1, pp. 122–128.

Chieregato A, Calzolari F, Trasforini G, Targa L and Latronico N (2003). *Normal jugular bulb oxygen saturation*, J. Neurol. Neurosur. Ps., Vol. 74, no. 6, pp. 784–786.

Chu SC, Xu Y, Balschi JA and Springer CS Jr. (1990). *Bulk magnetic susceptibility shifts in NMR studies of compartmentalized samples: use of paramagnetic reagents*, Magn. Reson. Med., Vol. 13, no. 2, pp. 239–262.

Conturo TE and Smith GD (1990). *Signal-to-noise in phase angle reconstruction: dynamic range extension using phase reference offsets*, Magn. Reson. Med., Vol. 15, no. 3, pp. 420–437.

de Rochefort L, Brown R, Prince MR and Wang Y (2008a). *Quantitative MR susceptibility mapping using piece-wise constant regularized inversion of the magnetic field*, Magn. Reson. Med., Vol. 60, no. 4, pp. 1003–1009.

de Rochefort L, Nguyen T, Brown R, Spincemaille P, Choi G, Weinsaft J, Prince MR and Wang Y (2008b). *In vivo quantification of contrast agent concentration using the induced magnetic field for time-resolved arterial input function measurement with MRI*, Med. Phys., Vol. 35, no. 12, pp. 5328–5339.

de Rochefort L, Liu T, Kressler B, Liu J, Spincemaille P, Lebon V, Wu J and Wang Y (2010). *Quantitative susceptibility map reconstruction from MR phase data using bayesian regularization: validation and application to brain imaging*, Magn. Reson. Med., Vol. 63, no. 1, pp. 194–206.

Farrell DE, Allen CJ, Whilden MW, Kidane TK, Baig TN and Tripp JH (2007). *A new instrument designed to measure the magnetic susceptibility of human liver tissue in vivo*, IEEE Trans. Magn., Vol. 43, no. 9, p. 12.

Fernandez-Seara MA, Techawiboonwong A, Detre JA and Wehrli FW (2006). *MR susceptometry for measuring global brain oxygen extraction*, Magn. Reson. Med., Vol. 55, no. 5, pp. 967–973.

Feynman RP, Leighton RB and Sands M (1965). *Lectures on Physics, Volume II*, Addison-Wesley, Boston, MA.

Ghiglia DC and Pritt MD (1998). *Two-dimensional Phase Unwrapping: Theory, Algorithms, and Software*, Wiley, New York.

Gibbs EL, Lennox WG, Nims LF and Gibbs FA (1942). *Arterial and cerebral venous blood—Arterial-venous differences in man*, J. Biol. Chem., Vol. 144, no. 2, pp. 325–332.

Gleich B and Weizenecker J (2005). *Tomographic imaging using the nonlinear response of magnetic particles*, Nature, Vol. 435, pp. 1214–1217.

Greenberg SM, Vernooij MW, Cordonnier C, Viswanathan A, Al-Shahi Salman R, Warach S, Launer LJ, Van Buchem MA and Breteler MMB (2009). *Cerebral microbleeds: a guide to detection and interpretation*, Lancet Neurol., Vol. 8, no. 2, pp. 165–174.

Haacke EM, Brown RW, Thompson MR and Venkatesan R (1999). *Magnetic Resonance Imaging — Physical Principles and Sequence Design*, Wiley-Liss, New York.

Haacke EM, Cheng NY, House MJ, Liu Q, Neelavalli J, Ogg RJ, Khan A, Ayaz M, Kirsch W and Obenaus A (2005). *Imaging iron stores in the brain using magnetic resonance imaging*, Magn. Reson. Imag., Vol. 23, no. 1, pp. 1–25.

Haacke EM, Mittal S, Wu Z, Neelavalli J and Cheng YC (2009). *Susceptibility-weighted imaging: technical aspects and clinical applications, part 1*, AJNR, Vol. 30, no. 1, pp. 19–30.

Hämäläinen M, Hari R, Ilmoniemi RJ, Knuutila J and Lounasmaa OV (1993). *Magnetoencephalography-theory, instrumentation, and applications to non-invasive studies of the working human brain*, Rev. Mod. Phys., Vol. 65, no. 2, 413 LP - 97.

Hanke M and Hansen PC (1993). *Regularization methods for large-scale problems*, Surveys Math Indust., Vol. 3, pp. 253–315.

Hestenes MR and Stiefel E (1952). *Methods of conjugate gradients for solving linear systems*, J. Res. Nat. Bur. Stand., Vol. 49, no. 6, p. 409.

Heyn C, Bowen CV, Rutt BK and Foster PJ (2005). *Detection threshold of single SPIO-labeled cells with FIESTA*, Magn. Reson. Med., Vol. 53, no. 2, pp. 312–320.

Holt RW, Diaz PJ, Duerk JL and Bellon EM (1994). *MR Susceptometry — an external-phantom method for measuring bulk susceptibility from field-echo phase reconstruction maps*, J. Magn. Reson. Im., Vol. 4, no. 6, pp. 809–818.

Jackson JD (1999). *Classical Electrodynamics*, Third edition, John Wiley and Sons, New York.

Kidwell CS, Chalela JA, Saver JL, Starkman S, Hill MD, Demchuk AM, Butman JA, Patronas N, Alger JR, Latour LL, Luby ML, Baird AE, Leary MC, Tremwel M, Ovbiagele B, Fredieu A, Suzuki S, Villablanca JP, Davis S, Dunn B, Todd JW, Ezzeddine MA, Haymore J, Lynch JK, Davis L and Warach S (2004). *Comparison of MRI and CT for detection of acute intracerebral hemorrhage*, JAMA, Vol. 292, no. 15, pp. 1823–1830.

Kressler B, De Rochefort L, Spincemaille P, Liu T and Wang Y (2008). *Estimation of sparse magnetic susceptibility distributions from MRI using non-linear regularization*, Proc ISMRM 2008, Toronto, p. 1514.

Kressler B, de Rochefort L, Liu T, Spincemaille P, Jiang Q and Wang Y (2010). *Nonlinear regularization for per voxel estimation of magnetic susceptibility distributions from MRI field maps*, IEEE Trans. Med. Imag., Vol. 29, no. 2, pp. 273–281. PMCID: 2874210.

Langham MC, Magland JF, Floyd TF and Wehrli FW (2008). *Retrospective correction for induced magnetic field inhomogeneity in measurements of large-vessel hemoglobin oxygen saturation by MR susceptometry*, Magn. Reson. Med., Vol. 61, no. 3, pp. 626–633.

Li J, Chang S, Liu T, Wang Q, Cui D, Chen X, Jin M, Wang B, Pei M, Wisnieff C, Spincemaille P, Zhang M and Wang Y (2012a). *Reducing the object orientation dependence of susceptibility effects in gradient echo MRI through quantitative susceptibility mapping*, Magn. Reson. Med., Vol. 68, no. 5, pp. 1563–1569.

Li L (2001). *Magnetic susceptibility quantification for arbitrarily shaped objects in inhomogeneous fields*, Magn. Reson. Med., Vol. 46, no. 5, pp. 907–916.

Li L and Leigh JS (2004). *Quantifying arbitrary magnetic susceptibility distributions with MR*, Magn. Reson. Med., Vol. 51, no. 5, pp. 1077–1082.

Li W, Wu B and Liu C (2011). *Quantitative susceptibility mapping of human brain reflects spatial variation in tissue composition*, Neuroimage, Vol. 55, no. 4, pp. 1645–1656.

Li W, Wu B, Avram AV and Liu C (2012b). *Magnetic susceptibility anisotropy of human brain in vivo and its molecular underpinnings*, Neuroimage, Vol. 59, no. 3, pp. 2088–2097.

Li X, Vikram DS, Lim IA, Jones CK, Farrell JA and van Zijl PC (2012c). *Mapping magnetic susceptibility anisotropies of white matter in vivo in the human brain at 7 T*, Neuroimage, Vol. 62, no. 1, pp. 314–330.

Lifshitz EM, Berestetskii VB and Pitaevskii LP (1982). *Quantum Electrodynamics*, Butterworth-Heinemann, Oxford, UK.

Liu C (2010). *Susceptibility tensor imaging*, Magn. Reson. Med., Vol. 63, no. 6, pp. 1471–1477.

Liu C, Li W, Wu B, Jiang Y and Johnson GA (2012). *3D fiber tractography with susceptibility tensor imaging*, Neuroimage, Vol. 59, no. 2, pp. 1290–1298.

Liu J, Liu T, de Rochefort L, Ledoux J, Khalidov I, Chen W, Tsiouris AJ, Wisnieff C, Spincemaille P, Prince MR and Wang Y (2012). *Morphology enabled dipole inversion for quantitative susceptibility mapping using structural consistency between the magnitude image and the susceptibility map*, Neuroimage, Vol. 59, no. 3, pp. 2560–2568.

Liu T, Spincemaille P, de Rochefort L, Kressler B and Wang Y (2009). *Calculation of susceptibility through multiple orientation sampling (COSMOS): a method for conditioning the inverse problem from measured magnetic field map to susceptibility source image in MRI*, Magn. Reson. Med, Vol. 61, no. 1, pp. 196–204.

Liu T, Khalidov I, de Rochefort L, Spincemaille P, Liu J and Wang Y (2010). *Improved background field correction using effective dipole fitting*, Proc. ISMRM 2010, p. 141.

Liu T, Liu J, de Rochefort L, Spincemaille P, Khalidov I, Ledoux JR and Wang Y (2011). *Morphology enabled dipole inversion (MEDI) from a single-angle acquisition: comparison with COSMOS in human brain imaging*, Magn. Reson. Med, Vol. 66, no. 3, pp. 777–783.

Liu T, Xu W, Spincemaille P, Avestimehr AS and Wang Y (2012a). *Accuracy of the morphology enabled dipole inversion (MEDI) algorithm for quantitative susceptibility mapping in MRI*, IEEE Trans. Med. Imag., Vol. 31, no. 3, pp. 816–824.

Liu T, Surapaneni K, Lou M, Cheng L, Spincemaille P and Wang Y (2012b). *Cerebral microbleeds: burden assessment by using quantitative susceptibility mapping*, Radiology, Vol. 262, pp. 269–278.

Liu T, Wisnieff C, Lou M, Chen W, Spincemaille P and Wang Y (2013). *Nonlinear formulation of the magnetic field to source relationship for robust quantitative susceptibility mapping*, Magn. Reson. Med., Vol. 69, no. 2, pp. 467–476.

Lustig M, Donoho D and Pauly JM (2007). *Sparse MRI: The application of compressed sensing for rapid MR imaging*, Magn. Reson. Med., Vol. 58, no. 6, pp. 1182–1195.

Marques JP and Bowtell R (2005). *Application of a Fourier-based method for rapid calculation of field inhomogeneity due to spatial variation of magnetic susceptibility*, Concept. Magnetic Res. B: Magnetic Resonance Engineering, Vol. 25B, no. 1, pp. 65–78.

Moon TK and Stirling WC (2000). *Matrix Condition Number, Mathematical Methods and Algorithms for Signal Processing*, Marsha Horton, Upper Saddle River, NJ, pp. 253–255.

Neelavalli J, Cheng YC, Jiang J and Haacke EM (2009). *Removing background phase variations in susceptibility-weighted imaging using a fast, forward-field calculation*, Magn. Reson. Imaging, Vol. 29, no. 4, pp. 937–948.

Nielsen P, Engelhardt R, Duerken M, Janka GE and Fischer R (2000). *Using SQUID biomagnetic liver susceptometry in the treatment of thalassemia and other iron loading diseases*, Transfus. Sci., Vol. 23, no. 3, pp. 257–258.

Paige CC and Saunders MA (1982). *LSQR: An algorithm for sparse linear equations and sparse least squares, ACM Trans. Math. Software*, Vol. 8, no. 1, pp. 43–71.

Pauling L (1977). *Magnetic properties and structure of oxyhemoglobin, Proc. Natl. Acad. Sci. USA*, Vol. 74, no. 7, pp. 2612–2613.

Riederer P, Sofic E, Rausch WD, Schmidt B, Reynolds GP, Jellinger K and Youdim MB (1989). *Transition metals, ferritin, glutathione, and ascorbic acid in parkinsonian brains, J. Neurochem.*, Vol. 52, no. 2, pp. 515–520.

Salomir R, De Senneville BD and Moonen CTW (2003). *A fast calculation method for magnetic field inhomogeneity due to an arbitrary distribution of bulk susceptibility, Concept. Magn. Reson. B*, Vol. 19B, no. 1, pp. 26–34.

Sati P, Silva AC, van Gelderen P, Gaitan MI, Wohler JE, Jacobson S, Duyn JH and Reich DS (2012). *In vivo quantification of T(2) anisotropy in white matter fibers in marmoset monkeys, Neuroimage*, Vol. 59, no. 2, pp. 979–985.

Schweser F, Deistung A, Lehr BW and Reichenbach JR (2010). *Differentiation between diamagnetic and paramagnetic cerebral lesions based on magnetic susceptibility mapping, Med. Phys.*, Vol. 37, no. 10, pp. 5165–5178.

Schweser F, Deistung A, Sommer K and Reichenbach JR (2012a). *Toward online reconstruction of quantitative susceptibility maps: Superfast dipole inversion, Magn. Reson. Med.*, Vol. 69, no. 6, pp. 1581–1593.

Schweser F, Sommer K, Deistung A and Reichenbach JR (2012b). *Quantitative susceptibility mapping for investigating subtle susceptibility variations in the human brain, Neuroimage*, Vol. 62, no. 3, pp. 2083–2100.

Seo JK and Woo EJ (2012). *Nonlinear Inverse Problems in Imaging*, Wiley Press, Hoboken, NJ.

Sepulveda NG, Thomas IM and Wikswo JP Jr. (1994). *Magnetic susceptibility tomography for three-dimensional imaging of diamagnetic and paramagnetic objects, IEEE Trans. Magn.*, Vol. 30, no. 6, pp. 5062–5069.

Shmueli K, de Zwart JA, van Gelderen P, Li TQ, Dodd SJ and Duyn JH (2009). *Magnetic susceptibility mapping of brain tissue in vivo using MRI phase data, Magn. Reson. Med.*, Vol. 62, no. 6, pp. 1510–1522.

Sukstanskii AL and Yablonskiy DA (2013). *On the role of neuronal magnetic susceptibility and structure symmetry on gradient echo MR signal formation, Magn. Reson. Med.*, 24629.

Tang J, Liu S, Neelavalli J, Cheng YC, Buch S and Haacke EM (2012). *Improving susceptibility mapping using a threshold-based K-space/image domain iterative reconstruction approach, Magn. Reson. Med.*, Vol. 69, no. 5, pp. 1396–1407.

Vogel CR and Oman ME (1996). *Iterative methods for total variation denoising, SIAM J. Sci. Comput.*, Vol. 17, no. 1, pp. 227–238.

Wang JJ, Li S and Haselgrove JC (1999). *Magnetic resonance imaging measurement of volume magnetic susceptibility using a boundary condition, J. Magn. Reson.*, Vol. 140, no. 2, pp. 477–481.

Weisskoff RM and Kiihne S (1992). *MRI susceptometry: image-based measurement of absolute susceptibility of MR contrast agents and human blood, Magn. Reson. Med.*, Vol. 24, no. 2, pp. 375–383.

Werring DJ (2011). *Cerebral microbleeds: Pathophysiology to Clinical Practice,* Cambridge University Press, Cambridge, UK.

Wharton S and Bowtell R (2010). *Whole-brain susceptibility mapping at high field: a comparison of multiple- and single-orientation methods, Neuroimage,* Vol. 53, no. 2, pp. 515–525.

Wharton S, Schafer A and Bowtell R (2010). *Susceptibility mapping in the human brain using threshold-based k-space division, Magn. Reson. Med.,* Vol. 63, no. 5, pp. 1292–1304.

Wisnieff C (2013). *Magnetic susceptibility anisotropy: cylindrical symmetry from macroscopically ordered anisotropic molecules and accuracy of MRI measurements using few orientations, Neuroimage,* Vol. 70, pp. 363–376.

Yao B, Li TQ, Gelderen Pv, Shmueli K, de Zwart JA and Duyn JH (2009). *Susceptibility contrast in high field MRI of human brain as a function of tissue iron content, Neuroimage,* Vol. 44, no. 4, pp. 1259–1266.

Index

Printed in the United States
By Bookmasters